Textbook of
Two-Dimensional Echocardiography

Textbook of
Two-Dimensional Echocardiography

Edited by

James V. Talano, M.D.

Chief, Cardiac Graphics Laboratory
Northwestern Memorial Hospital
Associate Professor of Medicine
Northwestern University Medical School
Chicago, Illinois

Julius M. Gardin, M.D.

Acting Chief, Cardiovascular Section
Long Beach Veterans Administration Medical Center
Long Beach, California
Director, Cardiology Noninvasive Laboratory and
Assistant Professor of Medicine
University of California, Irvine
Irvine, California

Grune & Stratton
A Subsidiary of Harcourt Brace Jovanovich, Publishers
New York   London
Paris   San Diego   San Francisco   São Paulo
Sydney   Tokyo   Toronto

Library of Congress Cataloging in Publication Data
Main entry under title:

Textbook of two-dimensional echocardiography.

Includes bibliographical references and index.
1. Ultrasonic cardiography.   2. Heart—Diseases—Diagnosis. I. Talano, James V.
II. Gardin, Julius M.   [DNLM: 1. Echocardiography.   WG 141.5.E2 T355]
RC683.5.U5T5   1983   616.1'207544   83—5638
ISBN 0–8089–1556–8

Grune & Stratton, Inc.
111 Fifth Avenue
New York, New York 10003

Distributed in the United Kingdom by
Academic Press Inc. (London) Ltd.
24/28 Oval Road, London NW 1

Library of Congress Catalog Number 83-5638
International Standard Book Number 0-8089-1556-8

Printed in the United States of America

To my wife, Joan, a woman of understanding and devotion.

J.V.T.

To the memory of my beloved parents, Abram and Fania Toba Gardin, and to my wife, Susan, and my sister, Sherri, two women of valor.

J.M.G.

Contents

Acknowledgments

We have numerous debts of gratitude—only some of which we can acknowledge in this space. We would first like to thank all our contributing authors who gave their time and expertise in the formulation of this book.

Thanks are also due to the editors at Grune & Stratton for their helpful suggestions and timely review. It was a pleasure working with them at every juncture.

To our colleagues at Northwestern University and the University of California at Irvine who shouldered additional responsibilities during our preparation of this text, especially Drs. David Mehlman, Edward J. Winslow, Michael Lesch, Walter Henry, Ali Dabestani, and Samuel Butman we offer our deepest thanks.

We are most grateful to Sharon Joseph whose efforts and expertise were responsible for the major preparation and organization of the text and to Jean Salomon, Lynne Miller, Judy Kinkaid, Janie Zimring, and Susan Leutheuser in Chicago and Cora Burn, Alice Allfie, Marypaull Quick, Dan Russell, William Childs, Peggy Trigg, Connie Barnes, Regina Lee, Ellen Mansour, Cynthia McDaniel, Estelle Cohen, Peggy Knoll, Nancy Haggerty Futty, Wilma Mottin, and Caroline West in Irvine and Long Beach, all of whom assisted in obtaining the illustrations and preparing the manuscript.

Many of the drawings and illustrations are the result of the artistic efforts of Joan Talano in Chicago. Jack Newby and his staff at the Medical Media Service of the Long Beach Veterans Administration Medical Center were also extremely helpful in preparing many figures.

We would like to express our gratitude to our mentors and teachers—Drs. W. Proctor Harvey, Joseph Perloff, Herbert Levine, Stephen Epstein, Michael Lesch, and Walter Henry—who have been a source of constant inspiration to us throughout our professional careers.

Finally, we offer our sincere appreciation and thanks to our wives, who provided the scholarly environment at home and the understanding and vision to allow us to complete this work.

Preface

The widespread application of two-dimensional echocardiography has expanded the practice of cardiac ultrasound dramatically since 1978. The two-dimensional technique has been incorporated into many aspects of the noninvasive evaluation of patients with known or suspected heart disease; in addition, new areas of application are being developed, such as tissue characterization, three-dimensional spatial reconstruction, and Doppler and contrast echocardiography. With two-dimensional echocardiography gaining such acceptance as a noninvasive imaging technique, we felt it important to include in one textbook both the many established clinical uses and the more recently developed aspects of the technique.

To be most effective in presenting the large volume of information now available about two-dimensional echocardiography, we invited additional experts in the field to prepare chapters about the state of the art. Although differences in style are unavoidable in chapters written by different authors, we have attempted through diligent editing and updating to maintain a uniformity of purpose and style throughout the text. Any shortcomings resulting from differences in style, however, are more than compensated by the knowledge and experience contributed by these authors.

The book begins with a discussion of the historical development of two-dimensional echocardiography. We believed it was important to begin with an overview of the early development of two-dimensionl echocardiography and to include descriptive and graphic material that outline basic principles used in its daily application. A detailed discussion of the principles and physics of ultrasound is not included, since it is outside the scope of this text and has been well described in other books.

In Chapter 2 anatomic slice specimens of normal hearts are presented and compared with tomographic slices of standardized two-dimensional views. Although references are made to other conventions of nomenclature and display, Chapter 3 lists in detail the standards published by the American Society of Echocardiography (ASE).

The next three chapters systematically consider the normal and abnormal two-dimensional echocardiographic findings related to the mitral valve (Chapter 4), the aortic valve and thoracic aorta (Chapter 5), and the right heart, including the tricuspid and pulmonic valves, right atrium, and right ventricle (Chapter 6). The discussion of echocardiography of valvular heart disease concludes with a chapter on the usefulness of two-dimensional echocardiography in evaluating prosthetic heart valves (Chapter 7).

Two-dimensional echocardiography is then considered in terms of its efficacy in assessing normal and abnormal myocardium. Specifically, there are clear and concise discussions about measuring right and left ventricular volumes (Chapter 8), ischemic heart disease and its complications (Chapter 9), and the hypertrophic, congestive, and restrictive cardiomyopathies (Chapter 10). These discussions are followed by chapters on diseases of the pericardium (Chapter 11); cardiac masses, tumors, and thrombi (Chapter 12); and the use of echocardiography in congenital heart disease (Chapter 13).

Since no serious discussion of two-dimensional echocardiography is complete without presenting the newer developments, we have included chapters that focus on new applications in contrast echocardiography (Chapter 14), the principles and uses of Doppler echocardiography (Chapter 15), three-dimensional echocardiography (Chapter 16), and tissue characterization (Chapter 17). The last chapter discusses the role of two-dimensional echocardiography in the context of other established and newer cardiac imaging techniques, including digital subtraction angiography, computerized axial tomography, and radionuclide imaging techniques, particularly positron emission tomography and nuclear magnetic resonance.

Although there are references to M-mode echocardiography and appropriate M-mode figures are used throughout the text, this work deals primarily with two-dimensional echocardiography. We have not attempted to present a comprehensive review of M-mode echocardiography, as this has already been well covered in other textbooks of echocardiography. It should be noted that a companion workbook—*Cardiac Ultrasound Workbook,* edited by James V. Talano, M.D., New York, Grune & Stratton, 1982—is designed to be of assistance to those who would like more instruction about the technique of properly performing and interpreting M-mode and two-dimensional echocardiograms.

We hope that the numerous illustrations and bibliographic references presented in this work will be useful to the reader as a reference source and as a stimulus to additional study of two-dimensional echocardiography.

Contributors

William J. Bommer, M.D. Director, Echocardiography Laboratory, and Assistant Professor of Medicine, Division of Cardiovascular Medicine, University of California, Davis, Medical Center, Sacramento, California

Samuel Butman, M.D. Director, Cardiology Noninvasive Laboratory, Long Beach Veterans Administration Medical Center, Long Beach, California; Assistant Professor of Medicine, University of California, Irvine, Irvine, California

P. A. N. Chandraratna, M.D., M.R.C.P. Professor of Medicine, Division of Cardiology, University of Southern California School of Medicine, Los Angeles, California

Ivan A. D'Cruz, M.D., F.A.C.C., F.R.C.P.E. Director, Echocardiography Section, Cardiovascular Institute, Michael Reese Hospital and Medical Center; Associate Professor of Medicine, Pritzker School of Medicine, University of Chicago, Chicago, Illinois

Anthony DeMaria, M.D. Chief of Cardiology, Cardiovascular Division, and Professor of Medicine, University of Kentucky Medical Center, Lexington, Kentucky

Elizabeth A. Fisher, M.D. Director, Pediatric Cardiology, and Professor of Clinical Pediatrics, University of Illinois College of Medicine at Chicago, Chicago, Illinois

Edward D. Folland, M.D. Director, Cardiac Catheterization Laboratory, West Roxbury Veterans Administration Medical Center, West Roxbury, Massachussetts; Associate in Medicine, Brigham and Women's Hospital; Assistant Professor of Medicine, Harvard Medical School, Boston, Massachussetts

Harsha Gandhi, B.S. Research Associate, Division of Cardiovascular Medicine, University of California, Davis, Medical Center, Sacramento, California

Charles Ganote, M.D. Professor of Pathology, Northwestern University Medical School, Chicago, Illinois

Julius M. Gardin, M.D. Acting Chief, Cardiovascular Section, Long Beach Veterans Administration Medical Center, Long Beach, California; Director, Cardiology Noninvasive Laboratory, and Assistant Professor of Medicine, University of California, Irvine, Irvine, California

Edward A. Geiser, M.D.   Assistant Professor of Medicine, Division of Cardiovascular Diseases, J. Hillis Miller Health Center, University of Florida, Gainesville, Florida

Thomas Jackson   Echocardiography Technician, Division of Cardiovascular Medicine, University of California, Davis, Medical Center, Sacramento, California

Mark Keown, R.D.M.S.   Echocardiography Technician, Division of Cardiovascular Medicine, University of California, Davis, Medical Center, Sacramento, California

Richard E. Kerber, M.D.   Professor of Medicine, University of Iowa College of Medicine; Associate Director, Cardiovascular Division, University of Iowa Hospitals, Iowa City, Iowa

Robert Kieso, M.S.   Research Assistant, Department of Internal Medicine, University of Iowa Hospitals, Iowa City, Iowa

David I. Koenigsberg, M.D.   Instructor in Medicine, Section of Cardiology, Northwestern University Medical School, Chicago, Illinois

Randall Mapes, B.S.   Medical Student, Division of Cardiovascular Medicine, University of California, Davis, Medical Center, Sacramento, California

Dean T. Mason, M.D.   Director, Cardiac Center, Cedars Medical Center, Miami, Florida

David J. Mehlman, M.D.   Assistant Professor of Medicine, Northwestern University Medical School; Associate Director, Cardiac Graphics Laboratory, Northwestern Memorial Hospital, Chicago, Illinois

Joel Morganroth, M.D.   Director, Sudden Death Prevention Program, Likoff Cardiovascular Institute; Professor of Medicine and Pharmacology, Hahnemann University, Philadelphia, Pennsylvania

Natesa G. Pandian, M.D.   Clinical Assistant in Medicine (Cardiology), Massachusetts General Hospital; Instructor in Medicine, Harvard Medical School, Boston, Massachusetts

Alfred F. Parisi, M.D.   Chief, Cardiology Section, West Roxbury Veterans Administration Medical Center, West Roxbury, Massachusetts; Senior Associate in Medicine, Brigham and Women's Hospital; Associate Professor of Medicine, Harvard Medical School, Boston, Masachusetts

Gerald Pohost, M.D.   Director, Cardiac Nuclear Imaging and Nuclear Magnetic Imaging Research, Massachusetts General Hospital; Associate Professor of Medicine, Harvard Medical School, Boston, Massachusetts

James B. Seward, M.D.   Associate Professor of Medicine and Assistant Professor of Pediatrics, Mayo Medical School; Consultant, Division of Cardiovascular Diseases and Internal Medicine, Mayo Clinic and Mayo Foundation, Rochester, Minnesota

David J. Skorton, M.D.   Assistant Professor of Medicine and Electrical and Computer Engineering, University of Iowa College of Medicine, and Iowa City Veterans Administration Medical Center, Iowa City, Iowa

Abdul J. Tajik, M.D.   Professor of Medicine and Associate Professor of Pediatrics, Mayo Medical School; Consultant, Division of Cardiovascular Diseases and Internal Medicine, Mayo Clinic and Mayo Foundation, Rochester, Minnesota

James V. Talano, M.D.   Chief, Cardiac Graphics Laboratory, Northwestern Memorial Hospital; Associate Professor of Medicine, Northwestern University Medical School, Chicago, Illinois

CHAPTER 1

History and Instrumentation

Julius M. Gardin and James V. Talano

EARLY HISTORY OF CARDIAC ULTRASOUND

The engineering principles used for diagnostic ultrasound have their origins in the latter half of the 19th century and the early part of this century. An early development was Galton's ultrasonic whistle in 1883, which was capable of generating vibrations with frequencies as high as 25,000 cycles per second. The advent of submarines during World War I became the impetus for developing ultrasound devices that were capable of detecting underwater objects. Langevin, in France, using a quartz crystal, developed a method of generating and transmitting ultrasound waves through water. The First World War, however, ended before an ultrasound device capable of detecting submarines could be built.

Between the First and the Second World War, much basic research into the properties and applications of ultrasound technology was performed. The speed of ultrasound transmission was determined in various human tissues. Ultrasound technology was applied to underwater depth measurements, to monitoring movement of dolphins and whales, and to detecting flaws in metal. The Second World War spurred the development of electronic instrumentation for military use. Radar applications required advanced technology in recording brief energy pulses and measuring extremely short transit times. An outgrowth of this technology was the adaptation of the oscilloscope to measure brief electronic events. In addition, the widespread use of ultrasound or sonar in detecting submarines was responsible for the increased knowledge of ultrasonic transducer technology.[1]

After World War II, nonmilitary use of ultrasound expanded rapidly. Firestone, in the United States, developed the first nondestructive flaw-detector for testing of metals.[2,3] His utilization of pulsed–reflected ultrasound for material-testing stimulated much interest in ultrasound for medical diagnostic use. In the late 1940s and early 1950s, American and European investigators began imaging cross-sections of the human body, including the heart. Keidel transmitted and recorded ultrasound waves through the heart in an attempt to determine cardiac volumes.[4] Hertz and Edler were the first investigators to examine the heart utilizing Firestone's pulsed–reflected ultrasound. Initially they used the Firestone device to record echoes from the back wall of the heart,[5] but eventually they were able to record an echo signal returning from the anterior mitral valve leaflet.[6,7]

The detection of mitral stenosis, pioneered by Edler and associates, was the foremost early clinical application of single-dimensional (both A-mode and M-mode) echocardiography. Other uses included detecting left atrial tumors, anterior pericardial effusion and aortic stenosis.[6,8] Effert and associates,[9,10] in Germany, and Joyner and Reid,[11] in the United States, confirmed the utility of single-dimensional ultrasound in detecting mitral stenosis. Other significant early advances in the use of single-dimensional echocardiography were the detection of pericardial effusion, described by Feigenbaum and associates,[12,13] and visualization of intracardiac echoes utilizing indocyanine green dye, reported by Gramiak and associates.[14]

DEVELOPMENT OF TWO-DIMENSIONAL ECHOCARDIOGRAPHY

Several different methods of producing two-dimensional (cross-sectional) echocardiograms were developed beginning in the late 1960s. Each technique reconstructed the two-dimensional cardiac image from multiple B-mode scan lines. In B-mode scans the reflected ultrasound signal is converted from a spike to a dot—the brightness of the dot reflecting the amplitude of the echo spike. With electronic tracking of the transducer, a spatially oriented two-dimensional image can then be created.

One classification categorizes two-dimensional systems as to their transducer location and beam angle, e.g., sector, linear, arc, or compound scans (Figure 1-1).

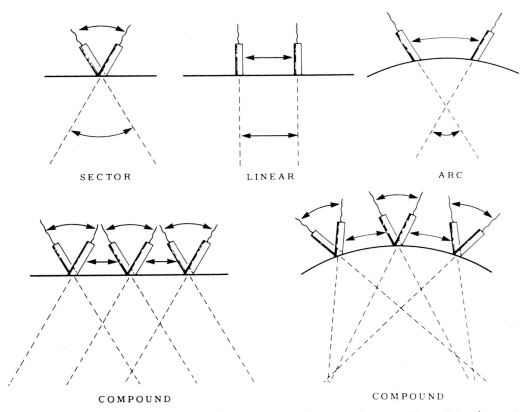

SECTOR   LINEAR   ARC

COMPOUND   COMPOUND

Figure 1-1. Types of scans utilized to obtain two-dimensional images. (From Feigenbaum H (ed): Echocardiography (ed 2). Philadelphia, Lea & Febiger, 1976. With permission.)

The most common scan used in examining the heart is the sector scan, where the transducer itself remains stationary with only the angle of the emitted ultrasound beam being changed. A linear scan, on the other hand, involves changing the transducer position but holding the beam angle constant. An arc scan is similar to a linear scan except that the transducer surface is curved so that the individual ultrasonic beams are not parallel and eventually cross within the organ being scanned. This type of scan is rarely used in echocardiography but is frequently used in ultrasound examination of the breast. Compound scanning is merely a combination of two or more of these basic scan types—e.g., a sector scan with a linear scan.[15]

Another classification for two-dimensional systems divides them into (1) composite—in which the two-dimensional image is a compilation of B-mode scan lines obtained from a number of cardiac cycles[15]; and (2) real-time—in which individual scans of the heart are obtained so rapidly that cardiac motion can be viewed directly.

A number of earlier approaches to two-dimensional echocardiography involved the use of composite B-mode scanning.[16–18] In this technique, the image produced is not real-time, since multiple cardiac cycles are required to develop an image. Ultrasound signals from cardiac structures are obtained by utilizing a standard M-mode echocardiographic system whose transducer is attached to a potentiometer capable of indicating the orientation of the transducer in space. The signals obtained are displayed vertically as dots whose depth and brightness are proportional to the distance of the target from the transducer and the amplitude of the signal, respectively. In M-mode echocardiography, these vertical ultrasound signals are swept across the horizontal axis with time. Conversely, in B-mode scanning, the multiple scan lines obtained are displayed at a position analogous to their spatial orientation and then combined to form a composite cardiac image.

During a cardiac cycle, however, there is significant translation of the heart in space. It is therefore necessary in the B-mode technique to obtain ultrasound signals only at a selected period during the cardiac cycle. This selection of images at specific times during the cardiac cycle is made possible by electrocardiographic gating—i.e., triggering the collection of images at specific intervals during the QRS and T waves of the EKG. Teichholz and associates[18] demonstrated the utility of B-mode scans in evaluating left ventricular anatomy and function.

Real-time two-dimensional sector scans can be performed by either mechanically or electronically steering the ultrasound beam through an arc ranging from 30° to 90°. A historical approach will be utilized to describe first the mechanical sector scanners and then the electronic linear-array and phased-array scanners. Figure 1-2 depicts the more common real-time scanners that are in use.

MECHANICAL SECTOR SCANNERS

The water bath and mirror system scanners were early types of mechanical sector scanners. One of the first attempts at clinical two-dimensional mechanical cardiac imaging was described by Ebina and associates in 1967.[16] Their approach utilized a water bath B-scanner that obtained either compound B-scans gated at a portion of the cardiac cycle or a real-time sector scan obtained by mechanically rotating the transducer within the water bath. Figure 1-3 demonstrates this early water bath real-time mechanical scanner and Figure 1-4 demonstrates images that were obtained utilizing this system.

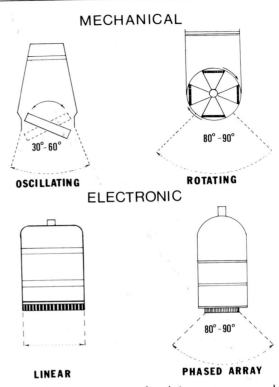

Figure 1-2. Diagrammatic representation of four common types of real-time scanners used in two-dimensional echocardiography.

Another early attempt at sector scanning was the cinematographic technique described by Asberg in 1967.[19] This approach involved a reciprocating mirror system containing two reflectors and two transducers that resulted in a two-dimensional image at a rate of seven frames per second. A different method of mechanical sector scanning, developed by Flaherty and associates, used an ultrasonic scanner in conjunction with a fluoroscopic image.[20] The system was capable of locating both the ultrasonic transducer and the anatomic cross-section being explored; furthermore, this unit was capable of framing rates of 40 frames per second and generated ultrasonic sectors up to 30°. Patzold and associates developed a device that rotated a sound source around the focal lines of a cylindrical parabolic mirror and produced

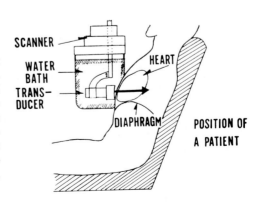

Figure 1-3. Early real-time sector scanner that obtained images by mechanically rotating a transducer within a water bath. Either gated compound B-scan images and real-time sector scan images could be obtained. (From Ebina T, Oka S, Tanaka M, et al: The ultrasonotomography of the heart and great vessels in living human subjects by means of the ultrasonic reflection technique. Jpn Heart J 8:331, 1967. With permission.)

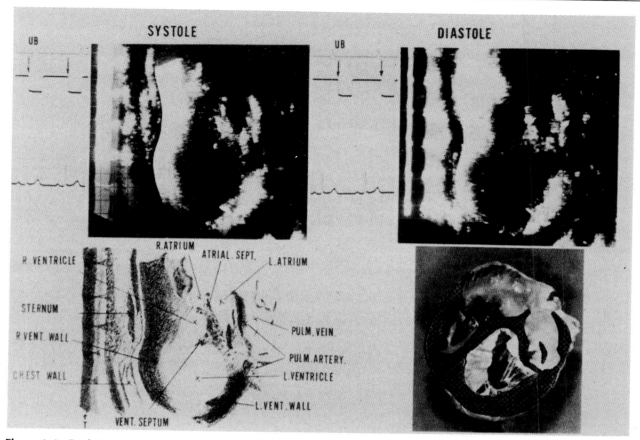

Figure 1-4. Real-time two-dimensional images obtained with a water bath mechanical sector scanner as seen in Figure 1-3. (From Ebina T, Oka S, Tanaka M, et al: The ultrasono-tomography of the heart and great vessels in living human subjects by means of ultrasonic reflection technique. Jpn Heart J 8:331, 1967. With permission.)

a rectangular ultrasound scan at a framing rate of 15 frames per second.[21] Hertz and Lindstrom reported the use of a water bath sector scanner that allowed cardiac imaging at a rate of 16 frames per second.[22]

The next major development was Griffith and Henry's mechanical sector scanner, which utilized a single transducer that oscillated rapidly through a 30° sector.[23] Thirty frames or sectors, each containing two fields, were produced each second. Since the pulse repetition frequency was 2000 Hz, each of the 30 separate frames consisted of 66 ultrasound scan lines. Eggleton and associates[24] developed a 30° sector scanner capable of producing 60 frames per second. As in B-mode scanning, electric potentiometers were attached to the transducer to depict the orientation of the individual B-mode scan lines analogous to their spatial orientation.

The advantages of the single transducer mechanical sector scanners include their relative inexpensiveness, portability, simplicity in engineering, compatibility with high-frequency transducers, excellent signal-to-noise ratio, and high line density (Table 1-1).[40] The disadvantages are the minor discomfort experienced by the patient from the oscillation of the transducer on the chest wall and the limited 60° sector scan. The narrow sector is due to the limitation of the arc through which the ultrasonic

Table 1-1
Comparison of Mechanical and Phased-Array Real-Time Sector Scanners

	Mechanical	Phased-Array
Simultaneous M-mode and 2-D echo	No*	Yes
Sequential M-mode and 2-D echo	Yes	Yes
Dual M-mode echo	No	Yes
Simultaneous 2-D and Doppler	No*	Yes
Sequential 2-D and Doppler	Yes	Yes
Small acoustic window for wide-angle scan	No	Yes†
Can be electronically focused in lateral (y) axis	No	Yes
Compatible with ring or annular phased-array transducer technology	Yes	No
Minimal side-lobe artifacts	Yes	No
Easily compatible with 4 MHz or above	Yes	Yes
Portable	Yes	Yes
Relatively inexpensive	Yes	No

Adapted from Feigenbaum H: Echocardiography (ed 3). Philadelphia, Lea & Febiger, 1981, p 18. With permission.
*Near-simultaneous M-mode/2-D echo and Doppler are possible.
†Size of phased-array transducer depends on whether it is dynamically focused and on the frequency of the transducer.

transducer can be driven while still maintaining skin contact. Thus, single-crystal mechanical scanners are less widely used today.

More recently, "wide-angle" mechanical sector scanners have been developed which produce sectors in excess of 80°. The relatively narrow scan angle of a single-crystal mechanical sector scanner has been improved by utilizing three or four ultrasound crystals that are motor driven through a 360° rotational arc.[25] Each of the individual transducers provides ultrasonic scan lines for only a quarter segment of its 360° rotation—i.e., 80°–90°. The crystals are not in contact with the skin; they are enclosed within a plastic housing in oil. In addition to providing a wider scan angle than does a single oscillating crystal, this device has the advantage of not producing any vibratory discomfort for the patient. It also provides a wider imaging angle and more evenly distributed line density. Potential disadvantages of such a multitransducer system are (1) the plastic housing may result in inferior ultrasound images due to attenuation of the ultrasound signal by the plastic or the air bubbles within the oil, (2) reverberation artifacts may also be produced from the plastic housing, and (3) image degradation may occur from "cross-talk" interference between transducer elements that are mismatched—i.e., have different acoustic properties.

LINEAR-ARRAY TECHNIQUES

The linear-array ultrasound scanner was another early development in real-time two-dimensional cardiac imaging.[26–31] The first linear-array scanner, described by Bom and associates in Holland in 1971, featured a row of 20 standard M-mode piezoelectric crystals electronically excited to emit ultrasound in a sequential manner.[26] Later systems utilized up to 64 single transducers producing a rectangular two-dimensional image whose overall size was dependent on the size of each transducer.

One transducer element produced a single B-mode scan line of data by emitting and receiving an independent ultrasound signal. The multiple elements were fired sequentially, providing a linear scan. This multi-element linear-array unit, called the Multiscan system, has recently undergone further improvements, including electronic focusing of the ultrasound beam.[32]

The main disadvantage of the linear-array transducer is its large size, requiring a large acoustic window, which is impeded by the ribs. As this transducer must overlie the ribs and intercostal space simultaneously, it cannot be easily angled in the proper imaging planes of the heart. Furthermore, the ultrasound image recorded tends to be incomplete because of linear "gaps" due to the space between individual transducer elements. Finally, there may also be distortion due to "cross-talk" or interference between individual transducer elements.[33] An advantage of the linear array system is its capability of producing an M-mode echocardiogram from any portion of the two-dimensional image by utilizing a single transducer. In addition, the linear-array system, because of electronic scanning and the relatively small number of scan lines, permits a relatively high frame rate. Finally, because the ultrasound scan lines are parallel rather than divergent from the source, the linear-array system permits good resolution in the near as well as far field.

PHASED-ARRAY TECHNIQUES

The most recently developed technique for real-time ultrasound cardiac imaging utilizes the phased-array transducer configuration.[34–37] The high speed and excellent resolution that can be achieved with phased-array scanning is related to techniques originally developed for radar. Thurstone and vonRamm described a high-resolution ultrasound scanner in which a multi-element transducer composed of 16 individual crystals was used to produce a single ultrasound beam.[34,35] The ultrasound beam emitted from each individual element fired by itself would diverge at much too shallow a depth to provide good image resolution. By firing each individual crystal simultaneously or nearly simultaneously, the resultant beam formed is nearly identical to a beam formed by a single large transducer of the same area with a single transmitter.[38]

The phased-array technique combines aspects of both linear-array and mechanical sector scanning.[33] As with linear-array, phased-array technique utilizes multi-element transducers to transmit and receive the ultrasound signal. However, rather than each crystal transmitting and receiving separate ultrasound beams, the elements in the phased-array system are activated and electronically steered in such a manner as to produce a single ultrasound beam with a circular sector arc and a fixed axis—similar to that produced in mechanical sector scanners. The direction of the beam is controlled by the time of firing of the individual elements (Figure 1-5).

The phased-array technique depends on Huygen's principle, which dictates that multiple small wavefronts of ultrasound will invariably combine to form a single large ultrasound wave whose direction is determined by the component wavefronts. Furthermore, the direction and angle of the resultant ultrasound wave is determined by the timing of the individual wavefronts. Thus, by altering the time-delay of activation of the individual transducers, the ultrasound beam can be rapidly steered electronically through a sector arc (see Figure 1-5A).

The phased-array transducer can also focus the ultrasound beam by altering the timing of the individual elements. The leading edge of the individual element wave

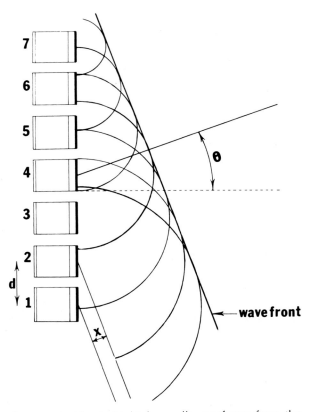

Figure 1-5A. Seven-element phased-array wavefront. Multiple small wavefronts from the individual elements are activated in a specific sequence: 1, 2, then 3, etc., in order to electronically steer the resultant ultrasound beam. The time required for each wavelet to travel a distance (x) is measured in nanoseconds. This is the delay between adjacent transducer elements, where Θ is the off-axis angle of the wavefront and $\sin \Theta = x/d$; d is the interelement distance. (Adapted from Hillard W, Weyns A: Basic physics of ultrasound, in Schapira J, Charuzi, Davidson (eds): Two-Dimensional Echocardiography. Baltimore, Williams & Wilkins, 1982. With permission.)

can form a concentrically curved wavefront so that the resultant ultrasound beam focuses at a given distance from the transducer (see Figure 1-5B). In addition to the capability of electronically focusing the transmitted beam, phased-array systems employ a microprocessor to focus the received ultrasound signal throughout its range depth. This dynamic focusing can provide excellent depth as well as lateral resolution.[36] Phased-array systems in general can produce wide-angle sector images (up to 90°) with relatively high line density and frame rate.

Advantages of the phased-array system over the mechanical sector scanner are the ability to obtain simultaneous (dual M-mode) echocardiograms from different portions of the sector image and the ability to obtain simultaneous two-dimensional and Doppler ultrasound recordings. These advantages are partially due to the fact that the phased-array transducer is stationary. Also, there should theoretically be less breakdown of an electronic than a mechanical transducer. However, in practice, both are prone to malfunction and often the availability of timely service is a more important consideration than the type of transducer. Finally, the phased-array trans-

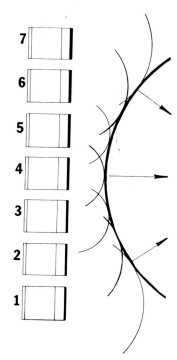

Figure 1-5B. Seven-element phased-array transducer sequenced to fire and electronically focus the resultant wavefront. The leading edge of the wavefront produces a curved front so that the ultrasound beam focuses at a given focal zone. (Adapted from Feigenbaum.[40])

ducer generally requires a smaller acoustic window than a mechanical scanner for a wide-angle scan (see Table 1-1).

The disadvantages of the phased-array system include its relatively large size and its complex and expensive technology. Newer developments, however, continue to diminish both the size and cost of these systems. Ultrasound artifacts known as "side lobes" or "grating lobes" (discussed later in this chapter) are seen only with phased-array scanners (see Table 1-1).

The size of the phased-array transducer depends on whether it is electronically focused and the frequency of the transducer. Unfocused or fixed-focus electronic sector scanners have a relatively small aperture (about 1 cm^2) from which the ultrasound scan is generated[38] (Figure 1-6A). Dynamically focused phased-array transducers (Figure 1-6B) are generally larger than mechanical transducers. However, more recently introduced focused transducers are smaller, partially because of their higher frequency (3.0–3.5 MHz range).[39]

ULTRASOUND BEAM CHARACTERISTICS

Electronic Beam Steering

A typical 32-element phased array transducer face measures approximately 13 mm by 12 mm, with each individual element measuring 0.4 mm by 12 mm.[39] The method of controlled-timed firing of the multiple elements is called electronic beam steering. A single element cannot image a target well because the beam diverges at too shallow a depth. Therefore, each element is used to form a large wavefront that measures the total width of the transducer. When the desired direction of the beam is at an angle other than directly forward, the time of firing of each element will

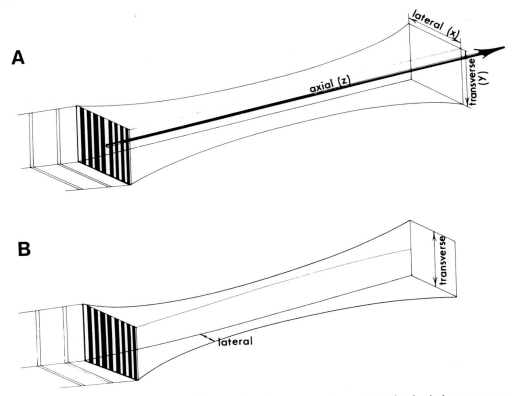

Figure 1-6. A: Diagram of a fixed-focus phased-array transducer. Note that both the transverse and lateral dimensions are fixed-focused. B: Diagram of a dynamically focused phased-array transducer. Note that only the lateral dimension is dynamically focused. The transverse beam is fixed-focused, allowing for unequal transverse and lateral dimensions.

determine the angle of the beam. Figure 1-5A depicts a seven-element phased-array transducer steering at an angle 20° off-axis. The first element fires first; the second element, second; the third element, third; etc. The off-axis angle Θ is calculated from the distance each wavelet propagates before the next element fires (x) and the interelement distance (d). The equation for the off-axis angle Θ is:

$$\text{Sin } \Theta = \frac{x}{d}$$

For each off-axis angle the delay can be calculated; thus, by altering the time-of-firing delay the angle of steering can be changed.

Beam Width

To understand beam width and beam focusing, it is important to review the longitudinal characteristics of the ultrasound beam. The ultrasound beam is a series of longitudinal waves that remain parallel for a given distance and then begin to diverge (Figure 1-7A). The portion of the ultrasound beam that is close to the transducer and parallel to it is known as the "near-field" or "Fresnel" zone. The divergent portion of the beam is known as the "far-field" or "Fraunshofer" zone.[40] It is in the near field where ultrasound waves are most diagnostic (Figure 1-7A). The length of

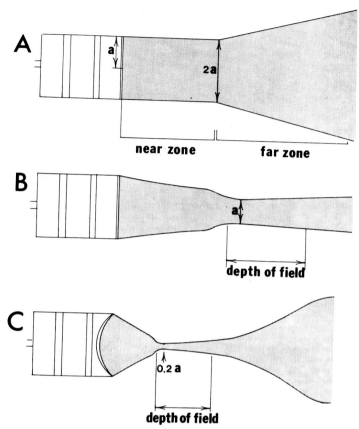

Figure 1-7. A: Beam profiles of a simplified beam-width transducer. B: A more accurate or true beam profile. C: An acoustically focused beam profile. Note that in the simplified beam profile, the beam width is twice (2a) the transducer radius (a), whereas in an accurate profile the beam width (a) equals the radius of the transducer. (Adapted from Hillard.[42])

the near field is directly related to the square of the radius (r) of the ultrasound crystal and inversely related to its wavelength (λ). The near-field length (l) can be calculated from the equation:

$$ 1 = \frac{r^2}{\lambda} $$

Thus, to increase the near field, it would be necessary to increase the diameter of the transducer or decrease the wavelength of the emitted ultrasound (i.e., increase the transducer frequency).

Actually, the ultrasound beam is not simply a beam whose width is equal to that of the transducer in the near field and then diverges, as in Figure 1-7A. Weyns has shown that the near-field portion of the ultrasound beam narrows down to as little as half the width of the transducer before it starts to diverge, as shown in Figure 1-7B.[41] With beam focusing, even smaller beam widths—as little as 10 percent of the diameter of the transducer—can be obtained. However, the smaller the beam width at the focal zone, the sooner the beam diverges beyond this point, resulting in a shallower depth of field (Figure 1-7C).

Beam Focusing

Far-field divergence of the ultrasound beam can be attenuated (1) by focusing the transducer with use of an acoustic lens, (2) by altering the curvature of the transducer head (see Figure 1-7C), or (3) electronically, by using multiple small elements as in a phased-array transducer (see Figure 1-5B). Using a concave acoustic lens or transducer head, the ultrasound beam can be made to converge at a focal zone at a known distance from the transducer, thereby diminishing the divergence of the beam in the far field.

Electronic focusing uses a multiple-element transducer, with each element fired at different time intervals, as in Figure 1-5B. The outside elements (i.e., 1 and 7) are fired first, then elements 2 and 6, 3 and 5, and finally element 4. The developed wavefront becomes concave, which results in an ultrasound beam converging at a focal zone, similar to what is seen with a single-element transducer with an acoustic lens. The curve can be electronically altered to change the focal zone by changing the time of firing of the individual elements.

Dynamic Versus Fixed Focusing

The three measurable components of a rectangular ultrasound beam used in most phased-array transducers are its lateral axis (x axis), its transverse axis (y axis), and its axial length (z axis) (Figure 1-6A,B). The phased-array ultrasound beam can be either fixed-focused or dynamically focused.[34–36] Fixed-focus phased-array transducers use a concave spherical lens to focus the beam at a fixed depth in both the lateral and transverse axes (Figure 1-6A). Dynamically focused phased-array systems use a cyclindrical lens to focus the ultrasound beam at a fixed depth only in the transverse (y) axis (Figure 1-6B). The focusing of the lateral dimensions (x axis) is performed electronically by creating a curved wavefront in transmission as discussed earlier. Dynamic focusing refers to the ability to electronically change the depth of focus. The advantages of a dynamically focused system are that it has a longer focal zone and that this zone can be quickly changed when necessary. Also, the lateral beam width focusing is improved over the transverse beam.

An important limitation of dynamic focusing is that the dynamic alteration in the beam is made not during transmission but during reception. Once the wavefront is transmitted, the transmitted focal zone is fixed and cannot be altered; only during reception can the focal zone be altered. In dynamic focusing, therefore, the beam is not focused in either the lateral or transverse dimension during transmission, nor is it focused in the transverse dimension during reception. Thus, only one of four beam dimensions is dynamically focused. Since lateral and transverse beam resolutions are both displayed in the image as lateral resolution, the poorer of the two dominates without visible improvement in display. Only when imaging single-dimension objects (such as pacing wires or catheters) perpendicular to the image plane can improved imaging ability in the lateral dimension be perceived.[42]

Mechanical sector scanners currently cannot be electronically focused. They can utilize acoustic focusing, employing a lens or shaped ultrasound crystal head that focuses the transverse and lateral axes equally. Although an annular or "ring beam" phased-array transducer has been developed,[37] it is not currently utilized in echocardiography[40] because of the difficulties inherent in electronic steering of an annular phased-array beam. If annular phased-array technology is perfected, electronic dynamic focusing of the ultrasound beam may be possible in the transverse as well as the lateral axis. This would be an advantage over the acoustically focused single-crystal mechanical sector scanner, since a dynamically focused beam has a longer focal zone and therefore better lateral resolution[40] (see Figure 1-6).

RESOLUTION

Resolution is defined as the capacity of an instrument to produce separate images of two similar close objects. In phased-array technology resolution cannot be described by one or two measurements, since the object or target lies in three dimensions but is displayed in only two. The radial or depth resolution of the phased-array image is directly related to the acoustic pulse length. Lateral resolution of an image is determined by the width of the ultrasound beam. The transverse beam width may also affect either the radial or lateral resolution depending on the object being imaged.[42]

Axial or Depth Resolution

The frequency or wavelength of the emitted ultrasound is the most important factor in axial or depth resolution. To define small targets, a short wavelength or high-frequency transducer is required. The longer the wavelength of the ultrasonic pulse the further apart must be the targets to be resolved, hence the poorer the depth resolution. Another factor that influences axial resolution is the processing of the

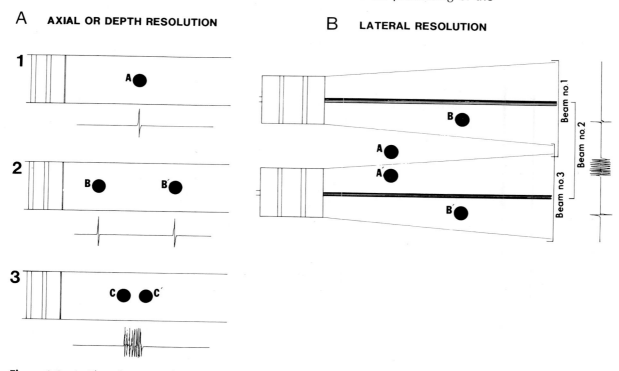

A   AXIAL OR DEPTH RESOLUTION   **B   LATERAL RESOLUTION**

Figure 1-8. A: Three beam profiles and their reception signals from two closely placed targets illustrate depth or axial resolution. Note that in profile 3 the closely placed targets are unresolved. B: Beam profiles and their reception signals from two closely placed targets illustrate lateral resolution. Targets A and A' in the same beam width are unresolved. Targets B and B' in separate beam widths are resolved.

reflected ultrasound signal. If, for instance, the reflected signal is displayed on a storage oscilloscope without a gray scale, two individual echoes cannot be resolved as two targets. If two small targets are closely spaced (as in Figure 1-8A), a typical pulse length of 1 microsecond will yield a depth resolution of 1.5 mm. Any two small targets closer together than 1.5 mm will not be resolved in their axial or depth axis.

Lateral Resolution

Beam width is the most important factor in lateral resolution. As discussed earlier, the beam width will vary with depth; therefore, lateral resolution will also vary with depth. In phased-array technology, lateral resolution varies not only with depth but also with beam angle. As larger off-axis angles are steered, the effective area of the transducer is reduced (see Figure 1-5A), resulting in increased beam width and decreased resolution.[42] If two targets are enveloped by a single beam at the same time, then the system cannot resolve them as separate objects. If, however, they are in separate beams, they can be laterally resolved (Figure 1-8B).

Image quality is not only a function of resolution but is also related to sensitivity of receivers, dynamic range, imaging rate, signal processing, scan conversion, display quality, and artifacts. Other factors that play a role are proper gain setting, noise level, and the target's acoustic reflectivity.[42] Some of these factors are discussed in the following sections.

IMAGING RATES

The factors limiting imaging rate are related to the physical properties of ultrasound. The imaging rate is determined by the depth of the image, the lines per image, and the machine set-up time.[42] The time to gather information from the target is related to the depth of the image. If the target depth is 22.5 cm, then sound must travel a total of 45 cm. Since the speed of ultrasound in tissues is approximately 1540 m/second, the time required to generate one line or transmit–receive cycle of ultrasound information is 0.29 millisecond. Thus, for an image made up of 128 lines of imaging data, 37 milliseconds would be required. Allowing for machine set-up time of 5 milliseconds, an imaging rate of 24 frames per second is calculated. The line rate or pulse repetition frequency would be 24 frames per second by 128 lines per frame, or approximately 3070 lines per second (3 kHz).

If all other variables remain constant, increasing the scan angle from 30° to 90° will decrease the line density (lines per degree) by two-thirds, leading to a significant degradation in image quality. Improvement in line density could be accomplished by decreasing the imaging depth or the sweep or frame rate.[40]

SIGNAL PROCESSING

Digital Scan Converter and Display Formats

The addition of a digital scan converter to many of the currently available two-dimensional ultrasound systems has resulted in major advances in image processing, display, and storage. The digital scan converter changes the reflected pulsed ultrasound signal from analog to digital format. The digital data is then placed in the

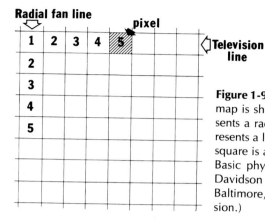

Figure 1-9. Digital scan converter memory. A memory map is shown in which each column (vertical) represents a radial scan line and each horizontal row represents a line of television information. Note that each square is a pixel. (Adapted from Hillard W, Weyns A: Basic physics of ultrasound, in Schapira J, Charuzi, Davidson (eds): Two-Dimensional Echocardiography. Baltimore, Williams & Wilkins, 1982. With permission.)

memory of a microprocessor frame by frame and can be read out in real-time television format to a video monitor and tape recorder.

The digital scan converter quantitizes the information from the two-dimensional scan lines into a regular matrix of small picture elements known as *pixels* (Figure 1-9). This matrix typically can be either a square with 512 elements or pixels on each side or a rectangle in which each radial fan line is represented by a column (e.g., 128 columns), and each television line is represented by a row (e.g., 480 rows). The former image matrix would be described by 262,144 pixels and the latter by 61,000 pixels, each of which is encoded by a number, or *word,* in the random-access memory of a microprocessor. The brightness of each pixel corresponds to this number. In the absence of a digital scan converter, the unprocessed ultrasound data appears in analog format and is displayed on an x-y oscilloscope. A television camera monitors the oscilloscope to develop an image that is displayed on the video monitor and recorded on a videotape recorder. Some image degradation occurs when the unprocessed ultrasound data is processed through the television camera for a video image.

Digital scan converters have the capacity to store large amounts of data. Depending on the "bit" (binary digit) capacity of the scan converter, varying levels of gray scale can be stored. For example, a digital scan converter with a 10-bit capacity allows storage of 2^{10}, or 1024, shades of gray in each pixel. Another option for the 10-bit memory digital scan converter is to store two images simultaneously, each image being represented by 5 bits of information per pixel. Although the human eye cannot distinguish more than 32 shades of gray (5 bits), the additional bit capacity is useful for various signal manipulations.

In addition to producing better image quality, the digital scan converter can manipulate, measure, and store images. Since the gray scale is stored in digital form, the scan converter has the capability to "freeze" image frames that display the appropriate gray scale. Furthermore, an EKG trigger permits freezing images in preselected portions of the cardiac cycle. The ability to "freeze" frames also allows two-dimensional images to be recorded directly onto a strip chart record. Furthermore, measurements of such parameters as mitral valve orifice area or left ventricular volume may be made electronically from the frozen image.

The digitized ultrasound data may be manipulated in a number of ways. Manipulations may be performed when the ultrasound data is being recorded ("preprocessing") or at some future time ("postprocessing"). Pre- and postprocessing changes in gray scale may be accomplished by manipulating the absolute range of echoes with an acoustic window, i.e., by rejecting echoes at either edge of the gray scale spectrum. In addition, amplification or suppression of echoes of different amplitude may be accomplished utilizing various linear or logarithmic functions to enhance certain portions of the gray scale. Incoming ultrasound data may be averaged temporally to increase the definition of the image and to reduce "noise." For example, three frames may be added together and displayed at 10 frames per second, providing a relatively "flicker-free" image when compared to an image displayed at 30 frames per second. Furthermore, spatial averaging may be performed to produce smoother images and eliminate individual scan lines seen in the analog television format. In this technique, new pixels are created to fill in between pixels by interpolating the values of the surrounding pixels.

Effects of Controls

The *transmission level control,* or *gain control,* adjusts the energy output in the transmission pulse, which may be varied depending on the echogenicity of the subject. The two types of gain control are the *overall gain* and the *time depth compensation* (TGC) controls. The overall gain adjusts the gain uniformly over the entire transmission range. The time depth compensation controls usually adjust gain at fixed depth intervals, thus allowing the operator to vary the gain at various depths and compensate for attenuation of the ultrasound signal in the heart or other structure.[42]

The *reject control* adjusts the level below which noise and signal will not be displayed. As reject is increased, more noise is removed from the image, but at the expense of low-level signals. This control is best set at its minimum level while other controls are set appropriately. It should be utilized only to eliminate noise and a minimal amount of signal.

Compression Transfer Functions

The compression control adjusts the assignment of gray scale to the received echo signal. The various echo signal amplitude data to gray scale assignments are called transfer functions. The logarithmic compression transfer function (log) can amplify low-level signals, such as from endocardium, *or* reduce the high-level signals from pericardium (Figure 1-10A). Using this display, the low-level signals such as from endocardium receive a greater amount of emphasis (more intense shades) than in the linear setting (Figure 1-10B). An expanded compression transfer function allows the operator to de-emphasize low-level signals and noise (Figure 1-10C).

The S-curve transfer function allows the operator to image low-level signals and high-level signals in a different manner. One can expand the high-level data and logarithmically compress the low-level data, as in Figure 1-10D, or expand low-level signals and compress high-level signals, as in Figure 1-10E. The window transfer function allows the operator to select a range of echo amplitude data and assign the entire gray scale to that range. The low- or midlevel amplitude signal could have the entire gray scale assigned, as shown in Figure 1-10F.[42]

Despite the advantages of digital scan conversion over a standard analog format, recording of ultrasound signals onto videotape can result in image quality degradation with either technique. In some videotape systems, only half of the scan lines displayed in real time (i.e., a *field*) are exhibited during stop-frame imaging. Furthermore, when viewing stop-frame images, the viewer loses information available from watching the target in motion. Advances in display technology have solved some

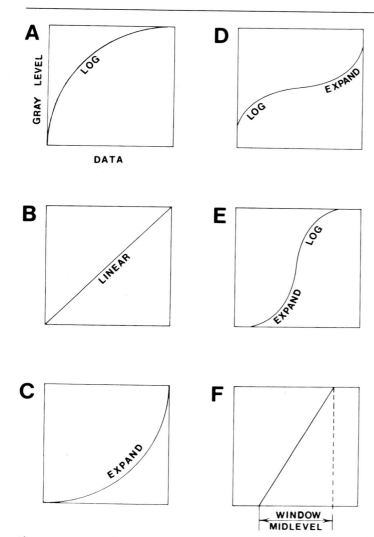

Figure 1-10. Six different compression transfer functions (A–F) in which echo data can be compressed into various levels of gray scale. (Adapted from Hillard W, Weyns A: Basic physics of ultrasound, in Schapira J, Charuzi, Davidson (eds): Two-Dimensional Echocardiography. Baltimore, Williams & Wilkins, 1982. With permission.)

of these problems. For example, use of a video disc allows stop-frame display of a full frame, rather than merely a field, and permits improved slow-motion analysis in both forward and reverse modes.

ARTIFACTS

One difficulty that frequently arises in the interpretation of echocardiographic images relates to differentiating ultrasonic artifacts from true intracardiac masses, such as those due to calcification, vegetation, tumor, or clot. There are a number of potential artifacts in a two-dimensional echocardiographic examination that may be related to the ultrasound instrument or to the performance or interpretation of the study.[33,40]

Reverberations

Reverberations may be seen in both M-mode and two-dimensional echocardiograms. Figure 1-11 illustrates the mode of genesis of a reverberation artifact. In this example, the ultrasound beam travels through the chest wall and right ventricular structures to strike the catheter. A relatively strong signal (B) is displayed on the echocardiogram at a distance behind the transducer echo (T) that is directly proportional to the distance of the catheter from the transducer. The returning signal is weaker than the transmitted ultrasound signal because of attenuation and backscatter of the signal that has occurred en route to its target—i.e., the catheter. In the absence of any rereflection signal the normal echocardiographic appearance of the structure is maintained. If, however, the transducer or another intracardiac structure reflects the ultrasound beam on its return path, a portion of the ultrasound beam may then move in its original path but with markedly diminished intensity. When this reflected beam strikes the catheter again and returns once more to the transducer, a second signal (B') will be recorded at twice the distance from the transducer as the original catheter signal.[40] This second signal (B'), or reverberation, is generally weaker than the original echo (B) because of attenuation. If the original echo (B) is in motion, the reverberation echo (B') will appear to be moving at twice the speed of the original echo. If the sampling depth of the instrument is less than twice the depth of the structure being imaged, the reverberating echo will appear on the screen at a shallower depth than the original structure. For example, a strong pericardial echo at 8 cm from the transducer may give rise to a weaker "wrap-around" reverberation at 4 cm if the sampling depth is only 12 cm.

Figure 1-12A demonstrates an instance in which reverberation echoes are seen within the left ventricular cavity. The origin of these echoes is not immediately obvious, and echoes such as these could be confused with a pathologic entity such as a thrombus.[33,43,44] Often, readjusting the angle of the transducer can eliminate these artifacts. Reverberations are commonly recorded from intracardiac catheters or prosthetic valves. Figure 1-12B shows a reverberation echo from the transducer and its housing in the right ventricular cavity.

An interesting form of reverberation artifact can be observed with a specific ul-

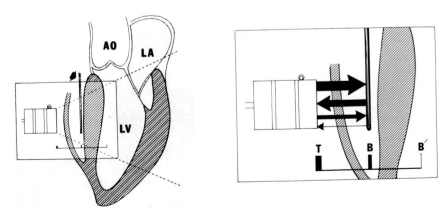

Figure 1-11. Diagrammatic representation of genesis of a reverberation artifact from a catheter in the right ventricle. An artifactual echocardiographic signal due to reverberation (B') which is weaker than the original echo may be recorded at twice the distance from the transducer (T) as the original catheter echo (B).

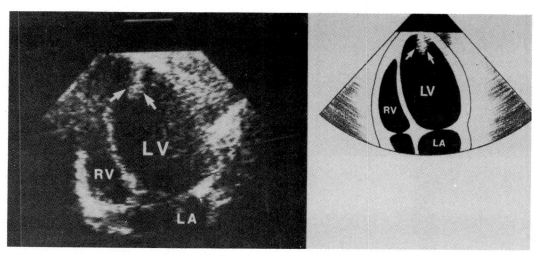

Figure 1-12A. Apical four-chamber view demonstrating a reverberation artifact from the apex of the left ventricle (arrows) that simulates a protruding intracavity thrombus. LA denotes left atrium; LV, left ventricle; RV, right ventricle. (From Asinger RW, Mikel FL, Sharma B, et al: Observations on detecting left ventricular thrombus with two-dimensional echocardiography: Emphasis on avoidance of false positive diagnoses. Am J Cardiol 47:145, 1981. With permission.)

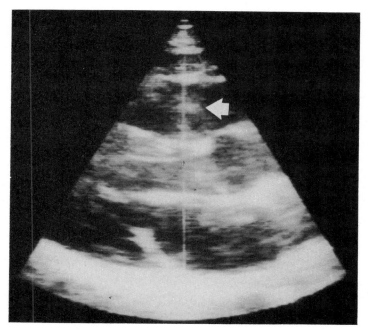

Figure 1-12B. Parasternal long-axis view demonstrating reverberation echoes in the right ventricle (solid arrow) arising from the transducer.

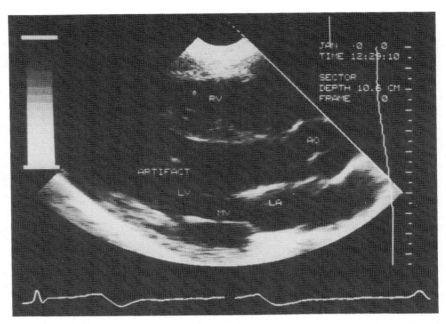

Figure 1-13. Parasternal long-axis view of a "Herbie" artifact in the left ventricle produced by a mechanical four-element rotating transducer. The system gain is artificially high, and the depth setting has been reduced to enhance the artifact. AO denotes aorta; MV, mitral valve. (Courtesy of Martha Ann Fulton, Advanced Technological Laboratories, Bellevue, WA.)

trasound system that utilizes a two-dimensional multi-element rotary mechanical transducer. This particular artifact, nicknamed "Herbie," is apparently caused by an ultrasound signal returning on a pulse–listen cycle later than the one during which it was transmitted. For example, if a signal is emitted into a very echogenic heart, part of the signal may be reflected all the way back to the scanhead and part may also be reflected off an anterior heart structure. The reflected signal may then reverberate within a cardiac chamber to be received on a later pulse–listen cycle. This artifact usually appears as a linear, rapidly oscillating signal, which can often be eliminated by changing depth settings. Figure 1-13 is an example of such an artifact.

Acoustic Shadowing

A target that strongly reflects or attenuates ultrasound slows the transmission of ultrasound through its area. Since little ultrasound is transmitted through the target, structures behind or in the shadow of the target may not be recorded on the echocardiogram. Figure 4-21 is an example of how calcification located behind the posterior mitral leaflet may produce an acoustic shadow that does not permit the left ventricular endocardium to be recorded.

Excessive Gain Settings

The apparent size of an imaged target is dependent upon the amount of the beam width being displayed. For example, if only 10 percent of the beam intensity is being displayed, the target will appear narrow or thin. On the other hand, when 90 percent of the beam intensity is displayed, targets will appear larger and more distorted than

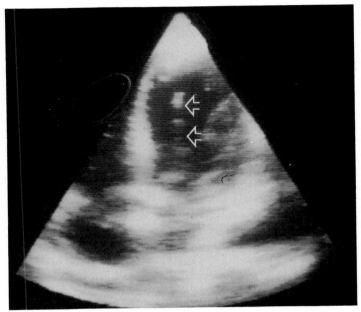

Figure 1-14. Apical four-chamber view demonstrating the artifactual production of masslike echoes (arrows) arising from blood within the left ventricular cavity in a normal subject. These artifactual echoes disappeared after reducing the gain settings.

their actual size and shape; valve orifices, on the other hand, will appear reduced when compared to their actual dimensions. This artifact is sometimes called "blooming."

Artifactual echoes may be produced by inappropriately high gain settings. Figure 1-14 is an example of an artifact produced by masslike echoes arising from intra-cavitary blood in a normal subject. This artifact disappeared after reducing the gain settings. Similarly, Figure 4-12 demonstrates the effect of excessive gain settings on mitral valve orifice measurement in a patient with mitral stenosis. The use of an inappropriately high gain setting results in the recording of a mitral valve orifice area that is artifactually smaller.[45]

Lobe Artifacts

All transducers have beam patterns that contain "side lobes."[40,42] These weaker beams of ultrasound energy are adjacent to the main beam and are generated from the edges of the individual transducer elements (Figure 1-15). Unfortunately, these auxiliary beams or side lobes can be reflected from intracardiac targets as if they were in the main ultrasound beam. Although these "phantom echoes" are generally weaker in intensity than those reflected from the main beam, they may occasionally be confused with a true anatomic structure. Generally, side-lobe artifacts originate from strong reflecting surfaces such as calcification or fibrous tissue that is present within the fibrous skeleton of the heart. Often a curved line known as a "smile artifact" is generated by multiple side-lobe artifacts from a single object.[42] Figures 1-16 and 1-17A demonstrate examples of side-lobe artifacts. Side-lobe artifacts can usually be diminished or eliminated by decreasing the gain settings or increasing the reject level of the ultrasound instrument.

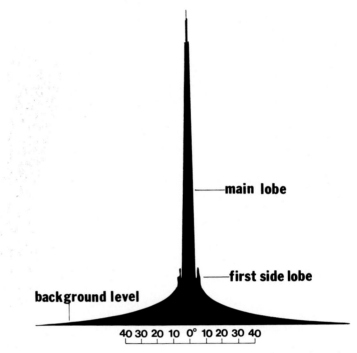

Figure 1-15. Lateral beam pattern profile shown to illustrate "side lobes" originating from the main lobe. The ultrasound beam profile is shown versus the angle from beam center at a constant depth from the transducer. (Adapted from Hillard W, Weyns A: Basic physics of ultrasound, in Schapira J, Charuzi, Davidson (eds): Two-Dimensional Echocardiography. Baltimore, Williams & Wilkins, 1982. With permission.)

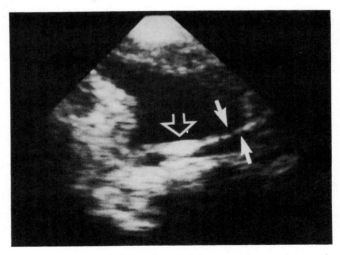

Figure 1-16. Apical four-chamber view of a side-lobe artifact (solid arrows) in a patient with a prosthetic Beall caged-disc mitral valve (open arrow).

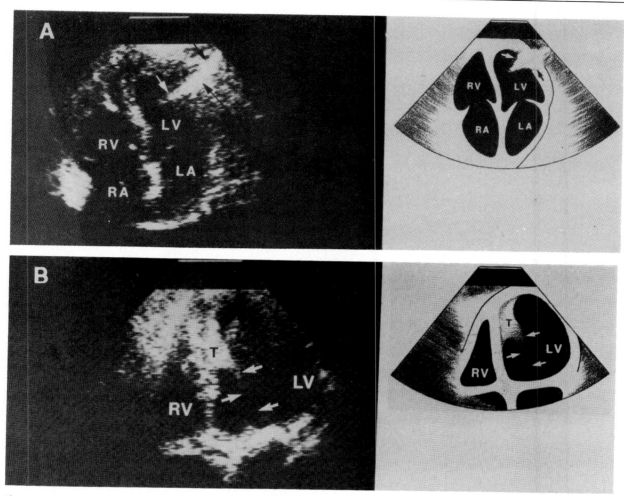

Figure 1-17. A. Apical four-chamber view demonstrating a spurious side-lobe artifact along the lateral wall of the left ventricle (arrows) which simulates a thrombus. B: In contrast, an apical septal thrombus (T) is present with a thrombus tail (arrows). (From Asinger RW, Mikell FL, Sharma B, et al: Observations on detecting left ventricular thrombus with two-dimensional echocardiography: Emphasis on avoidance of false positive diagnoses. Am J Cardiol 47:145, 1981. With permission.)

Another type of lobe artifact occasionally produced by phased-array transducers is known as a "grating-lobe" artifact. Grating-lobe artifacts may occur when there are gaps between individual transducer elements of greater than one wavelength. Since more than one beam is present simultaneously, a single object may be imaged at two locations.[42]

Confusing Structures

Sometimes, echoes from normal cardiac structures may be erroneously confused with an intracardiac mass. For example, a prominent papillary muscle may be mistaken for a left ventricular clot or tumor, especially when it is imaged in an

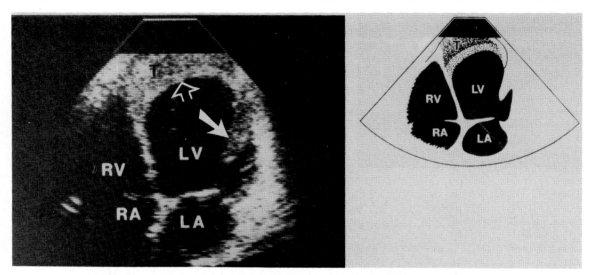

Figure 1-18. Apical four-chamber view demonstrating a prominent left ventricular papillary muscle (solid arrow) in the anterior lateral region of the apex. The echocardiographic appearance of a papillary muscle, especially when imaged tangentially, may sometimes be confused with the appearance of an intraventricular thrombus (as in Figure 1-17B). There is also a layered thrombus (open arrow) in the left ventricular apical region. (From Asinger RW, Mikell FL, Sharma B, et al: Observations on detecting left ventricular thrombus with two-dimensional echocardiography: Emphasis on avoidance of false positive diagnoses. Am J Cardiol 47:145, 1981. With permission.)

unusual way. Figure 1-18 demonstrates an example of a prominent papillary muscle simulating an intracardiac thrombus.

DeMaria and coworkers[43] and Asinger and associates[44] have stressed a number of guidelines for distinguishing the echocardiographic appearance of a cardiac mass from that of an artifact. First, it has been noted that most true masses exhibit some motion during the cardiac cycle, either in association with or independent of the motion of a cardiac structure. Second, virtually all true masses demonstrate a relatively circumscribed border, rather than an amorphous accumulation of echoes. Third, cardiac masses must demonstrate some attachment to a cardiac structure; otherwise, a true intracavitary mass would be propelled out of the heart. Failure to demonstrate such an attachment to a cardiac surface suggests that the accumulation of echoes is an artifact. Fourth, a true mass or other pathologic lesion should be capable of being imaged in multiple projections in the same anatomic region. Finally, intraventricular thrombi that occur in the context of an acute myocardial infarction or a dilated cardiomyopathy have all been noted to reside adjacent to an area of abnormally contracting left ventricular wall.[46]

REFERENCES

1. Feigenbaum H: Echocardiography (ed 2). Philadelphia, Lea & Febiger, 1976, pp 1–4
2. Firestone FA: The supersonic reflectoscope, an instrument for inspecting the interior of solid parts by means of sound waves. J Acoust Soc Am 17:287, 1945
3. Firestone FA: The supersonic reflectoscope for interior inspection. Metal Prog 48:505, 1945

4. Keidel WD: Uber eine methode zur reistriering der volumanderungen des herzens am menschen. Z Kreislaufforsch 39:257, 1950
5. Edler I, Hertz CH: Use of ultrasonic reflectoscope for continuous recording of movements of heart walls. Kung Fysiograf Sallsk Lund Fordhandl 24:40, 1954
6. Edler I, Hertz CH, Gustafson A, et al: The movements of the heart valves recorded by ultrasound. Nord Med 64:1178, 1960
7. Edler I, Gustafson A, Karlefors T, et al: Ultrasound cardiography. Acta Med Scand (suppl) 370:68, 1961
8. Edler I, Gustafson A, Karlefors T, et al: The movements of aortic and mitral valves recorded with ultrasonic echo techniques. Film presented at Third European Congress of Cardiology, Rome, 1960
9. Effert S, Erkens K, Grossebrockhoft F: Ultrasonic echo method in cardiological diagnosis. German Med Monthly 2:325, 1957
10. Effert S: Pre- and post-operative evaluation of mitral stenosis by ultrasound. Am J Cardiol 19:59, 1967
11. Joyner CR, Reid JM, Bond JP: Reflected ultrasound in the assessment of mitral valve disease. Circulation 27:506, 1963
12. Feigenbaum H, Waldhausen JA, Hyde LP: Ultrasound diagnosis of pericardial effusion. JAMA 191:107, 1965
13. Feigenbaum H, Zaky A, Waldhausen JA: Use of ultrasound in the diagnosis of pericardial effusion. Ann Intern Med 65:443, 1966
14. Gramiak R, Shah PM, Kramer DH: Ultrasound cardiography: Contrast studies in anatomy and function. Radiology 92:939, 1969
15. Feigenbaum H: Echocardiography (ed 2). Philadelphia: Lea & Febiger, 1976, pp 30–33
16. Ebina T, Oka S, Tanaka M, et al: The ultrasono-tomography of the heart and great vessels in living human subjects by means of the ultrasonic reflection technique. Jpn Heart J 8:331, 1967
17. King DL: Cardiac ultrasonography: Cross-sectional ultrasonic images of the heart. Circulation 47:843, 1973
18. Teichholz L, Cohen MV, Sonnenblick EM, et al: Study of left ventricular geometry and function by B-scan ultrasonography in patients with and without asynergy. N Engl J Med 291:1220, 1974
19. Asberg A: Ultrasonic cinematography of the living heart. Ultrasonics 6:113, 1967
20. Flaherty JJ, Clark JW, Walgren HN: Simultaneous fluoroscopic and rapid scan ultrasound imaging. Proceedings of the Second International Conference of Medical Biology and Engineering 7:221, 1967
21. Patzold J, Krause W, Resse H: Present state of ultrasonic cross section procedure with rapid image rate. IEEE Trans Biomed Eng 17:263, 1970
22. Hertz CH, Lindstrom K: A fast ultrasonic scanning system for heart investigation, in Proceedings of the Third International Conference on Medical Physics, Gothenburg 35:6, 1972
23. Griffith JM, Henry WL: A sector scanner for real-time two-dimensional echocardiography. Circulation 49:1147, 1974
24. Eggleton RC, Feigenbaum H, Johnston KW: Visualization of cardiac dynamics with real-time B mode ultrasonic scanner. Ultrasound Med Biol 1:385, 1975
25. vonRamm OT, Thurstone FL: Thauma-scan: Design considerations and performance characteristics, in White D (ed): Ultrasound in Medicine. New York, Plenum Press, 1975
26. Bom N, Lancee CT, Honkoop J, et al: Ultrasonic viewer for cross-sectional analyses of moving cardiac structures. Biomed Eng 6:500, 1971
27. Bom N, Lancee CT, Van Zwieten G et al: Multiscan echocardiography. I. Technical description. Circulation 48:1066, 1973
28. Kloster FE, Roelandt J, ten Cate FJ, et al: Multiscan echocardiography. II. Technique and initial clinical results. Circulation 48:1075, 1973
29. King DL: Real-time cross-sectional ultrasonic imaging of the heart using a linear array multi-element transducer. JCU 1:196, 1973
30. Yoshikawa J, Owaki T, Kato H, et al: Electroscan echocardiography: Application to the cardiac diagnosis. J Cardiogr 7:33, 1977
31. Pederson JF, Northeved A: An ultrasonic multitransducer scanner for real-time heart imaging. JCU 5:11, 1977
32. Vogel J, Bom N, Ridder J, et al: Transducer design considerations in dynamic focusing. Ultrasound Med Biol 5:187, 1979
33. DeMaria AN, Bommer W, Joye JA, et al: Cross-sectional echocardiography: Physical principles, anatomic planes, limitations, and pitfalls. Am J Cardiol 46:1097, 1980

34.   vonRamm OT, Thurstone FL: Cardiac imaging using a phased array ultrasound system: I. System design. Circulation 53:258, 1976

35.   Kisslo J, vonRamm OT, Thurstone FL: Cardiac imaging using a phased array ultrasound system: II. Clinical technique and application. Circulation 53:262, 1976

36.   Morgan CL, Trought WS, Clark WM, et al: Principles and applications of a dynamically focused phased array real-time ultrasound system. JCU 6:385, 1978

37.   Melton HE, Thurstone FL: Annular array design and logarithmic processing for ultrasonic imaging. Ultrasound Med Biol 4:1, 1978

38.   Somer J: Electronic sector scanning for ultrasonic diagnosis. Ultrasonics 6:153, 1968

39.   Anderson W, Arnold J, Clark L, et al: A new real-time phased-array sector scanner for imaging the entire adult human heart, in White D, Brown R (eds): Ultrasound in Medicine, vol. 3B. New York: Plenum Press, 1977, p 1547

40.   Feigenbaum H: Echocardiography (ed 3). Philadelphia, Lea & Febiger, 1981, pp 1–50

41.   Weyns A: Radiation field calculations of pulsed ultrasonic transducers. Ultrasonics 18:183, 1980

42.   Hillard W: Basic physics of ultrasound, in Schapira J, Charuzi, Davidson (eds): Two-Dimensional Echocardiography. Baltimore, Williams & Wilkins, 1982, pp 319–334

43.   DeMaria AN, Bommer W, Neuman A: Left ventricular thrombi identified by cross-sectional echocardiography. Ann Intern Med 90:14, 1979

44.   Asinger RW, Mikell FL, Sharma B, et al: Observations on detecting left ventricular thrombus with two dimensional echocardiography: Emphasis on avoidance of false positive diagnoses. Am J Cardiol 47:145, 1981

45.   Martin R, Rakowski H, Kleiman J, et al: Reliability and reproducibility of two-dimensional echocardiographic measurement of stenotic mitral valve orifice area. Am J Cardiol 43:560–568, 1979

46.   Asinger RW, Mikell FL, Elsperger J, et al: Incidence of left ventricular thrombosis after acute myocardial infarction. Serial evaluation by two-dimensional echocardiography. N Engl J Med 305:297, 1981

CHAPTER 2

Anatomy of the Heart

David I. Koenigsberg and Charles Ganote

The heart obtained at postmortem examination is not the same size or configuration of the heart during life because normal intravascular and intracavity pressures are not present. With cessation of blood flow, the heart becomes globally ischemic, undergoes ischemic contracture, and enters a state analogous to rigor mortis in skeletal muscles. Because of ischemic contracture and rigor after death, the heart assumes a ventricular cavity size and wall thickness approximate to that of cardiac systole during life. It may therefore be said that the heart "dies" in systole and that anatomic measurements made at postmortem examination most closely approximate those of ventricular systole obtained by echocardiography. The heart in failure or with elevated end-systolic intracavity volumes during life retains a dilated atrium and ventricle after death and apparently resembles a normal heart in diastole. Only fortuitous circumstance generates a heart that at postmortem examination duplicates the atrial and ventricular chamber size and configuration of a living heart. Although the measurements of the living and fixed heart differ, the anatomic structures of both remain similar.

It is often difficult or impossible to section a heart specimen so that it exactly corresponds to an analogous echocardiographic "cut" of a living heart. Nonetheless, attempts to correlate sectional views of fixed hearts with M-mode or two-dimensional echocardiograms can lead to a greater understanding of anatomic relationships among structures in the normal and diseased heart. Although a still-frame image of a two-dimensional echocardiogram does not do justice to real-time imaging of cardiac motion, sufficient information is present on still photographs of two-dimensional echocardiograms for comparison with pathologic specimens.

Two-dimensional echocardiography allows multiple tomographic views of the living heart that are similar to those obtained in pathologic specimens. Cineangiography provides a positive contrast image of the left ventricular cavity and allows analysis of segmental wall disease, left-to-right shunts, intracardiac masses, and stenotic or regurgitant lesions. On the other hand, two-dimensional echocardiography is noninvasive and allows better definition of valvular, myocardial, and pericardial anatomy than does cineangiography. In addition, several views of the heart obtained with echocardiography cannot be obtained with cineangiography. Never-

---

Some of the figures in this chapter are reprinted with permission from Talano JV: Cardiac Ultrasound Workbook. New York, Grune & Stratton, 1982.

theless, left ventriculographic and two-dimensional echocardiographic views of the heart are frequently analogous in their orientations; the apical two-chamber two-dimensional echocardiogram and the 30° right anterior oblique left ventriculogram are similar.

This chapter focuses on the standard two-dimensional echocardiographic views of the heart. In each instance the anatomic view is presented first, followed by the corresponding tomographic echocardiographic view. Where instructive, the two-dimensional echocardiograms in both systole and diastole are demonstrated. The American Society of Echocardiography recommendations for standard terminology are used.[1] In addition, the tomograms are cross-referenced to those obtained by Tajik et al.[2]

PARASTERNAL LONG-AXIS VIEW, LEFT VENTRICLE

Anatomic Specimen

The section in Figures 2-1A and B, oriented to correspond to an echocardiographic parasternal long-axis view (see also Tajik et al.[2] section 1), shows the heart sliced from apex to base. The anterior wall of the right ventricle (RV) is at the top of the photograph and this view looks toward the tricuspid valve. The plane crosses the interventricular septum (IVS), the left coronary cusps (LCC), the posterior aorta and anterior left atrial wall. The membranous septum (MS) is located at the junction of the right coronary cusp (RCC) and the noncoronary cusp (NCC) of the aortic valve.

The section crosses near the middle of the anterior and posterior leaflets of the mitral valve (AML and PML). The posteromedial papillary muscle (PPM) lies at the junction of the septum (IVS) and the posterior wall (PW) of the left ventricle. The chordae tendineae are attached to the medial halves of both the anterior and posterior mitral leaflets (AML and PML). The posterior wall of the left atrium (LA) is continuous with the posterior mitral leaflets; there is good continuity between the cavities of the left atrium and left ventricle. The posterior wall of the left ventricle forms a rounded shelf which bulges posteriorly to the wall of the left atrium. The atrioventricular sulcus (junction) is filled with adipose and contains the coronary sinus (CS). A pulmonary vein (PV) enters the posterior wall of the left atrium.

Two-Dimensional Echocardiogram

The heart is seen in long-axis view during systole with both leaflets of the mitral valve forming a "Y" coaptation pattern (Figures 2-1C, D, E). The anterior and posterior mitral valve leaflets (AML and PML) form the two arms of the "Y"; the chordae tendineae form the leg. The anterior leaflet of the mitral valve is contiguous with the posterior aortic wall (PAW). The leaflets of the mitral valve can be seen to open in their full excursion during diastole (Figure 2-1C). The left atrium (LA) is posterior to the posterior wall of the aorta. At the junction of the posterior left atrial wall and posterior mitral leaflet, the atrioventricular sulcus can be seen. Only the right curonary cusp (RCC) and the noncoronary cusp (NCC) of the aortic valve are seen during systole. The cusps of the aortic valve can be seen to coapt in a single line (Figure 2-1D) during diastole. The right ventricular outflow tract (RVOT) is anterior to the aorta (AO). The left ventricular cavity is seen in its long axis. The interventricular septum (IVS) and right ventricle (RV) are located anteriorly, and the left ventricular posterior wall (PW) and posterior papillary muscle (PPM) are located posteriorly. The apex of the left ventricle (LV) is identified as the rounded tip at the left of the image (Figure 2-1C). Note the enlargement of the left ventricle and contraction of the left atrium during diastole. The difference in left ventricular cavity size in systole and diastole is particularly noteworthy in Figure 2-1D. The apex may not be easily visualized in this view; the apical four-chamber view and the apical two-chamber view may be useful for demonstrating it.

PARASTERNAL LONG-AXIS VIEW, RIGHT VENTRICLE

Anatomic Specimen

To view the right atrium and right ventricle in long axis, a section is made from base to apex tangential to the heart (Figures 2-2A, B). This view of the heart (seen from the right side looking toward the left) shows the plane of section. Lateral and medial to the plane of section are the aorta, the right atrial appendage, the superior vena cava, the coronary sinus, and the septal leaflet of the tricuspid valve. The section cuts across the anterior and posterior tricuspid valve leaflets, the inferior vena cava, and the right coronary artery.

The long-axis view of the right ventricle (Figures 2-2B, C) looks toward the right side of the atrium (RA) and ventricle (RV); this corresponds to the tomographic long-axis view no. 2 described by Tajik et al.[2] The section passes across the anterior and posterior leaflets of the tricuspid valve (ATL and PTL) and the opening of the inferior vena cava (IVC). The anterior and posterior papillary muscles (APM and PPM) of the tricuspid valve are present. The right coronary artery (RCA) lies in adipose in the atrioventricular sulcus. It should be noted that in the long-axis view of the right ventricle commonly obtained during two-dimensional echocardiography, the interventricular septum, as opposed to the posterior wall of the right ventricle, forms the inferior border of the right ventricle. Consequently, Figure 2-2D is an alternate description of the corresponding echocardiographic tomogram. Here the interventricular septum (IVS) is cut tangentially; the section passes through the septal and anterior leaflets of the tricuspid valve (STL and ATL) rather than the posterior and anterior leaflets of the tricuspid valve, as in Figures 2-2A and B. Although the posterior leaflet of the tricuspid valve is seen in Figure 2-2D, it is commonly not visualized in the corresponding two-dimensional echocardiogram (Figures 2-2E, F) since it is parallel to the ultrasound beam.

Two-Dimensional Echocardiogram

The right atrium (RA) is at the bottom of the echocardiogram (Figures 2-2E, F). The anterior and septal leaflets of the tricuspid valve (ATL and STL) are seen to coapt during systole. During diastole the leaflets of the tricuspid valve move outside the tomographic plane owing to rotation of the heart. The right ventricle (RV), with its anterior and septal wall (RVW), is seen at the top of the echocardiogram. This section cuts across the interventricular septum (IVS) and images the left ventricle (LV) obliquely.

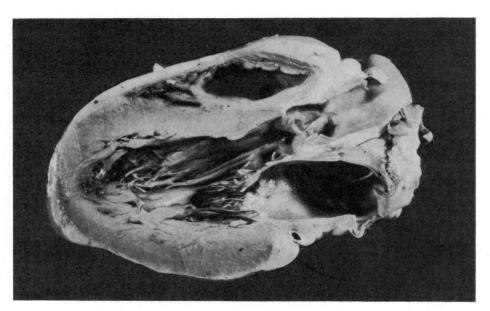

Figure 2-1A. Parasternal long-axis view of the heart, anatomic specimen.

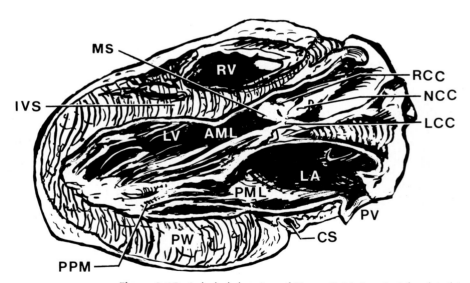

Figure 2-1B. Labeled drawing of Figure 2-1A (see text for details).

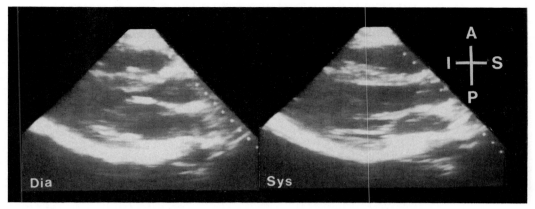

Figure 2-1C. Parasternal long-axis views of the heart in diastole and systole demonstrating mitral valve motion, two-dimensional echocardiogram.

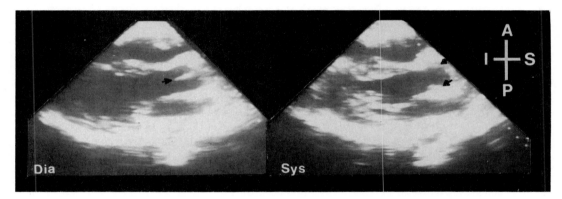

Figure 2-1D. Parasternal long-axis views of the heart in diastole and systole demonstrating aortic valve motion, two-dimensional echocardiogram.

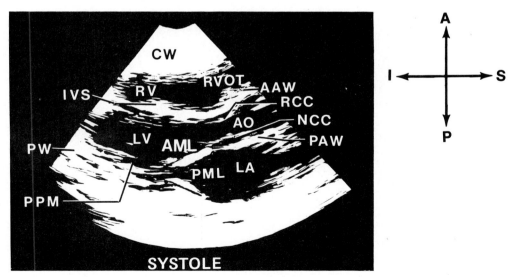

Figure 2-1E. Labeled drawing of the heart in systole from echocardiograms in Figures 2-1C and D (see text for details).

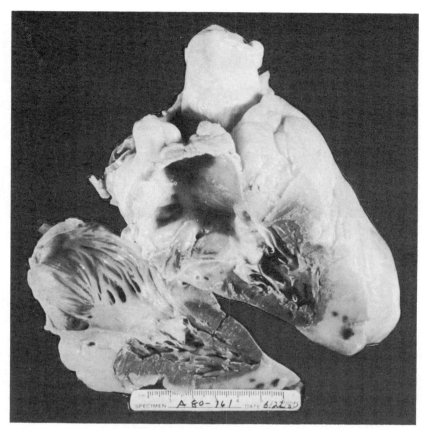

Figure 2-2A. Whole heart opened to show the plane of sector along the axis of the right ventricle. The heart is viewed from the right toward the left, as in a right anterior oblique angiographic view.

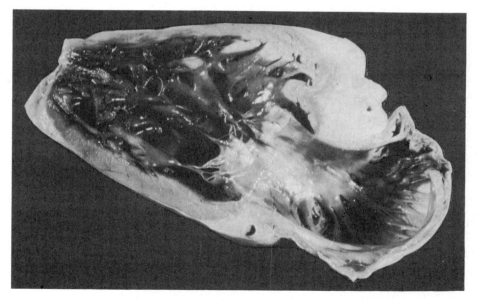

Figure 2-2B. Long-axis section of right ventricle oriented with the anterior wall at the top of the picture and the posterior wall of the right ventricle at the bottom. The view is of the free wall of the right ventricle, showing the large anterior papillary muscle and one of the smaller posterior papillary muscles.

32

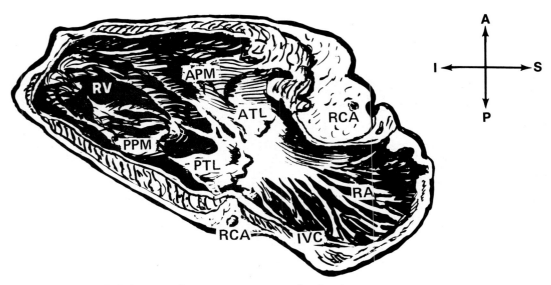

Figure 2-2C. Labeled drawing of Figure 2-2B (see text for details).

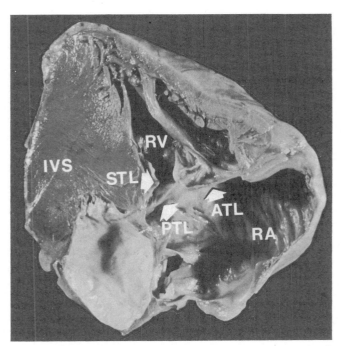

Figure 2-2D. Anatomic section that corresponds somewhat better than Figures 2-2A and B with the echocardiographic tomogram.

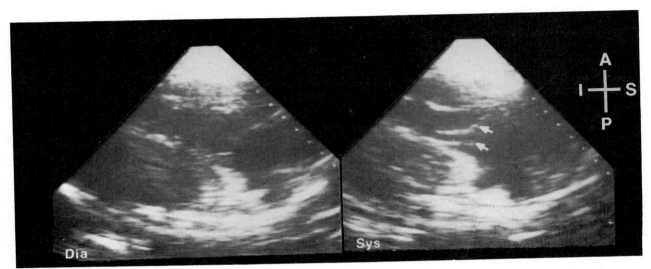

Figure 2-2E. Parasternal long-axis views of the right ventricle in diastole and systole, two-dimensional echocardiogram.

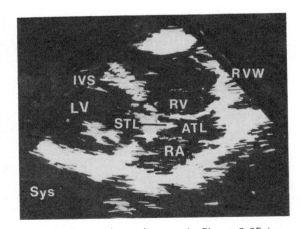

Figure 2-2F. Labeled drawing of heart in systole from echocardiogram in Figure 2-2E (see text for details).

PARASTERNAL SHORT-AXIS VIEW, AORTIC VALVE LEVEL

Anatomic Specimen

The heart shown in Figure 2-3A has been sectioned for short-axis views and then reassembled as shown. The superior section has been laid back, as though opening a book, and is viewed from the apex toward the base of the heart. The most common echocardographically performed tomograms will be described.

The short-axis section through the base of the heart (Figure 2-3B) follows the pulmonary artery outflow tract and cuts through several major cardiac structures. In this photograph of the reconstructed heart the following structures are seen: the right ventricular outflow tract, the left circumflex coronary artery (as it passes beneath the left atrial appendage), and the left anterior descending coronary artery lying near the pulmonic valve. Also seen are the coronary sinus and the septal leaflet of the tricuspid valve.

The section shown in Figures 2-3C and D is the same as that in Figure 2-3B but has been rotated to correspond to the two-dimensional echocardiographic tomogram (compare with Tajik et al[2] section 9). It passes through the right ventricular outflow tract (RVOT) and includes portions of the pulmonic valve (PV), the right, left, and noncoronary cusps of the aortic valve (RCC, LCC, and NCC), and the anterior leaflet of the tricuspid valve (ATL). Other structures seen are the coronary sinus (CS), the left atrium (LA), the right atrium (RA), and the left atrial appendage (LAA). The circumflex and left anterior descending (LAD) coronary arteries are seen to pass near the left atrial appendage (LAA) and the pulmonic valve, respectively.

Two-Dimensional Echocardiogram

In Figures 2-3E and F the aortic valve is seen as an inverted "Mercedes Benz" sign, with the cusps of the aortic valve (RCC, LCC, NCC) forming the three components during diastole. The left atrium (LA) is located posteriorly. The right atrium (RA) with the interatrial septum is anatomically to the right of the left atrium (left in figure). The posterior cusp of the pulmonic valve (PV) is seen to the anatomic left of the aorta (right in figure) and the anterior tricuspid leaflet (ATL) to the right of the aorta (left in figure). The left atrium, right atrium, and interatrial septum (IAS) appear at the bottom of the echocardiogram. The right ventricular outflow tract is located anteriorly. The interatrial septum is not always imaged in the same plane as the aortic valve leaflets. Minimal shifting of the transducer will usually demonstrate the IAS.

PARASTERNAL SHORT-AXIS VIEW, MITRAL VALVE LEVEL

Anatomic Specimen

A section passing near the base of the heart below the great vessels (Figures 2-4A, B) demonstrates the tricuspid valve (TV) and the anterior and posterior mitral valve leaflets (AML and PML). The interventricular septum (IVS) separates the right ventricle (RV) from the left ventricle. The left anterior descending coronary artery

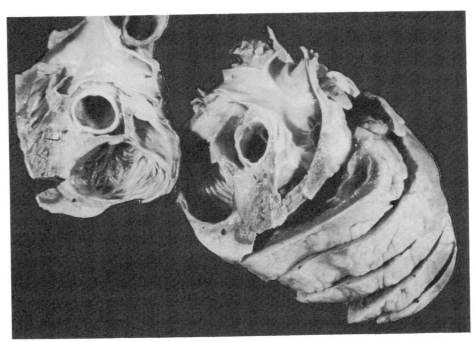

Figure 2-3A. Whole heart in short-axis plane, anatomic section.

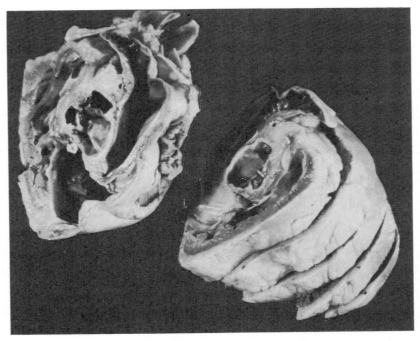

Figure 2-3B. Whole heart in short-axis plane, aortic valve level, anatomic specimen.

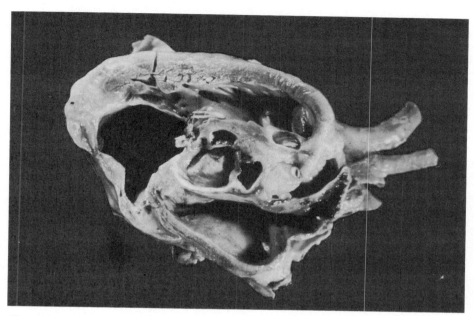

Figure 2-3C. Parasternal short-axis view of the heart, aortic valve level, anatomic specimen.

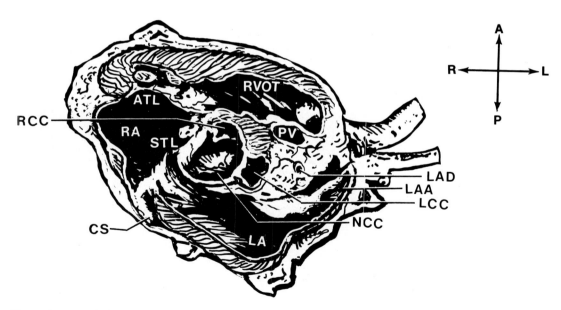

Figure 2-3D. Labeled drawing of Figure 2-3C (see text for details).

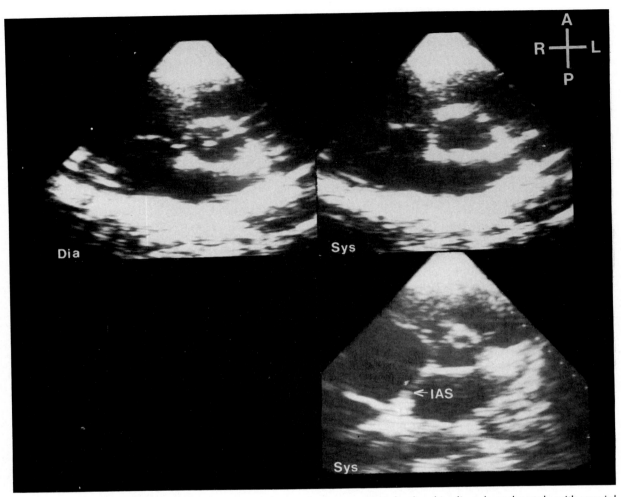

Figure 2-3E. Parasternal short-axis view, aortic valve level in diastole and systole with special demonstration of the interatrial septum, two-dimensional echocardiograms.

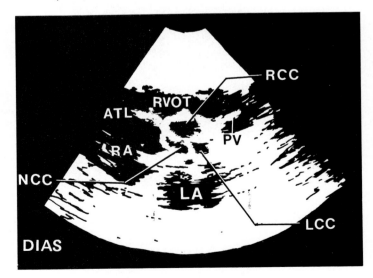

Figure 2-3F. Labeled drawing of heart in diastole from echocardiograms in Figure 2-3E (see text for details).

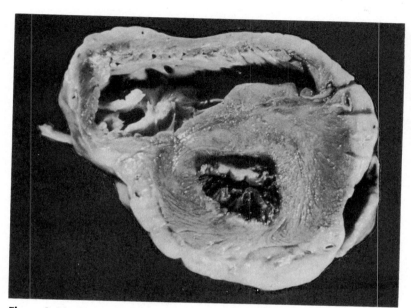

Figure 2-4A. Parasternal short-axis view of the heart, mitral valve level, anatomic specimen.

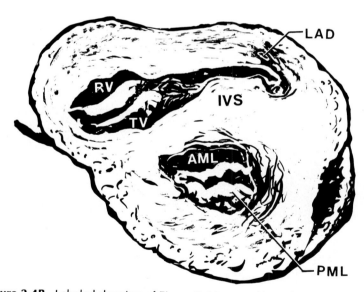

Figure 2-4B. Labeled drawing of Figure 2-4A rotated 30° clockwise (see text for details).

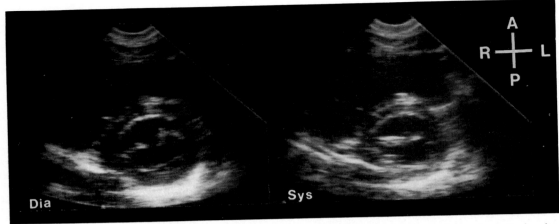

Figure 2-4C. Parasternal short-axis view of the heart in diastole and systole, mitral valve level, two-dimensional echocardiogram.

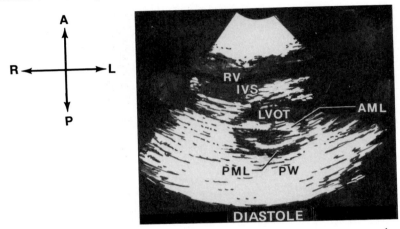

Figure 2-4D. Labeled drawing of heart from echocardiograms in Figure 2-4C (see text for details).

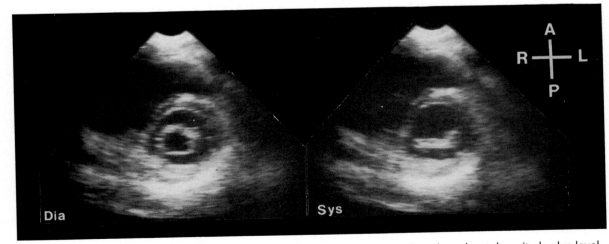

Figure 2-4E. Parasternal short-axis view of the heart in diastole and systole, mitral valve level, two-dimensional echocardiogram. Mild mitral stenosis.

(LAD) lies anterior to the septum near the junction of the right and left ventricles. (Compare Tajik et al.[2] section 7.)

Two-Dimensional Echocardiogram

The mitral valve is in the center of the echocardiograms in Figures 2-4C and E, with its two leaflets opening and closing like a "fish mouth." As shown in Figure 2-4D, the right ventricular outflow tract lies anterior to the left ventricle, separated from it by the interventricular septum (IVS). The septum and free posterior wall (PW) of the left ventricle surround the mitral valve (AML and PML). The left ventricular outflow tract (LVOT) lies anterior to the mitral valve. Figure 2-4E was obtained from a patient with mitral valve thickening from rheumatic mitral valve disease. Systolic and diastolic motions of the mitral valve are more easily appreciated.

PARASTERNAL SHORT-AXIS VIEW, PAPILLARY MUSCLE LEVEL

Anatomic Specimen

A section at the midportion of the ventricular cavities (Figures 2-5A, B) shows the anterior and posterior papillary muscles (APM and PPM) of the tricuspid valve (top of specimen) in the right ventricle and the anterolateral and posteromedial papillary muscles (APM and PPM) of the mitral valve in the left ventricle (LV). Note also the moderator band (MB) in the right ventricle. The specimen is oriented to correspond to an echocardiographic short-axis view taken with the subject supine; see also Tajik et al[2] section 6.

Two-Dimensional Echocardiogram

In the echocardiograms shown in Figure 2-5C and D, the posteromedial papillary muscle (PPM) of the mitral valve is seen in the right posterior portion of the left ventricle (LV) (left in figure), next to the interventricular septum (IVS). The anterolateral papillary muscle (APM) is seen in the left posterior portion of the left ventricle (right in figure). The interventricular septum, right ventricular cavity (RV), and anterolateral free wall of the left ventricle (ALW) are seen near the top of the echocardiogram. The posterior wall of the left ventricle (PW) is seen in the lower portion of the echocardiogram. The difference in size of the left ventricle during systole and diastole is easily visualized.

APICAL FOUR-CHAMBER VIEW (OPTION 2)

Anatomic Specimen

The orientation of the apical four-chamber view shown in Figures 2-6A and B corresponds to option 2 of the American Society of Echocardiography's Committee on Nomenclature and Standards in Two-Dimensional Echocardiography.[1] The specimen is viewed with the posterior portion of the heart removed, looking toward the anterior surfaces of the cardiac chambers (compare Tajik et al[2] section 11; note that

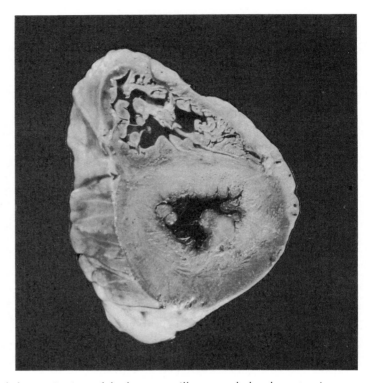

Figure 2-5A. Parasternal short-axis view of the heart, papillary muscle level, anatomic specimen.

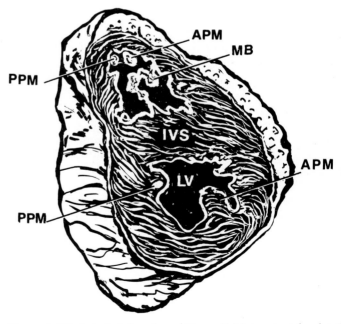

Figure 2-5B. Labeled drawing of Figure 2-5A (see text for details).

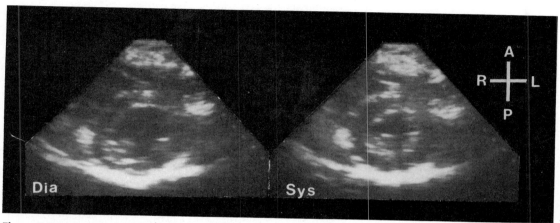

Figure 2-5C. Parasternal short-axis view of the heart in diastole and systole, papillary muscle level, two-dimensional echocardiogram.

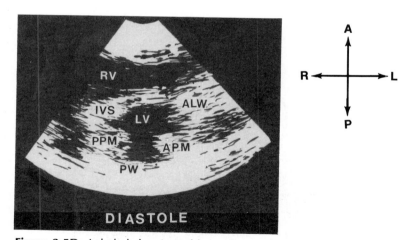

Figure 2-5D. Labeled drawing of heart from echocardiogram in Figure 2-5C (see text for details).

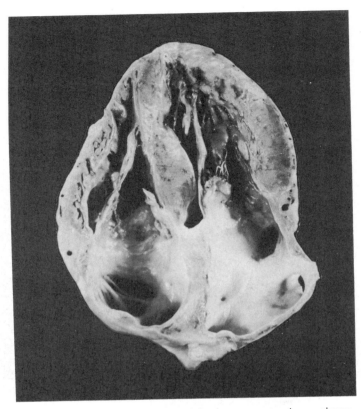

Figure 2-6A. Four-chamber view of the heart, anatomic specimen.

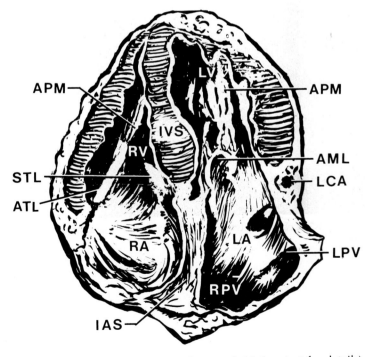

Figure 2-6B. Labeled drawing of Figure 2-6A (see text for details).

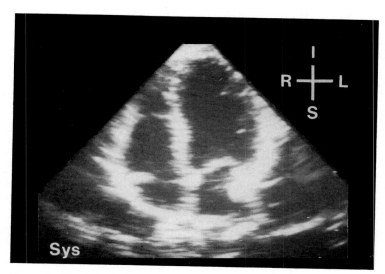

Figure 2-6C. Apical four-chamber view (option 2) in systole, two-dimensional echocardiogram.

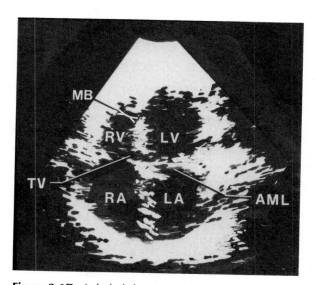

Figure 2-6D. Labeled drawing of Figure 2-6C (see text for details).

right and left are reversed). The right atrium (RA) and right ventricle (RV) are displayed to the left and the left atrium (LA) and left ventricle (LV) to the right. The section cuts across the septal leaflet of the tricuspid valve (STL), the interatrial and interventricular septa (IAS and IVS), and the anterior mitral leaflets (AML). Fat is present in the interatrial septum. The anterior leaflets of the tricuspid valve (ATL), portions of the mitral valve, and its anterolateral papillary muscle (APM) are anterior to the plane of section. The left circumflex coronary artery (LCA) and ostia of the pulmonary veins (RPV and LPV) are seen.

Two-Dimensional Echocardiogram

The echocardiogram in Figures 2-6C and D is also oriented according to option 2; the interventricular septum separates the right and left ventricles (RV and LV), and the interatrial septum separates the left and right atrium (LA and RA). Note that there is normally a "drop-out" of echoes in the interatrial septum. The anterior and septal leaflets of the tricuspid valve (TV) separate the right ventricle from the right atrium, and the anterior mitral valve leaflet (AML) separates the left ventricle from the left atrium. Note that the tricuspid valve attaches to the septum closer to the apex than does the mitral valve. The moderator band (MB) connects the interventricular septum with the right ventricular free wall.

APICAL FOUR-CHAMBER VIEW WITH AORTA (OPTION 2)

Anatomic Specimen

The section shown in Figures 2-7A and B is cut slightly anteriorly to the section shown in Figure 2-6A; see also Tajik et al[2] section 12 (note that right and left are reversed). In addition to the previously delineated structures, it demonstrates the left ventricular outflow tract located between the septum (IVS) and the anterior mitral valve leaflet (AML). The ascending aorta (AO), the ostium of the superior vena cava (SVC), and the left atrial appendage (LAA) are also seen. The section cuts across the anterolateral papillary muscle (APM) of the mitral valve, the anterior leaflet of the mitral valve (AML), and a portion of the membranous septum. This view is sometimes called the apical five-chamber view.

Two-Dimensional Echocardiogram

The view in Figure 2-7C is of similar orientation as the four-chamber view but is often labeled the five-chamber view because it includes the aorta. The aorta (AO) is seen at the junction formed by the interventricular septum, interatrial septum, anterior mitral leaflet, and septal leaflet of the tricuspid valve. The left atrial appendage and the superior vena cava are not visualized here. Frequently, when the aorta cannot be well imaged from a parasternal position, it can be adequately demonstrated using the apical five-chamber view.

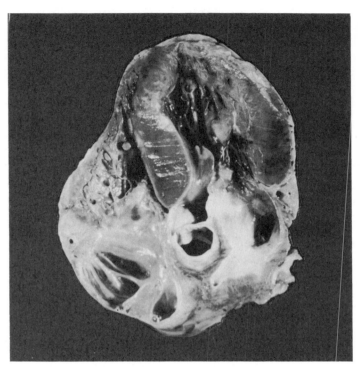

Figure 2-7A. Four-chamber view of the heart and aorta (five-chamber view), anatomic specimen.

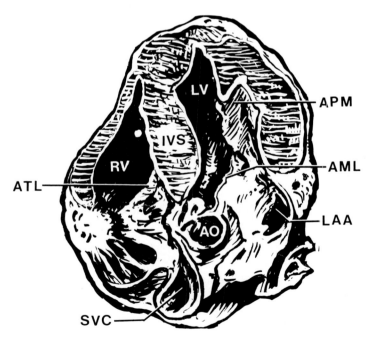

Figure 2-7B. Labeled drawing of Figure 2-7A (see text for details).

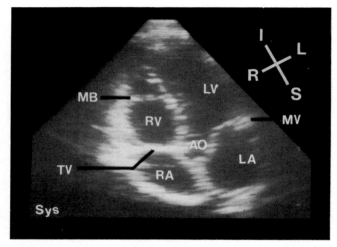

Figure 2-7C. Apical four-chamber view of the heart with aorta (option 2) in systole, two-dimensional echocardiogram (see text for details).

APICAL TWO-CHAMBER VIEW

Anatomic Specimen

The heart shown in Figure 2-8A is sectioned from its apex to base (compare Tajik et al[2] section 13). The orientation is similar to the previously described parasternal long-axis view of the left ventricle except that this section is more medial.

Two-Dimensional Echocardiogram

The view in Figure 2-8B is somewhat analogous to the 30° right anterior oblique angiographic view.[3,4] The left ventricular cavity (LV) in this view is bound by the interventricular septum (IVS), apex, and posterior wall (PW). It should be noted that in the right anterior oblique angiographic view the most anterior structure is the anterolateral wall rather than the interventricular septum. The anterior leaflet of the mitral valve (MV), the aorta (AO), and the left atrium (LA) are also visualized. The mitral valve can be seen to move in systole and diastole. This view, together with the apical four-chamber view, is frequently useful in examining the apical portion of the left ventricle in ischemic heart disease.

SUBCOSTAL FOUR-CHAMBER VIEW (OPTION 2)

Anatomic Specimen

The anatomic specimen shown in Figures 2-9A and B is the same as that previously described for the apical four-chamber view, but here it is seen from a subcostal approach (see also Tajik et al[2] section 15). This view is oriented 45° clockwise from the apical four-chamber view. The right atrium (RA) and right ventricle (RV) are at the top of the figure. Note that this view allows the right and left pulmonary veins (RPV and LPV) to be visualized.

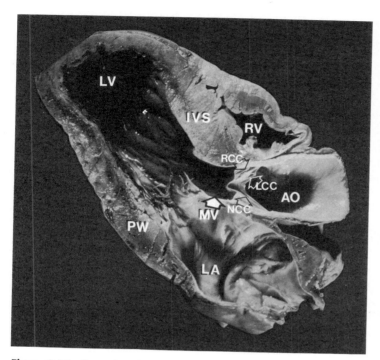

Figure 2-8A. Two-chamber view of the heart, anatomic specimen.

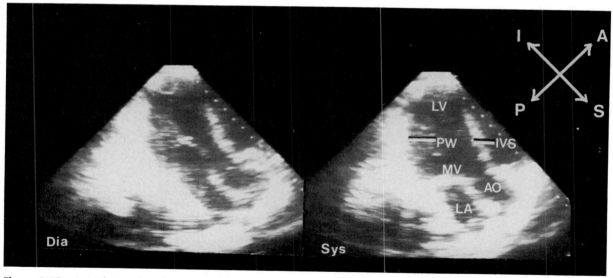

Figure 2-8B. Apical two-chamber view of the heart in diastole and systole, two-dimensional echocardiogram.

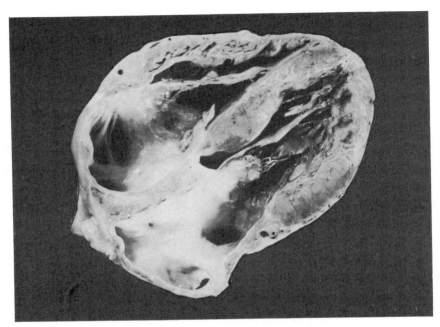

Figure 2-9A. Subcostal four-chamber view of the heart, anatomic specimen.

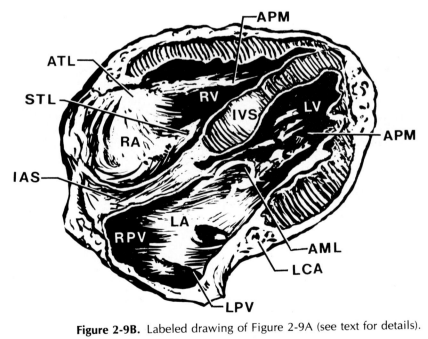

Figure 2-9B. Labeled drawing of Figure 2-9A (see text for details).

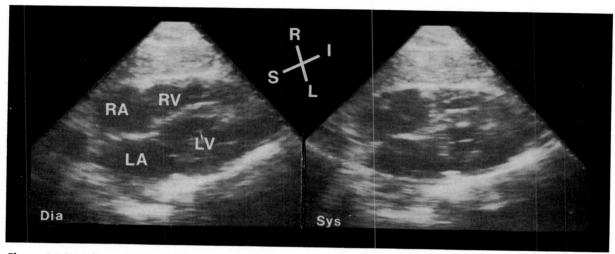

Figure 2-9C. Subcostal four-chamber view of the heart (option 2) in diastole and systole, two-dimensional echocardiogram.

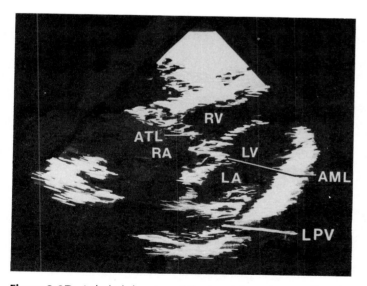

Figure 2-9D. Labeled drawing of the heart from the systolic echocardiogram in Figure 2-9C (see text for details).

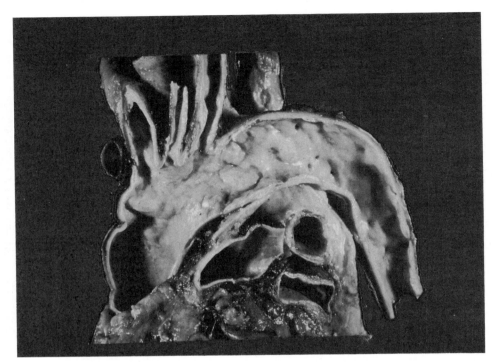

Figure 2-10A. Long-axis view of the aortic arch and great vessels, anatomic specimen.

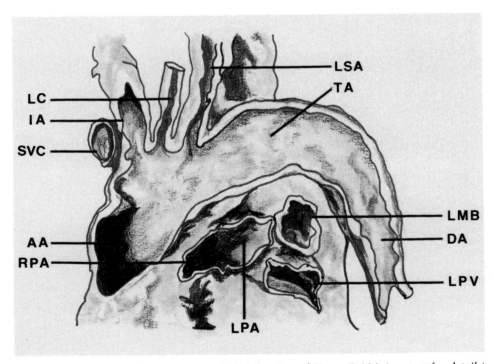

Figure 2-10B. Labeled drawing of Figure 2-10A (see text for details).

Two-Dimensional Echocardiogram

The view in Figures 2-9C and D is similar to the apical four-chamber view, with the following exception: a liver–diaphragm interface with the right ventricular free wall is seen anteriorly. The right and left superior pulmonary veins are seen superior and posterior to the left atrium (LA); more of the left atrium and right atrium (RA) are visualized in the subcostal four-chamber view than in the apical four-chamber view. This view is particularly useful in evaluating the interatrial septum. In addition, with slight manipulation of the transducer, the entry of inferior vena cava into the right atrium and hepatic veins can be seen; this view is particularly useful in assessing tricuspid regurgitation.

SUPRASTERNAL LONG-AXIS VIEW, LEVEL OF THE GREAT VESSELS

Anatomic Specimen

The view in Figures 2-10A and B reveals the transverse arch of the aorta (TA); note the innominate artery (IA) at the top left of the figure, which gives rise to the right subclavian and carotid arteries. The superior vena cava (SVC) is behind and to the left of the innominate artery. The left carotid and left subclavian arteries (LC and LSA) originate more distally from the arch of the aorta. The descending aorta (DA) can be seen to the right of the figure. The aorta is seen to encircle the pulmonary artery. The lumen of the right pulmonary artery (RPA) can be seen through the oblique section of the left pulmonary artery (LPA). The left pulmonary veins (LPV) and left mainstem bronchus (LMB) are labeled. Compare this view with Tajik et al[2] section 18.

Two-Dimensional Echocardiogram

The aortic arch and the innominate, left carotid, and left subclavian arteries are easily recognizable (Figure 2-10C). The right pulmonary artery is also faintly visualized.

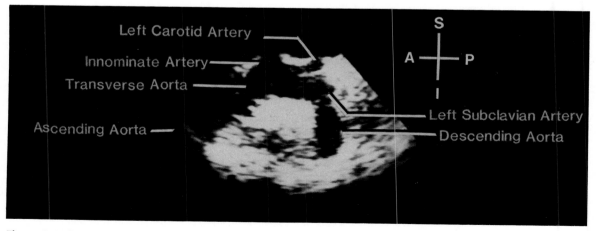

Figure 2-10C. Suprasternal long-axis view, level of the great vessels, two-dimensional echocardiogram.

REFERENCES

1. Henry WL, DeMaria A, Gramiak R, et al: Report of the American Society of Echocardiography Committee on Nomenclature and Standards in Two-Dimensional Echocardiography. Circulation 62:212–218, 1980
2. Tajik AJ, Seward JB, Hagler DJ, et al: Two-dimensional real-time ultrasonic imaging of the heart and great vessels: technique, image orientation, structure identification and validation. Mayo Clin Proc 53:271–303, 1978
3. Silverman NH, Schiller NB: Apex echocardiography of two-dimensional technique for evaluating congenital heart disease. Circulation 57:503–509, 1978
4. Schiller NB, Acquatella H, Ports TA, et al: Left ventricular volume from paired biplane two-dimensional echocardiography. Circulation 60:547–554, 1979

CHAPTER 3

Nomenclature and Standards

Julius M. Gardin

NOMENCLATURE

Many names have been proposed for the technique of real-time B-mode scanning of the heart. One of the first terms utilized, *ultrasonic cinematography,* described a rotating ultrasound transducer and a mirror system housed in a water tank.[1] Other names have included *ultrasonocardiotomography*[2] and *cardiac ultrasonography,*[3] while terms currently more popular include *real-time, cross-sectional,* and *two-dimensional* echocardiography. Although some echocardiographers prefer the term *cross-sectional echocardiography,*[4] the Committee on Nomenclature and Standards in Two-Dimensional Echocardiography of the American Society of Echocardiography has recommended that the term *two-dimensional echocardiography* be used to refer to the technique.[5] We utilize this recommended terminology throughout this book.

Transducer Location

Figure 3-1 depicts the nomenclature adopted by the American Society of Echo-cardiography to designate various transducer locations for examining the heart.[5] The traditional transducer position is located over the left precordium between the second and fifth intercostal spaces. This "echocardiographic window," called the *parasternal position,* generally lies within a few centimeters of the left sternal border. The heart can usually be examined from at least two precordial interspaces. The presence of a "barrel chest" or emphysema or a narrow intercostal space may make imaging difficult from this position. The *left parasternal position*—i.e., bounded by the sternum, the left clavicle, and the cardiac apex—is assumed when one uses the term *parasternal* alone. The *right parasternal position*—i.e., bounded by the sternum and right clavicle—may be useful in patients with dextrocardia or in imaging the right atrium and interatrial septum[6-8] or the ascending aorta.[9]

The *apical position* is found at the location of the apical impulse and thus is almost always on the left side of the sternum. The so-called apical four-chamber view allows simultaneous visualization of the right and left atria and ventricles and comparison of their relative sizes. This view is useful in evaluating the interatrial septum in identifying entry of the inferior pulmonary veins into the left atrium[10] and in demonstrating various congenital cardiac abnormalities.[11] In addition, the view has been helpful in diagnosing mitral valve prolapse,[12] as well as in evaluating left ventricular dimensions and wall motion—particularly of the apical portion. The apical two-chamber view or "right anterior oblique equivalent" is similar, but not identical, to

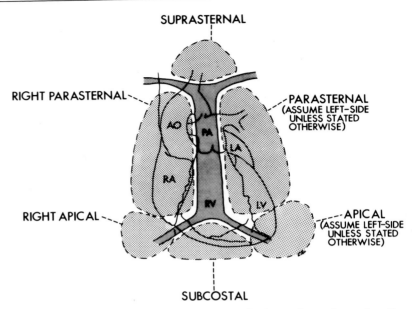

Figure 3-1. Nomenclature adopted by the American Society of Echocardiography to describe the various transducer locations for performing echocardiographic studies. (From Henry WL, DeMaria A, Gramiak R, et al: Report of the American Society of Echocardiography Committee on Nomenclature and Standards in Two-Dimensional Echocardiography. Circulation 62:212–217, 1980. By permission of the American Heart Association, Inc.)

the right anterior oblique view of the left ventricular angiogram (see Chapter 2).[13] This view is useful for visualizing the apex as well as the anterior and posterior walls of the left ventricle.

Two additional locations, produced with the transducer located cephalad and caudad to the sternum are known as the *suprasternal* and the *subcostal* or *subxiphoid positions,* respectively. Echocardiographic examination from the suprasternal notch has a number of useful applications[10]: (1) examination of transverse and descending portions of the thoracic aorta for detection of aortic dissection, coarctation, and other abnormalities of the aorta; (2) evaluation of the main pulmonary artery and its right and left branches for demonstration of patent ductus arteriosus and aorto-pulmonary anastomoses; and (3) evaluation of the superior vena cava for detection of tricuspid insufficiency and other abnormalities. The subcostal position is useful in patients with chronic obstructive pulmonary disease who have a barrel chest and low diaphragm and in whom the parasternal approach proves technically very difficult. In addition, the subcostal approach provides access to areas of the interatrial septum slightly different from that imaged in the apical four-chamber view; it also provides another method for investigating various congenital anomalies.[14,15] Furthermore, the subcostal approach allows for an improved ultrasonic examination of the right ventricular free wall.[16,17]

Echocardiographic Imaging Planes

A number of different schemes for transducer location and imaging plane orientation have been described.[5,10,18] Recently the American Society of Echocardiography (ASE) has standardized and simplified some of the proposed imaging approaches, designating all views by three orthogonal planes—i.e., long-axis, short-axis, and four-chamber[5] (Figure 3-2). The long-axis imaging plane is defined as that plane which transects the heart parallel to its long axis and perpendicular to the dorsal and ventral surfaces of the body (see Figure 2-1). The short-axis plane also transects the heart perpendicular to the dorsal and ventral surfaces of the body, but it is perpendicular (rather than parallel) to the long axis of the heart (see Figure 2-3). Finally, the four-chamber plane transects the heart almost parallel to the dorsal and ventral surfaces of the body. The ASE standards emphasize that each of the three orthogonal planes is actually a series of planes. Thus "long-axis" describes a family of planes parallel to the long axis of the heart and within 45° of the plane perpendicular to the dorsal and ventral surfaces of the body. In addition, the ASE recommends that two-dimensional images be identified by both transducer location and imaging plane—e.g., parasternal short-axis view, apical four-chamber view.

The ASE recognizes, however, that all current imaging views are not described unambiguously by its system without further information. It therefore recommends that views not corresponding to the standard orthogonal planes be designated by additional descriptive terms. For example, the two-chamber view described by Schiller and Silverman[11] is actually a variant of the long-axis view. In this view the transducer is positioned at the apex and rotated clockwise (when viewed from the handle), resulting in an image plane which transects the heart just lateral to the junction of the right ventricle and anterolateral left ventricular free wall (see Figures 2-8A, B). This view excludes the right ventricle and right atrium and, consequently, is called the two-chamber view; however, it could be described more precisely as an apical short-axis view (clockwise rotation) or, alternatively, as an apical long-axis (two-chamber) view.[5]

Another problem in the designation of imaging planes is related to imaging the apex in the parasternal long-axis view. Because the left ventricular outflow tract, left ventricular body, and apex are generally in slightly different long-axis planes,

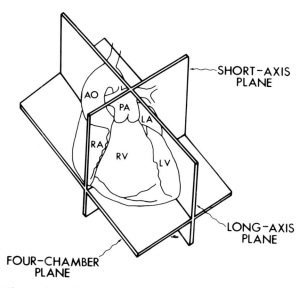

Figure 3-2. Diagram of the three orthogonal imaging planes utilized in two-dimensional echocardiography. (From Henry WL, DeMaria A, Gramiak R, et al: Report of the American Society of Echocardiography Committee on Nomenclature and Standards in Two-Dimensional Echocardiography. Circulation 62:212–217, 1980. By permission of the American Heart Association, Inc.)

the ultrasonic transducer must be angulated differently to record all of these structures. Imaging the true left ventricular apex from the standard parasternal long-axis view is difficult; frequently a "pseudo-apex" is recorded when the ultrasound beam transects the medial wall of the left ventricle, producing a foreshortened image. To record the apex in the parasternal long-axis view, the transducer often must be moved to a lower interspace.[19]

ASE STANDARDS FOR IMAGE ORIENTATION

Various groups have utilized different conventions for displaying their two-dimensional images.[5,10,18,20] For example, in the apical four-chamber view, some investigators have displayed the left atrium and left ventricle to the left,[10,18] whereas others have displayed these structures to the right of the screen.[5,18] In order to resolve the issue of image orientation, the ASE recommends that an index mark be placed on the side of each two-dimensional transducer to indicate the edge of the imaging plane—i.e., the direction in which the ultrasound beam is being angled (Figures

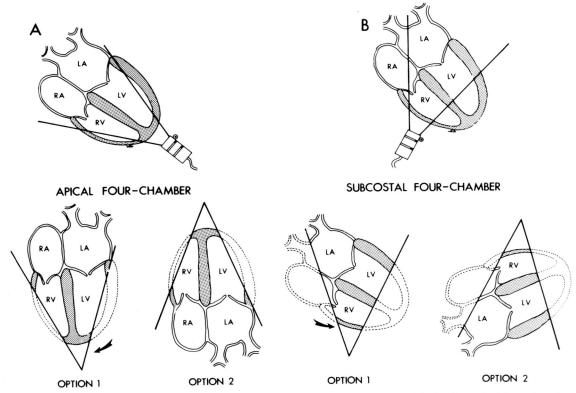

Figure 3-3. Diagram illustrating the two display options possible for the apical four-chamber view (A) and for the subcostal four-chamber view (B). Each of the images was obtained with the transducer index mark pointed toward the patient's left side. For each view, option 1 is produced by turning the image inversion switch to the "on" position, resulting in inversion of the "near signals" of the image from the top to the bottom of the display. (From Henry WL, DeMaria A, Gramiak R, et al: Report of the American Society of Echocardiography Committee on Nomenclature and Standards in Two-Dimensional Echocardiography. Circulation 62:212–217, 1980. By permission of the American Heart Association, Inc.)

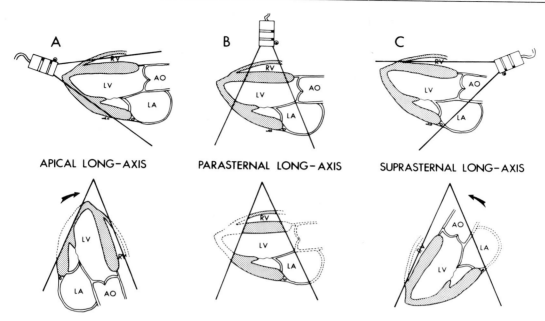

Figure 3-4. Diagram of the two-dimensional apical long-axis view (A), parasternal long-axis view (B), and suprasternal long-axis view (C). These images were obtained with the transducer index mark pointing toward the patient's head. (From Henry WL, DeMaria A, Gramiak R, et al: Report of the American Society of Echocardiography Committee on Nomenclature and Standards in Two-Dimensional Echocardiography. Circulation 62:212–217, 1980. By permission of the American Heart Association, Inc.)

3-3 and 3-4). The purpose of the index mark is to indicate the part of the image plane that will appear on the right side of the image display. Thus, if the index mark is pointed in the direction of the aorta in a parasternal long-axis view, the aorta will appear on the right side of the image display. The Society recommends that during performance of two-dimensional echocardiographic studies the index mark on the transducer always be pointed either in the direction of the patient's head or toward his left side.

The ASE also recommends that each ultrasound unit incorporate an image inversion switch so that the "near signals" present in an image can be inverted from the top to the bottom of the display without producing a change in the left–right orientation of the image (see Figure 3-3). This image inversion switch was designed solely for use with the four-chamber plane to allow two display options in both the apical and subcostal four-chamber views. It should be noted that both the apical and subcostal four-chamber views are obtained with the transducer index mark pointed toward the patient's left side so that it is possible simply to move from the apical four-chamber view to the subcostal four-chamber view without having to rotate the transducer 180°. A discussion of the image orientations that result from these ASE recommendations follows.

Long-Axis Views

It is possible to view the long axis of the heart from either the apical, the parasternal, or the suprasternal location (see Figure 3-4). By ASE convention, the index mark is pointed toward the patient's head in these three locations. In the parasternal long-axis view, the apex of the heart is displayed toward the left of the image. In the apical long-axis view, the apex of the heart is visualized at the top of the image and the left ventricle is displayed to the left of the image. Note how this display differs from the apical four-chamber view, in which the left ventricle in either of the two display options is always displayed to the right of the right ventricle. A suprasternal long-axis view would theoretically display the apex toward the bottom of the image with the left ventricle to the right of the right ventricle. In practice, however, it is difficult to image the left ventricle in an adult from this view. The long-axis views of the heart can be obtained from any of the three transducer locations simply by sliding the transducer from one location to the next without rotating the transducer 180°.

Short-Axis Views

Short-axis views can be obtained from the parasternal, subcostal, and suprasternal locations. Figure 3-5 demonstrates parasternal and subcostal short-axis views at the level of the papillary muscles. Note that the images were obtained with the transducer index mark pointing toward the patient's left side. This convention produces a

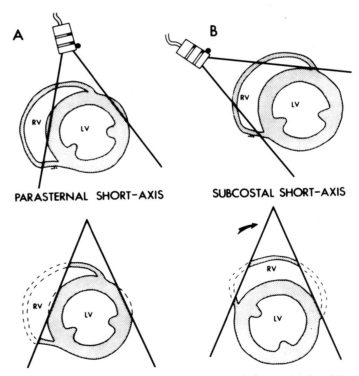

Figure 3-5. Illustrations of two-dimensional images in the parasternal short-axis view (A) and the subcostal short-axis view (B) obtained with the transducer index mark pointing toward the patient's left side. (From Henry WL, DeMaria A, Gramiak R, et al: Report of the American Society of Echocardiography Committee on Nomenclature and Standards in Two-Dimensional Echocardiography. Circulation 62:212–217, 1980. By permission of the American Heart Association, Inc.)

situation in the parasternal short-axis in which the left ventricle is to the right of the right ventricle on the image display. In the subcostal short-axis view, ASE guidelines result in an image with the right ventricle at the top and the left ventricle at the bottom. Again, since the transducer index mark is pointed toward the patient's left side in both views, it is not necessary to rotate the transducer 180° in order to move from the parasternal short-axis to the subcostal short-axis view.

Four-Chamber Views

Four-chamber views of the heart can be obtained with the transducer located in either the apical or subcostal location (see Figure 3-3). Both the apical and subcostal four-chamber views are obtained with the transducer index mark pointing toward the patient's left side. Two options exist for displaying either view. The first involves turning the image inversion switch on, resulting in inversion of the near signals of the image from the top to the bottom of the image display. In the apical four-chamber view, this option (option 1) allows the apex of the heart to appear at the bottom of the image, the left ventricle on the right of the display, the right ventricle on the left, and the atria at the top. For the subcostal four-chamber view, option 1 results in the near signals of the image—i.e., the right ventricle—appearing at the bottom of the display, while the apex of the heart is displayed on the right and the atria on the left.

Option 2 involves leaving the image inversion switch off, resulting, for the apical four-chamber view, in an image displaying the apex of the heart at the top and the atria at the bottom of the screen. As in the first display option, the left ventricle remains on the right side and the right ventricle on the left side of the image. For the subcostal four-chamber view, option 2 results in the near signals—i.e., the right ventricle—remaining at the top of the display, with the apex on the right and the atria on the left side (see Figure 3-3). Currently it appears that option 2 is more commonly used for both apical and subcostal four-chamber views.

DESIGNATION OF LEFT VENTRICULAR WALL SEGMENTS

There have been a number of different suggestions for naming the various segments of the left ventricle in the different imaging planes.[21–23] Figures 3-6 and 3-7A, B, and C detail two conventions that have been proposed. A committee of the American Society of Echocardiography has recently standardized the nomenclature for ventricular segmental anatomy; these recommendations are shown in Appendix C. One issue to be settled is the relationship of echocardiographic nomenclature for ventricular segments to angiocardiographic nomenclature. One must bear in mind that the echocardiographic planes of orientation are not precisely the same as those obtained from the traditional right anterior and left anterior oblique angiocardiographic views.[13] In any case, it is obviously important that different observers be able to communicate when comparing ventricular segmental findings, as in the evaluation of ischemic heart disease.

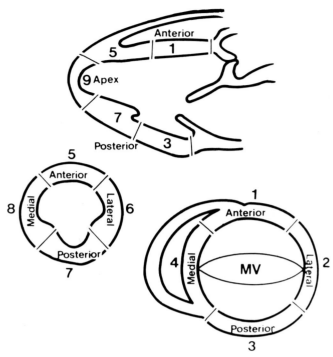

Figure 3-6. One proposed convention for identifying the segmental anatomy of the left ventricle and ventricular septum in the two-dimensional long-axis and short-axis views. The term *posterior* is considered in this proposed nomenclature to be synonymous with *inferior*. (From Wann LS, Faris JV, Childress RH, et al: Exercise cross-sectional echocardiography in ischemic heart disease. Circulation 60:1300–1308, 1979. By permission of the American Heart Association, Inc.)

Figure 3-7. A second system proposed for regional nomenclature of the heart. ANT denotes anterior, AO, aorta; INF, inferior; L, left; LA, left atrium; LAT, lateral; LV, left ventricle; POST, posterior; R, right, RV, right ventricle; SUP, superior; VS, ventricular septum. A: Parasternal long-axis view. Note that the long axis of the heart is designated as a line drawn from the site of mitral-aortic valvular continuity to the left ventricular apex. Two dividing lines perpendicular to this axis divide both the right ventricle and left ventricle into three sections. B: Short-axis view. Note that at the apical level, the right ventricular lateral segment is absent and the ventricular septum is not divided into anterior and inferior segments. C: Four-chamber view. Note that each level extends approximately one-third of the distance from the base to the apex. (From Edwards WD, Tajik AJ, Seward JB: Standardized nomenclature and anatomic basis for regional tomographic analysis of the heart. Mayo Clin Proc 56:479–497, 1981. With permission.)

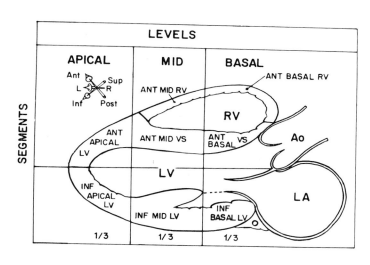

A

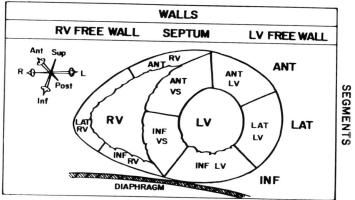

B

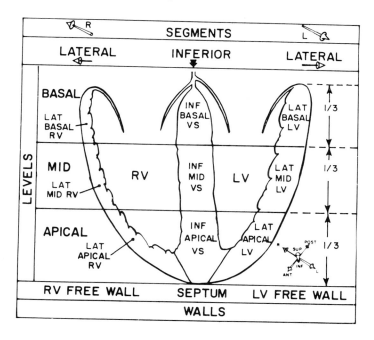

C

REFERENCES

1. Asberg A: Ultrasonic cinematography of the living heart. Ultrasonics 6:113–117, 1967
2. Ebina T, Oka S, Tanaka M, et al: The ultrasono-tomography of the heart and great vessels in living human subjects by means of the ultrasonic reflection technique. Jpn Heart J 8:331–353, 1967
3. King DL: Cardiac ultrasonography: cross-sectional ultrasonic imaging of the heart. Circulation 47:843–847, 1973
4. Feigenbaum H: Echocardiography (ed 3). Philadelphia, Lea & Febiger, 1981, pp 1–50
5. Henry WL, DeMaria A, Gramiak R, et al: Report of the American Society of Echocardiography Committee on Nomenclature and Standards in Two-Dimensional Echocardiography. Circulation 62:212–217, 1980
6. Gramiak R, Nanda NL: Structure identification in echocardiography, in Gramiak R, Waag R (eds): Cardiac Ultrasound. St. Louis, C V Mosby Co, 1975
7. Tei C, Tanaka H, Kashima T, et al: Real-time cross-sectional echocardiographic evaluation of the interatrial septum by right atrium–interatrial septum–left atrium direction of ultrasound beam. Circulation 60:539–546, 1979
8. Tei C, Tanaka H, Kashima T, et al: Echocardiographic analysis of interatrial septal motion. Am J Cardiol 44:472–477, 1979
9. D'Cruz IA, Jain DP, Hirsch L, et al: Echocardiographic diagnosis of dilatation of the ascending aorta using right parasternal scanning. Radiology 129:465–469, 1978
10. Tajik AJ, Seward JB, Hagler DJ, et al: Two-dimensional real-time ultrasonic imaging of the heart and great vessels: technique, image orientation, structure identification, and validation. Mayo Clin Proc 53:271–303, 1978
11. Silverman NH, Schiller NB: Apex echocardiography. A two-dimensional technique for evaluating congenital heart disease. Circulation 57:503–511, 1978
12. Morganroth J, Mardelli TJ, Naito M, et al: Apical cross-sectional echocardiography: Standard for the diagnosis of mitral valve prolapse syndrome. Chest 79:23–28, 1981
13. Schiller NB, Acquatella H, Ports TA, et al: Left ventricular volume from paired biplane two-dimensional echocardiography. Circulation 60:547–555, 1979
14. Bierman FZ, Williams RG: Subxyphoid two-dimensional imaging of the interatrial septum in infants and neonates with congenital heart disease. Circulation 60:80–90, 1979
15. Lange LW, Sahn DJ, Allen HD, et al: Subxyphoid cross-sectional echocardiography in infants and children with congenital heart disease. Circulation 59:513–524, 1979
16. Matsukubo H, Furukawa K, Watanabe T, et al: Echocardiographic measurement of right ventricular wall motion by subxyphoid echocardiography. J Cardiogr 6:15–23, 1976
17. Matsukubo H, Matsuura T, Endo N, et al: Echocardiography measurement of right ventricular wall thickness. A new application of subxyphoid echocardiography. Circulation 56:278–284, 1977
18. Popp RL, Fowles R, Coltart J, et al: Cardiac anatomy viewed systematically with two-dimensional echocardiography. Chest 75:579–585, 1979
19. Weyman AE, Peskoe SM, Williams ES, et al: Detection of left ventricular aneurysms by cross-sectional echocardiography. Circulation 54:936–944, 1976
20. Griffith J, Henry WL: A sector scanner for real-time two-dimensional echocardiography. Circulation 49:1147–1152, 1974
21. Kisslo JA, Robertson D, Gilbert BW, et al: A comparison of real-time, two-dimensional echocardiography and cineangiography in detecting left ventricular asynergy. Circulation 55:134–141, 1977
22. Wann L, Faris JV, Childress RH, et al: Exercise cross-sectional echocardiography in ischemic heart disease. Circulation 60:1300–1308, 1979
23. Edwards WD, Tajik AJ, Seward JB: Standardized nomenclature and anatomic basis for regional tomographic analysis of the heart. Mayo Clin Proc 56:479–497, 1981

CHAPTER 4

Mitral Valve Disease

Julius M. Gardin, Samuel Butman, and James V. Talano

Two-dimensional echocardiography supplements information gained by M-mode in the evaluation of the mitral valve by providing additional information on the location, spatial orientation, and motion of structures. In this chapter we review the two-dimensional echocardiographic appearance of the mitral valve and its supporting structures both under normal conditions and in disease states. In addition, we stress where the two-dimensional technique has advantages over M-mode echocardiography. Certain technical considerations in proper imaging of the valve and in measurement of its orifice area are outlined.

NORMAL MITRAL VALVE APPEARANCE

Figures 4-1 and 4-2 illustrate the normal mitral valve and surrounding structures from the parasternal long-axis position. Note that the anterior mitral valve leaflet is continuous with the posterior aortic wall and that the posterior mitral leaflet inserts into the posterior mitral annulus, which is at the junction of the posterior left atrial and left ventricular walls. The anterior and posterior mitral leaflets appear relatively thin and are attached to papillary muscles by thin structures—the chordae tendineae. In systole the anterior and posterior mitral leaflets coapt, or touch each other, within the left ventricular cavity—i.e., caudad to a line drawn from the junction of the anterior mitral leaflet and the mitral annulus. In diastole the mitral leaflets move apart in a relatively parallel fashion, with the tip of the anterior leaflet, at its maximal excursion, approaching the left side of the ventricular septum.

Figures 4-2 and 4-3 depict the normal parasternal short-axis mitral valve echocardiogram in systole and diastole. Note the relatively thin leaflets, which coapt in systole, touching each other completely. In diastole they separate to give a maximum diastolic mitral orifice area (Figure 4-2), which measures approximately 4.8 cm². The size and motion of the mitral valve annulus can also be appreciated by two-dimensional echocardiography.[1] Narrowing of the mitral annulus normally occurs during systole. Figure 4-4 demonstrates the two-dimensional apical four-chamber views of a normal mitral valve. Note that the anterior mitral leaflet inserts into the ventricular septum in a more basal position than does the septal leaflet of the tricuspid valve. During systole the anterior and posterior mitral leaflets coapt slightly caudad to the plane of the mitral annulus (i.e., within the left ventricle). In a normal individual coaptation generally occurs either within the left ventricle or in the plane of the

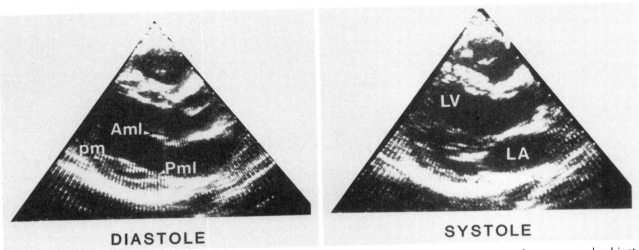

DIASTOLE **SYSTOLE**

Figure 4-1. Parasternal long-axis two-dimensional echocardiograms from a normal subject. The anterior mitral leaflet (Aml) is continuous with the posterior aortic wall, and the posterior leaflet (Pml) inserts into the junction of the posterior left atrial (LA) and left ventricular (LV) walls. Label pm denotes papillary muscle.

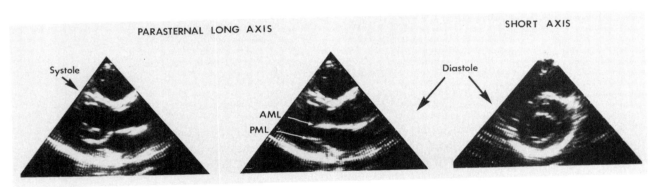

Figure 4-2. Parasternal long-axis and short axis echocardiograms from a normal subject. The mitral valve orifice measured in early diastole at normal leaflet excursion was 4.8 cm^2.

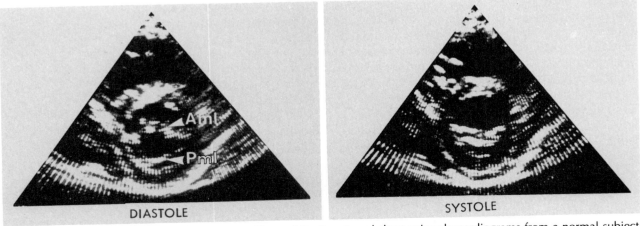

DIASTOLE **SYSTOLE**

Figure 4-3. Parasternal short-axis echocardiograms from a normal subject.

66

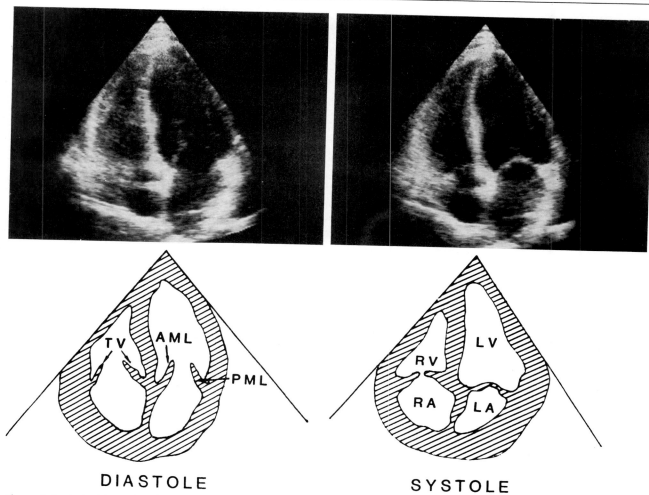

Figure 4-4. Apical four-chamber views from a normal subject. The anterior mitral valve leaflet inserts into the ventricular septum in a more basal position than the tricuspid leaflet and coaptation of the mitral leaflets in systole is within the left ventricle. RA denotes right atrium; RV, right ventricle; TV, tricuspid valve.

mitral annulus. In diastole the anterior and posterior mitral leaflets open toward the ventricular septum and the left ventricular free wall, respectively.

MITRAL STENOSIS

M-Mode Echocardiographic Findings

M-mode echocardiography was first applied clinically to detect mitral stenosis in 1957.[2] Through the years, M-mode echocardiography has been excellent in detecting mitral stenosis; it is not reliable, however, in estimating the severity of stenosis.[3–5] The M-mode echocardiographic criteria for detection of mitral stenosis include (1) thickening of the mitral leaflets, (2) reduced diastolic closing velocity (E-F slope), (3) abnormal posterior mitral leaflet motion, and (4) reduced diastolic excursion and separation of the leaflets. Increased thickness of the anterior and posterior leaflets from rheumatic fibrosis and calcification is seen and is relatively specific for the diagnosis of rheumatic mitral valve disease.[3] The decrease in the diastolic closing velocity is a function of the slow filling of the left ventricle and of the diastolic pressure gradient between the left atrium and the left ventricle, which tends to keep the mitral valve open. Although measurement of the E-F slope is still felt to be of value in serial followup of the extent of mitral stenosis or restenosis in a single individual, there is a poor correlation between the E-F slope and the degree of mitral stenosis in groups of patients.[3,4,6]

In most patients with mitral stenosis the posterior leaflet exhibits anterior motion during diastole; relatively normal or downward motion of the posterior leaflet has been described in approximately 10 to 20 percent of patients.[7,8] The anterior motion of the posterior leaflet in mitral stenosis is probably related to commissural fusion of the anterior and posterior leaflets, with the anterior leaflet pulling the posterior leaflet anteriorly as it domes toward the left ventricle during diastole. Fisher et al[9] used maximal diastolic separation of the anterior and posterior mitral leaflets to predict the degree of mitral stenosis. Narrow separation (less than 10 mm) was associated with severe mitral stenosis, and wide separation (more than 15 mm) was associated with relatively mild mitral stenosis. Unfortunately, many patients had intermediate values that were not predictive. Figure 4-5 reveals why M-mode estimates of the mitral valve orifice area may be erroneous. By angulating the M-mode beam laterally, the mitral valve leaflet separation is made to appear less than when the beam intersects the center of the valve orifice. The two-dimensional echocardiographic determination of mitral valve orifice area, to be discussed later, is now the noninvasive method of choice for accurate prediction of the degree of mitral stenosis.

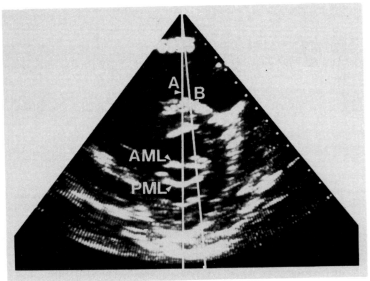

Figure 4-5. Parasternal short-axis image from a subject with mild mitral stenosis. Cursors A and B have been directed down the center of the mitral valve and lateral to the center, respectively. This figure demonstrates one possible limitation of M-mode echocardiography in estimating the severity of mitral stenosis.

Two-Dimensional Echocardiographic Findings

Mitral Leaflet Morphology and Motion

One of the characteristic findings of mitral stenosis in both M-mode and two-dimensional echocardiography is mitral leaflet thickening. In 25 patients with mitral stenosis, Nichol and associates[3] observed commissural fusion and nodularity of the leaflets in all; the greatest degree of thickening occurred at the leaflet tips. They noted no correlation between the degree of leaflet thickening and the severity of mitral stenosis determined at cardiac catheterization.

Although the diagnosis of mitral stenosis can be made in most patients from M-mode echocardiographic findings, two-dimensional echocardiography has been of help in some difficult cases. Figure 4-6 depicts two-dimensional parasternal long-axis views of the mitral valve in diastole in a normal subject, a subject with mitral stenosis, and a patient with congestive cardiomyopathy. Note that in addition to thickening of the anterior and posterior mitral leaflets in mitral stenosis there is also an anterior bowing or doming of the anterior mitral leaflet during diastole. This bowing occurs because the rheumatic process results in fusion primarily at the commissures or leaflet tips, while mobility in the body of the leaflets is preserved. In contrast, in the normal patient the mitral leaflets during diastole tend to be relatively parallel to each other without any significant bowing. In the patient with a dilated (congestive) cardiomyopathy and diminished cardiac output, the mitral valve also opens poorly; however, there is neither bowing of the anterior leaflet in diastole nor thickening of the leaflets (see Figure 10-3A). The two-dimensional parasternal long-axis view is generally diagnostic for rheumatic mitral valve disease, although the severity of stenosis is best determined by measuring the mitral valve orifice area in the parasternal short-axis view.

The two-dimensional echocardiogram also helps us to understand why the M-mode echocardiographic findings used to diagnose mitral stenosis may be variable in the same patient. Figure 4-7 shows the effect of recording an M-mode echocardiogram with the ultrasound beam traversing the mitral leaflets at their tips. Because the leaflets tend to be fused at their commissures, the posterior leaflet moves with the anterior mitral leaflet during diastole. This is the abnormal anterior diastolic motion of the posterior leaflet usually recorded in mitral stenosis by M-mode echocardiography. In all 25 patients studied by Nichol et al,[3] the tip of the posterior mitral leaflet was pulled toward the left ventricular outflow tract during diastole by the fused anterior mitral leaflet. Likewise, the separation of the anterior and posterior leaflets at the tip of the mitral valve is small. On the other hand, if the M-mode echocardiographic beam is directed through the bodies of the mitral leaflets, the leaflets tend to move in opposite directions during diastole, giving rise to the M-mode appearance of relatively normal motion of the posterior mitral leaflet. The excursion of the anterior and posterior mitral leaflets may also appear greater than that recorded through the tips of the mitral leaflets. Consequently, the M-mode echocardiographic findings may be distinctly different in the same patient with mitral stenosis, depending on the path of the ultrasound beam.

MITRAL STENOSIS AND MITRAL VALVE PROLAPSE   In mitral stenosis the anterior and posterior mitral leaflets are attached normally to the mitral annulus but are fused abnormally at the tips. The maximum amplitude of motion occurs in the midportion of the leaflets, giving rise in diastole to the convex or domed anterior mitral leaflet

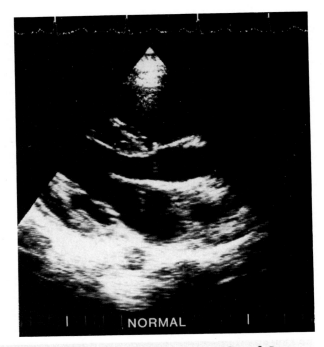

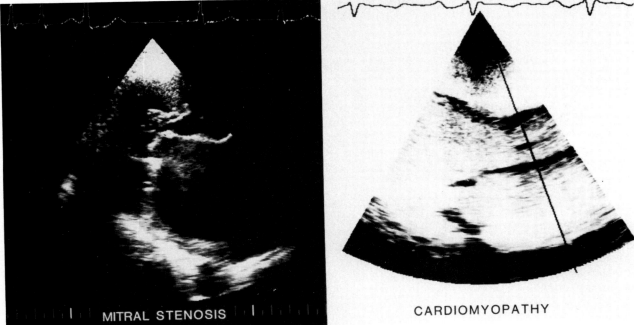

Figure 4-6. Parasternal long-axis two-dimensional echocardiograms in diastole from a normal subject, a patient with mitral stenosis, and a patient with a congestive cardiomyopathy. In mitral stenosis, the anterior mitral leaflet demonstrates diastolic anterior bowing in addition to the reduced opening seen in low output states.

70

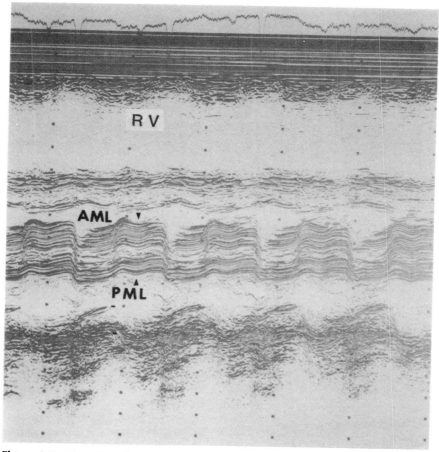

Figure 4-7. M-mode echocardiogram of a patient with mitral stenosis. The posterior leaflet is seen to move anteriorly during diastole. Note the dense echoes emanating from the anterior and posterior mitral leaflets.

into the outflow tract. In systole the anterior leaflet becomes convex toward the left atrium. Nichol and coworkers[3] noted no correlation between the degree of mobility of the midportion of the anterior mitral leaflets and the mitral valve area. Furthermore, they found that in 10 of their 25 patients (40 percent) the body of the anterior mitral leaflet bowed cephalad to the mitral annulus into the left atrium during systole— similar to the finding in patients with anterior mitral valve prolapse (Figure 4-8). Similarly, Beasley and Kerber[10] found two-dimensional echocardiographic criteria of mitral valve prolapse in 4 of 20 patients (20 percent) with mitral stenosis; M-mode echocardiographic criteria of holosystolic prolapse were found in 13 of the 20 patients (65 percent). Only 4 of the 20 patients had objective angiographic evidence of mitral valve prolapse. Pathologic specimens of the mitral valves from 3 of these 4 patients revealed myxomatous changes in two of the three valves. None of these three patients had clinical features of the mitral prolapse syndrome. These investigators concluded that the coexistence of mitral valve prolapse did not support the concept of a rheumatic etiology for mitral valve prolapse. Rather, the mitral valve prolapse associated with mitral stenosis appears to be an abnormal motion due to the mechanical distortion induced by the rheumatic process.[3]

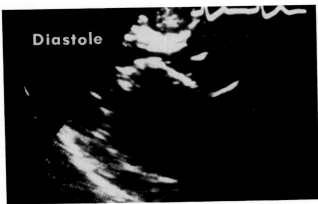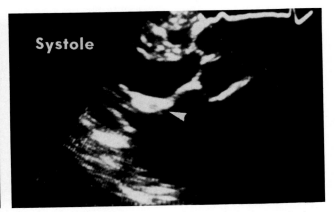

Figure 4-8. Parasternal long-axis two-dimensional echocardiograms from a patient with rheumatic mitral valve disease and prolapse of the mitral valve. The arrowhead points to the systolic bowing of the anterior leaflet into the left atrium.

Mitral Orifice Area

CORRELATIONS AT CARDIAC SURGERY AND CARDIAC CATHETERIZATION   Two-dimensional echocardiography has proven extremely useful in quantitating the degree of mitral stenosis. In fact, visualization and measurement of the mitral valve orifice area in the parasternal short-axis view is one of the first applications for the two-dimensional technique. Several investigators have now shown that the mitral valve orifice area, when planimetered properly from the parasternal short-axis view, correlates well with the orifice area determined at surgery or by the Gorlin formula at cardiac catheterization[11-14] (Table 4-1). Henry and colleagues,[11] utilizing a mechanical two-dimensional echocardiogram, were the first to demonstrate the usefulness of the two-dimensional technique in measuring the mitral valve orifice area. In 14 patients, 10 of whom had associated mitral regurgitation, mitral valve orifice area was measured directly at the time of operation utilizing a custom-built orifice sizer—a Delrin. The mitral valve orifice area was measured from a stop-frame image in early diastole by tracing the orifice outline onto a piece of transparent plastic and planimetering the orifice area. These investigators measured the mitral orifice (i.e.,

Table 4-1
Calculation of Mitral Valve Orifice Area

Investigators	Cath/Surg*	Regression Formula	No. of Patients	Correlation Coefficient (r)
Henry et al[11]	Surg	2D† = 0.91 (Surg) − 0.06	14	0.92
Henry et al [13]	Cath	2D = 0.89 (Gorlin) + 0.3	10	0.91
Nichol et al[3]	Cath	2D = 1.00 (Gorlin) + 0.1	25	0.95
Wann et al[4]	Cath	Not given	37	0.90
Martin et al[14]	Cath	2D = 0.92 (Gorlin)	24	0.92

*Echocardiographic orifice was compared to the orifice area (cm²) determined at heart catheterization by the Gorlin formula (Cath) or at surgery by an orifice sizer (Surg).
†Two-dimensional mitral valve area (cm²).

at the black–white interface) just within the reflected echoes of the orifice (personal communication from W.L. Henry, M.D.). They reported that the operative and echocardiographic data were related by the following equation:

Operative mitral area (cm²) = (1.1) × (2D mitral area) + 0.07

or inversely:

2D mitral area (cm²) = 0.91 (operative mitral area) − 0.06

The correlation coefficient was excellent (r = 0.92). Furthermore, in 12 (86 percent) of these 14 patients, the mitral orifice area measured by echocardiography was within 0.3 cm² of that measured at operation.

In a followup study, Henry and coworkers[13] measured mitral orifice area by the same two-dimensional echocardiographic technique in 10 patients before and after mitral commissurotomy. These data were compared with the mitral valve area calculated at cardiac catheterization by the Gorlin formula.[12] A good correlation (r = 0.91) was again found between the measurements of mitral orifice size, related by the following equation:

2D mitral area (cm²) = 0.98 (Gorlin mitral area) + 0.3

The results of this work have been confirmed by other investigators.[3,4] Utilizing stop-frame images of the mitral valve in short axis, Nichol and associates[3] planimetered the mitral valve orifice along their inner margins in 25 patients with pure mitral stenosis and compared the planimetered area with the area calculated by the Gorlin formula at cardiac catheterization. These workers found a strong correlation (r = 0.95) between the two methods of measurement, with their relationship being expressed by the following equation:

2D mitral area (cm²) = 1.0 (Gorlin mitral area) + 0.1

Wann and associates[4] studied 37 patients with mitral stenosis, 10 of whom had associated mitral regurgitation, and also found a strong correlation (r = 0.90) between the mitral valve area planimetered in the short-axis view at the innermost margin of the mitral orifice echoes and the mitral valve area calculated at cardiac catheterization by the Gorlin formula. The mitral valve area by two-dimensional echocardiography averaged 0.27 cm² larger than that calculated at cardiac catheterization, a finding similar to that of Henry and associates.[10,12] Differences found by Wann et al[4] between the echocardiographic and Gorlin measurements ranged from 0 to 0.9 cm². These investigators postulated that the differences might be related to the asymmetry inherent in the conical (funnel-shaped) narrowing of the mitral orifice or in the fused and thickened chordae tendineae which might also obstruct mitral valve flow. In using the mitral valve pressure gradient and forward flow to derive the area of the mitral valve orifice the Gorlin formula assumes an idealized valve orifice representing the total valvular apparatus. The two-dimensional echocardiographic method, on the other hand, measures the imaged valve area at its narrowest point. Nonetheless, the discrepancy between the two methods is slight and should not limit the clinical utility of two-dimensional echocardiography.

PROPER TECHNIQUE AND POTENTIAL ERRORS   It is essential that proper technique be adhered to in the imaging and measurement of the mitral valve orifice area, as a number of pitfalls and limitations have been described by several investigators.

ORIFICE LOCATION   There are a number of considerations associated with locating the true mitral valve orifice. First, one must be certain that the true minimal mitral valve orifice area is measured at the tips of the mitral leaflets. It is essential to perform a sweep in the parasternal short-axis view from the level of the papillary muscles to the origin of the great arteries so that the mitral orifice can be measured at the tips of the mitral leaflets. The mitral orifice should be imaged in a plane perpendicular to the long axis of the left ventricle.[11,14]

Figure 4-9 demonstrates a second potential problem in imaging the mitral orifice. By imaging the bowed anterior mitral leaflet in two areas, a falsely large orifice image may be created (Cursor C). The long-axis view in the figure shows the typical bowing or domed configuration of the anterior leaflet in diastole with the ultrasound beam intersecting the leaflet in two areas, rather than passing through the tips of both mitral leaflets at the orifice. A falsely large orifice image results from a higher transducer position on the chest wall—i.e., near the base of the heart (Cursor B). The ultrasound beam traverses the body rather than the tip of the anterior mitral leaflet to produce the misleading image.

Figure 4-10 demonstrates a fourth potential error—misinterpreting a calcified mitral annulus for the posterior mitral leaflet and including the annulus in measuring the mitral orifice. It cannot be overemphasized that the stenotic mitral valve assumes the shape of a funnel (the narrowest part being in the region of the commissural

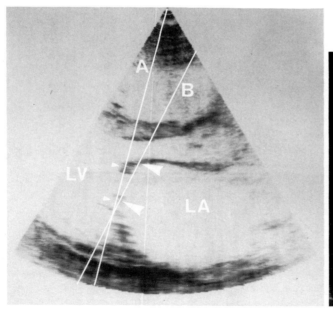
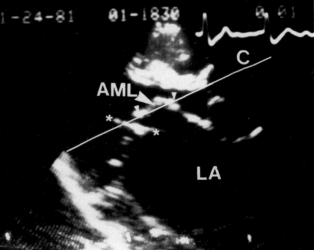

Figure 4-9. Parasternal long-axis diastolic views from patients with mitral stenosis. The typical exaggerated anterior bowing of the anterior mitral leaflet is seen. Cursors have been drawn through the leaflets to demonstrate potential errors in imaging the mitral valve orifice. Cursor A correctly intersects the anterior leaflet and posterior leaflets at their tips. Cursor B intersects the body of the anterior leaflet and the tip of the posterior leaflet. Cursor C intersects the anterior leaflet in two areas. The arrowheads point to the area(s) of the leaflet(s) intersected by the imaginary cursors. Note that the orifice generated by Cursor B would be larger than the true orifice generated by the Cursor A. The asterisks identify "side-lobe artifacts" that extend perpendicularly from the calcified tip of the posterior mitral leaflet.

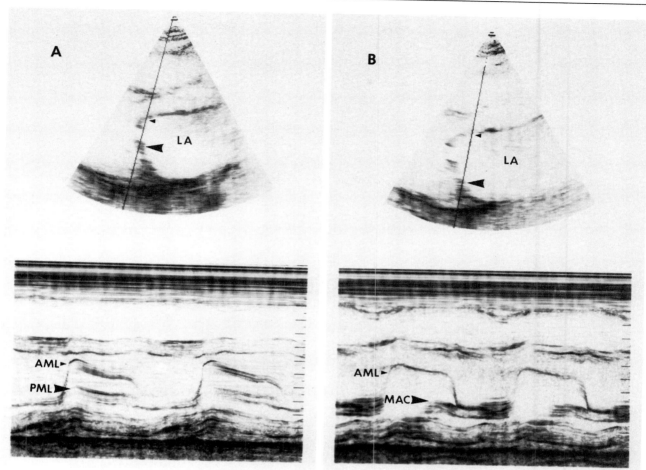

Figure 4-10. Parasternal long-axis frames from a patient with mitral stenosis and calcification of the mitral annulus (MAC). A: The cursor is positioned properly through the mitral leaflet tips. B: The cursor is positioned through the body of the anterior mitral leaflet and posterior mitral annulus. Simultaneous M-mode scans reveal how improper technique, as in B, can lead to falsely large mitral orifice measurements.

tips). It is important to image the mitral orifice in the parasternal short-axis at the level of the papillary muscles and to move the plane of examination gradually cephalad to locate the minimal mitral valve orifice. Martin and coworkers[14] point out a fifth potential source of error in locating the true mitral orifice in the short-axis view. These workers and others[3] note that the mitral valve apparatus moves in a cephalad and posterior direction during diastole. This movement causes the mitral valve orifice to move in a similar direction; thus, the orifice appears to decrease in size during diastole, as the ultrasound beam no longer intersects the true apex of the funnel. Hence, avoid measuring the orifice in mid- to late-diastole (Figure 4-11).

GAIN SETTINGS   Errors in measuring the mitral valve area may arise from improper selection of ultrasound receiver gain settings. The perceived mitral orifice is critically dependent on receiver gain settings at any transmitted power level.[13] If receiver

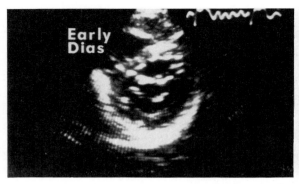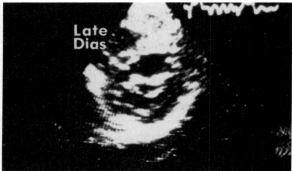

Figure 4-11. Parasternal short-axis frames from a patient with mitral stenosis. Visualization of the true mitral valve orifice must be made in early diastole in order to properly demonstrate the maximal orifice area. Note that in late diastole the orifice is smaller than in early diastole.

gains are set too high, image saturation and a falsely narrowed orifice image may occur (Figure 4-12). On the other hand, if gain settings are too low, signal drop-out may occur and result in measurement of a falsely large orifice. Another potential error relates to the phenomenon of acoustic shadowing (see Chapter 1). Intense reflections from calcium deposits on the anterior mitral leaflet can make this leaflet look thicker, causing the mitral orifice to appear smaller than its actual size.[10] In a patient with a very heavily calcified mitral valve, a clear mitral orifice may, in fact, not be visualized (Figure 4-13).

ORIFICE PLANIMETRY   Due to anterior bowing of the mitral leaflet in diastole (see Figure 4-6), the ultrasound beam can include a large portion of the body of the anterior leaflet. This gives a thickened appearance to the leaflet that makes accurate edge detection of the mitral orifice very difficult. Consequently, Martin and associates[14] investigated planimetry of the mitral valve orifice to include part of the anterior leaflet within the area drawn; they compared this method to simple planimetry of the black–white interface at the edges of the mitral orifice. The former method gave consistently larger values for the mitral valve, which resulted in less accurate mitral

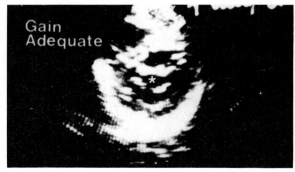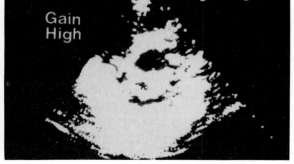

Figure 4-12. Parasternal short-axis echocardiograms at the mitral valve level in diastole. Inappropriate gain settings may result in orifice measurements that are either too high or too low. Note that on the left the apparent orifice is falsely decreased due to inappropriately high gain settings. An asterisk marks the orifice.

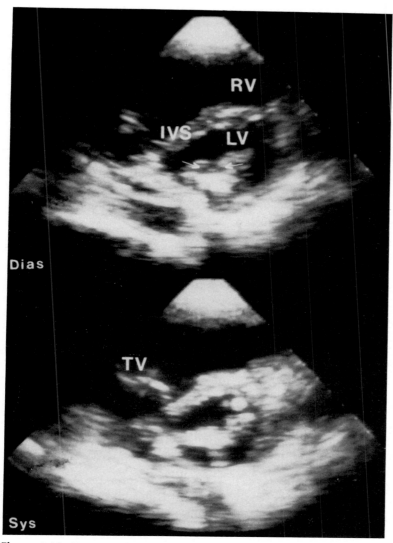

Figure 4-13. Parasternal short-axis view in a patient with severe calcific mitral stenosis in diastole and systole. The mitral valve orifice (arrows) measured 0.35 cm² in area. There is heavy calcification of the mitral leaflets and annulus. In addition, the tricuspid valve (TV) is thickened due to rheumatic disease.

valve area measurements when compared to the Gorlin formula. The mitral valve orifice should thus be drawn at, or near, the actual black–white interface.[11]

   To summarize, precautions must be taken to properly measure the mitral orifice area. These include (1) care in locating the true minimal mitral valve orifice, (2) utilization of the proper instrument gain settings, and (3) planimetry of the orifice drawn at the actual black–white interface (innermost margin of the echoes from the orifice) in early diastole. The reported rates of success in imaging the mitral valve orifice in the parasternal short-axis view for area measurement range from 83 to 95 percent.[3,4]

Left Ventricular and Septal Morphology

The left ventricular contour as seen in the parasternal short-axis view may be abnormal in patients with mitral stenosis. Nichol et al[3] reported that the systolic short-axis tomogram at the mitral valve or papillary muscles deviated from the normal round configuration in 19 of their 25 (76 percent) patients. These changes in left ventricular contour ranged from mild straightening of the ventricular septum to severe flattening of the ventricle, which correlated roughly with the elevation in mean pulmonary arterial pressure.

Abnormal ventricular motion, i.e., an exaggerated early diastolic septal dip, has been well described on M-mode echocardiography in mitral stenosis. The explanation for this distortion is that there is restriction to filling of the left ventricle during early diastole; the nonstenotic tricuspid valve allows normal filling of the right ventricle. Since the right ventricle fills more rapidly in early diastole than the left, the septum bulges toward the left ventricle.[5]

Calcification and Fibrosis

Two-dimensional echocardiography can be of help in the assessment of the degree of fibrosis and calcification of the mitral valve. Figure 4-14A illustrates a fibrotic but noncalcified (or relatively noncalcified) mitral valve. Notice that the body of the valve exhibits fairly good motion or pliability. In contrast, Figure 4-14B reveals a mitral valve that is highly calcified and exhibits little pliability of the bodies of the leaflets. Different areas of the same mitral valve may actually show different degrees of calcification and pliability.[5] Chandraratna and associates[15] have shown that preservation of the opening sound in calcific mitral stenosis depends on the distribution of calcification. Heavy calcification that is limited to the tips of the mitral valve leaflets allows the anterior leaflet to bow anteriorly in early diastole with preservation of the opening sound. On the other hand, heavy calcification of not only the tips but also the bodies of the leaflets reduces the pliability of the valve, which results in a diminished opening sound. Figure 4-15 is an example of just such a valve as seen in the apical four-chamber view.

Mitral Subvalvular Stenosis

There have been several reports of mitral stenosis primarily involving the papillary muscles and chordae tendineae.[5,15] In these cases the mitral leaflets can appear relatively normal, but the subvalvular structures may be fibrosed and fused in such a manner that surgical resection is difficult. In Figure 4-16 marked calcification and fibrosis of the chordae tendineae and papillary muscles, causing mitral stenosis, are shown.

Surgical Considerations

Two-dimensional echocardiography may be potentially useful to the surgeon in assessing the mitral valve; it can yield important information as to the degree of calcification or pliability of the mitral valve, and the presence or absence of mitral annular or subvalvular calcification. In addition, it can provide information as to left ventricular dimensions and function, left atrial size, and concomitant disease of the aortic or tricuspid valves. Finally, the mitral orifice index (mitral orifice area divided by body surface area) has been reported a useful parameter in determining whether a patient's symptoms can be attributed to the degree of mitral stenosis. Typical symptoms of mitral stenosis can be attributed to mitral valvular narrowing

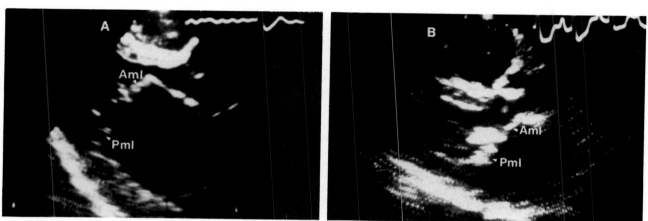

Figure 4-14. Parasternal diastolic long-axis frames from patients with rheumatic mitral disease and varying amounts of calcification and fibrosis of the mitral valvular apparatus. A: Fibrotic valve with well preserved motion of the body of the anterior leaflet. B: Heavily calcified commissures with the mitral leaflet exhibiting little motion during opening.

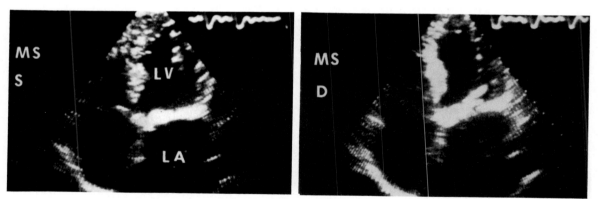

Figure 4-15. Apical four-chamber view from a subject with a heavily calcified and nonpliable valve. S denotes systole; D, diastole.

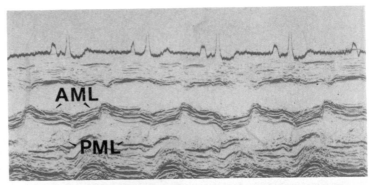

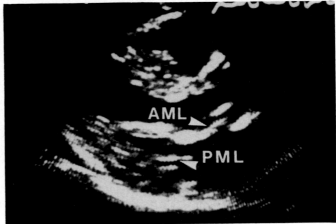

Figure 4-16. The M-mode echocardiogram reveals apparent thickening of the anterior mitral leaflet and a thin mobile posterior mitral leaflet. Real-time analysis in the parasternal long-axis view, however, revealed that the anterior mitral leaflet was in fact thin and pliable, whereas the submitral structures were densely fibrotic and/or calcified.

if preoperative symptoms are at least moderately severe and the mitral orifice index derived from two-dimensional echocardiography is less than 1.1 cm^2.[4,12]

MITRAL REGURGITATION

Various investigators have attempted to define sensitive and specific M-mode echocardiographic criteria for the diagnosis of mitral regurgitation, with generally poor results.[5,16–19] Two-dimensional echocardiography is superior to M-mode echocardiography in the detection of specific causes[19–21] but is less helpful in estimating the severity of mitral regurgitation. Useful hemodynamic information can be obtained by evaluating left ventricle size and systolic function. Combined Doppler and two-dimensional echocardiography has proved to be more useful in detecting and estimating the severity of mitral regurgitation than echocardiography alone (see Chapter 15). In this section, the echocardiographic findings of various etiologies of mitral regurgitation, including rheumatic mitral valve disease, ruptured chordae tendineae with flail mitral leaflets, papillary muscle dysfunction, and mitral annular calcification, are discussed. Mitral valve prolapse, which also gives rise to mitral regurgitation, is discussed at the end of this chapter. Other potential causes for mitral regurgitation—endocarditis, atrial myxoma, hypertrophic cardiomyopathy, mitral valve aneurysm,[22] and congenital causes—are discussed in more detail in later chapters.

Rheumatic Mitral Regurgitation

The two-dimensional echocardiographic features of rheumatic mitral regurgitation include (1) a bowing or doming of the anterior mitral leaflet toward the septum during diastole (parasternal long-axis view) similar to that seen in mitral stenosis; (2) thickening of the mitral valve leaflets; (3) a relatively immobile posterior mitral leaflet (parasternal long-axis view); (4) enlargement of both the left atrium and left ventricle with exaggerated motion of the ventricular septum and left ventricular free wall—i.e., left ventricular volume overload pattern; and (5) failure of coaptation of portions of the mitral valve (parasternal short-axis view).[19,21] In one large series[21] 80 of 289 patients undergoing two-dimensional echocardiography with a clinical diagnosis of mitral regurgitation exhibited findings suggestive of rheumatic mitral regurgitation. Fifty-six patients had mixed mitral stenosis and regurgitation, while 24 had pure mitral regurgitation. Patients with pure mitral regurgitation tended to have larger mitral valve areas (usually 3.0 cm² or greater). In pure rheumatic mitral insufficiency the midportion of the anterior mitral leaflet exhibits normal motion during diastole, even though the anterior leaflet has a right-angle diastolic bend.[20] Mintz and coworkers[20] found that patients in their series with pure mitral insufficiency had diastolic mitral valve orifice areas of at least 3.0 cm².

Wann and colleagues[19] utilized the parasternal short-axis view of the mitral valve orifice to differentiate mild from moderate or severe mitral regurgitation. Complete closure of the leaflets was detected in patients without mitral regurgitation; in patients with insignificant mitral regurgitation, there was failure of closure of portions of either the medial or lateral aspects of the mitral valve. In moderate or severe mitral regurgitation, two patterns of leaflet closure were detected: a central area of leaflet noncoaptation, or noncoaptation of both medial and lateral aspects of the mitral leaflets. The thickened leaflets of the mitral valve can easily be identified in all patients with significant mitral regurgitation. Closure of the mitral leaflets is best evaluated early in systole; during later portions of systole, ventricular contraction causes the mitral annulus to move in a caudal direction and results in the orifice moving out of the plane of the ultrasound beam. The observation that the severity of mitral regurgitation can be detected reliably by imaging the mitral valve orifice in the parasternal short-axis view has not been confirmed by other investigators. Technical difficulties result from a number of factors. First, lack of coaptation can only be evaluated during early systole; therefore, tedious frame-by-frame analysis is required to isolate these early systolic images. Second, the axial resolution of the ultrasound instrument must be of sufficient quality to allow accurate evaluation of the orifice.[5] Consequently, estimation of severity of mitral regurgitation by imaging of the early systolic mitral valve orifice will require further refinement before it can be clinically useful. Recent work by Gehl and associates[23] related left atrial systolic volume changes to the severity of mitral regurgitation; these changes may better reflect the severity of mitral regurgitation.

Papillary Muscle Dysfunction

Burch and colleagues proposed two possible mechanisms for papillary muscle dysfunction causing mitral regurgitation, mitral valve prolapse, and incomplete valve coaptation.[24,25] Mitral valve prolapse might occur if the normal sequence of myocardial contraction was delayed due to infarction or fibrosis of a papillary muscle or its neighboring myocardium. Incomplete valve leaflet coaptation could occur if ventricular dilatation, asynergy or dyssynergy resulted in an abnormal spatial orientation of the papillary muscles with malalignment of the mitral leaflets. Utilizing M-mode echocardiography, workers have been unable to distinguish between these two possible mechanisms in papillary muscle dysfunction.[5,17,26,27] More recent findings in papillary muscle dysfunction have been reported as abnormalities in coaptation of the mitral leaflets and in wall motion adjacent to one or both of the papillary muscles.[28,29] Godley and associates[29] described incomplete mitral leaflet closure in 20 of 22 patients studied with prior myocardial infarction and clinical evidence of papillary muscle dysfunction. In these patients, the leaflets remained partially retracted within the left ventricular cavity and failed to reach the atrioventricular ring during systole, resulting in incomplete mitral valve closure. Figure 4-17 is an apical four-chamber view of incomplete mitral leaflet closure in a patient with mitral regurgitation due to papillary muscle dysfunction. Note that in systole the mitral leaflets fail to coapt, presumably as a result of the fibrosed papillary muscles and/or a dyskinetic adjacent ventricular wall. The mitral apparatus is foreshortened, and incomplete leaflet closure occurs. This finding can also be seen in the parasternal long-axis view.[28] Some patients with a dilated cardiomyopathy may also demonstrate a similar pattern of incomplete mitral leaflet closure. In Kotler's series of 289 patients with presumed mitral regurgitation, 49 (17 percent) were diagnosed as having papillary muscle dysfunction.[21] Thirty-eight patients had clinical and electrocardi-

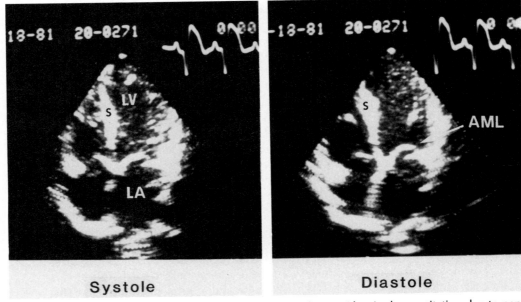

Systole   **Diastole**

Figure 4-17. Apical four-chamber views from a subject with mitral regurgitation due to papillary muscle dysfunction. There is little motion of the leaflets, which coapt abnormally within the ventricle in systole. S denotes septum.

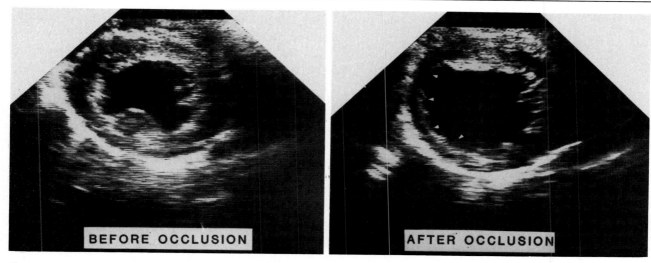

Figure 4-18. Parasternal short-axis systolic echocardiograms taken before and 8 hours after occlusion of the left anterior descending artery in a dog. There is thinning of the septum and absence of systolic thickening in the region of the posteromedial papillary muscle (arrowheads) after occlusion. (Courtesy of Dr. Steven Corday and William Childs.)

ographic evidence of coronary artery disease and 11 were felt to have dilated (congestive) cardiomyopathy. In addition to demonstrating incomplete mitral leaflet closure, Godley and coworkers[29] also noted dyskinesis in either the posteromedial or the anterolateral papillary muscle. Thus, abnormal segmental wall motion adjacent to a papillary muscle appears to be the more common mechanism of mitral regurgitation.

Papillary muscle motion and thickening are best assessed in the parasternal short-axis view.[20] Figure 4-18 depicts parasternal short-axis systolic frames from a dog who underwent ligation of his left anterior descending coronary artery. The echocardiograms taken before and after 8 hours of occlusion graphically reveal failure of the posteromedial papillary muscle to thicken appropriately in systole. In real time, there was also evidence of akinesis and absence of wall thickening adjacent to and involving the posteromedial papillary muscle. When motion of the papillary muscles is evaluated, the normal counterclockwise left ventricular rotation during systole must be taken into account.[30]

Papillary Muscle Rupture

Two-dimensional echocardiographic features of ruptured papillary muscle have been reported[31] (see Figure 9-7). The findings reported included (1) a mobile mass of echoes attached to normal-appearing chordae tendineae, (2) absence of the tip of the papillary muscle, and (3) mitral valve prolapse. These findings must await confirmation by other cases.

Flail Mitral Leaflet

M-mode echocardiography is very useful in evaluating patients with a suspected flail mitral leaflet secondary to ruptured chordae tendineae. Findings that appear to be relatively unique to this entity include intracavitary left atrial echoes in systole, coarse systolic anterior mitral leaflet fluttering, and chaotic diastolic anterior motion of the posterior mitral leaflet.[32–36] Severe mitral valve prolapse may, in certain circumstances, mimic a flail mitral leaflet; but the two conditions can generally be diagnosed separately.[33]

Mintz and associates[37] first described the two-dimensional echocardiographic findings in flail mitral leaflets. In their series of 280 patients undergoing two-dimensional echocardiography for evaluation of mitral regurgitation, 15 percent were diagnosed as having a flail mitral leaflet.[21] Characteristically there is a rapid systolic motion of the involved mitral leaflet beyond the point of coaptation into the left atrium. In addition, maximal abnormal systolic motion is greatest at the tip of the mitral leaflet with a loss of the normal coaptation. This latter finding is in contrast to the two-dimensional echocardiographic features of mitral valve prolapse, in which maximal abnormal mitral systolic motion is in the body of the leaflet while leaflet coaptation remains intact.

Child and coworkers[38] similarly reported patients with a flail posterior mitral leaflet studied by two-dimensional echocardiography: all showed a systolic whipping in the posterior mitral leaflet into the left atrium. Four of their 10 patients also demonstrated a mass of systolic left atrial echoes. The etiology of flail mitral leaflets includes active infective endocarditis, healed infective endocarditis, mitral annular calcification, spontaneous rupture, and myxomatous degeneration.[38,39,40] Figures 4-19 and 4-20 demonstrate the two-dimensional findings in a patient with ruptured chordae tendineae and a flail mitral leaflet. Note the loss of the normal mitral coaptation, which can be seen in both the parasternal long-axis and apical four-

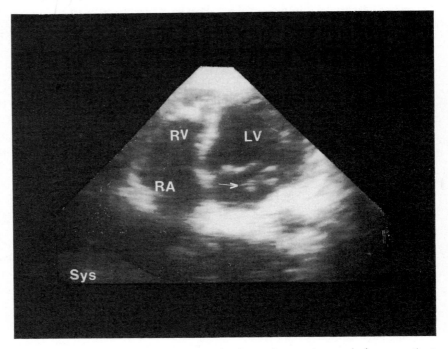

Figure 4-19. Apical four-chamber two-dimensional echocardiogram in systole from a patient with ruptured chordae tendineae and flail posterior leaflet. The arrow is adjacent to the flail posterior mitral valve leaflet in the left atrium.

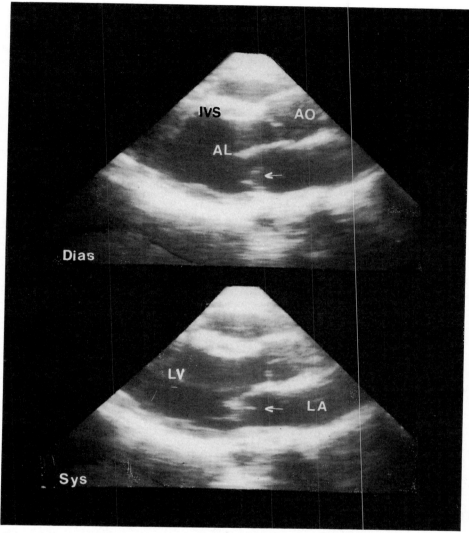

Figure 4-20. Parasternal long-axis view in diastole and systole from patient with a flail posterior mitral leaflet. This patient, with mitral valve prolapse, developed acute mitral regurgitation secondary to ruptured chordae tendineae. AL denotes anterior mitral valve. Arrows point to flail posterior mitral valve.

chamber views. Two-dimensional echocardiography appears to have a greater sensitivity, specificity, and predictive accuracy than does M-mode echocardiography in the diagnosis of flail mitral leaflets.[41]

Mitral Annular Calcification

There have now been published several reports demonstrating the utility of echocardiography in the detection of mitral annular calcification.[37–45] Both M-mode and two-dimensional echocardiography have been shown to be more sensitive and specific than radiographic techniques in detecting calcium in the mitral annulus.[46,47,51]

Echocardiography can better differentiate calcification of the annulus from that of the mitral leaflets and other structures[48,50] than can radiography.

The principal M-mode echocardiographic feature usually associated with calcification of the mitral annulus is a dense band of high-reflectance echoes located between the posterior mitral leaflet and the posterior left ventricular wall. The posterior band of echoes located behind the posterior mitral leaflet on M-mode echocardiography may actually extend from the region of the chordae tendineae to the left atrium.[42-52] Mitral annular calcification has also been associated pathologically with calcification of the aortic annulus and valve, the ventricular septum, the mitral valve leaflets, and the posterior left ventricular wall.[46,53,54] In one small series, aortic stenosis accompanied mitral annular calcification in about two-thirds of cases; in another series 44 percent of patients with hypertrophic cardiomyopathy had mitral annular calcification.[44,50]

Because dense mitral annulus echoes may be in close proximity to the posterior left ventricular endocardium, the annular echoes may partially or entirely obscure the endocardial echoes because of acoustic shadowing (Figure 4-21).[44] Furthermore, the highly reflective calcium may result in an effective ultrasound beam that is artificially wider than the true beam because the ultrasound beam travels more slowly through calcium than through muscle.[56]

Failure to differentiate the calcified mitral annulus from calcification of the posterior mitral leaflet may result in an erroneous diagnosis of mitral stenosis.[43-46] Generally, however, confusion with mitral stenosis is not a problem, as mitral leaflet thickening is generally not present in nonrheumatic mitral annular calcification.[45] Another common diagnostic problem in M-mode echocardiography is that the space between the calcified mitral annulus and the posterior left ventricular wall may be confused as the echo-free space of a pericardial effusion.[43-46,55]

The presence of calcification of the mitral annulus can result in false-negative or a false-positive diagnoses of asymmetric septal hypertrophy.[46,49] A false-positive diagnosis of asymmetric septal hypertrophy can occur when calcified aortic cusps, or the aortic annulus, protrudes downward into the left ventricular outflow tract.[46] In addition, pseudo-SAM (systolic anterior motion of the anterior mitral leaflet) may be present as the calcified ring elevates the anterior mitral leaflet during systole.[44] A false-negative diagnosis of asymmetric septal hypertrophy can occur when the thick annular echo behind the posterior mitral leaflet is misinterpreted as the endocardium of the left ventricle, resulting in an erroneously large measurement for left ventricular posterior wall thickness.[49]

The incidence of mitral annular calcification among 289 subjects undergoing two-dimensional echocardiography to elucidate the causes of mitral regurgitation was 5 percent.[21] Two-dimensional echocardiography has permitted a more precise localization of mitral annular calcification than possible by the M-mode technique. D'Cruz and associates[48] have suggested that the terms *anterior submitral calcification* and *posterior submitral calcification* are more appropriate than *mitral annulus calcification,* as in most instances the calcific deposits are not located in the true mitral annulus. We will use mitral annular calcification in this chapter as a generic term.

D'Cruz et al[48] studied 84 elderly patients with M-mode echocardiography, 35 of whom also underwent two-dimensional echocardiography. Posterior mitral annular calcification (located in the angle between the posterior mitral leaflet and the left ventricular posterior wall) was present in 82 patients. Anterior mitral annular calcification (located immediately anterior to the base of the anterior mitral cusp) was visualized in 12 patients, 10 of whom also had posterior mitral annular calcification. In 2 patients, however, the anterior mitral annular calcification was present between the aortic and mitral rings; in another patient, it was located solely in the mitral chordal region. M-mode echocardiographic scans from the left ventricle cephalad to the left atrium in posterior mitral annular calcification patients show that in some patients the dense band of echoes behind the posterior leaflet ends abruptly and becomes continuous with the posterior atrioventricular junction (true mitral annulus). In other patients, the posterior mitral annular calcification slopes anteriorly to merge with the posterior aortic root. Figure 4-21 depicts mitral annular calcification in an elderly patient without evidence of rheumatic heart disease. Note the dense band of echoes in the posterior region in the long-axis view.

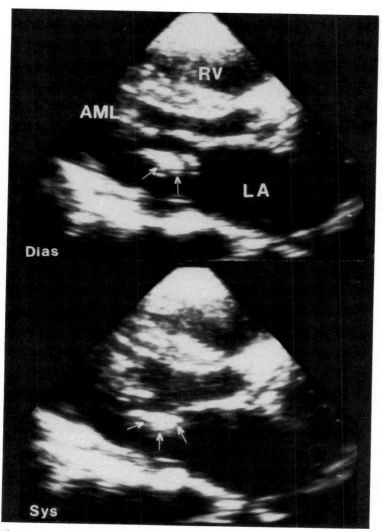

Figure 4-21. Parasternal long-axis echocardiogram in diastole and systole from a patient with heavy calcification of the posterior mitral annulus (arrows). The posterior mitral leaflet is obscured by the annular calcification.

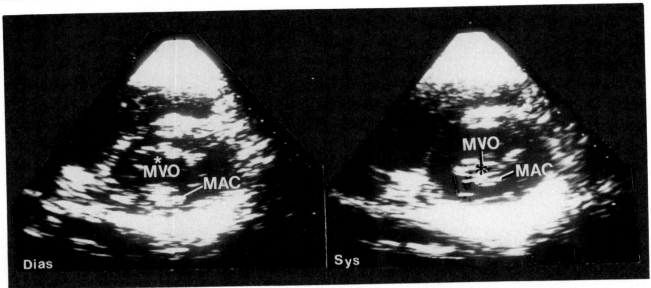

Figure 4-22. Parasternal short-axis two-dimensional echocardiogram from a patient with rheumatic mitral stenosis and calcification of the mitral annulus. MVO denotes mitral valve orifice (the asterisk is in the center of the orifice).

Figure 4-22 demonstrates posterior mitral annular calcification in a patient who also exhibits calcific mitral stenosis and a calcified aortic root. In the presence of severe mitral annular calcification, diastolic gradients may develop across the left ventricular inflow tract.[56–58] Mitral valve replacement may be warranted if the symptoms and findings at cardiac catheterization confirm the presence of a significant transmitral gradient.[59]

SYSTOLIC ANTERIOR MOTION OF THE MITRAL VALVE

Systolic anterior motion of the mitral valve (SAM) was initially described in conjunction with asymmetric septal hypertrophy as one of the two M-mode echocardiographic hallmarks of hypertrophic obstructive cardiomyopathy.[60–64] The presence of SAM was considered to be the M-mode echocardiographic manifestation of left ventricular outflow tract obstruction.[60–63] Moreover, the extent and duration of SAM was reported to correlate with the presence and the degree of left ventricular outflow obstruction.[63] More recently, SAM has been reported without asymmetric septal hypertrophy both in the presence[65–67] and in the absence[68,73–78] of subaortic obstruction. Conditions other than hypertrophic cardiomyopathy known to be associated with SAM include discrete subaortic stenosis,[69] dextrotransposition of the great vessels with subpulmonic obstruction,[70] pulmonary hypertension,[71] concentric left ventricular hypertrophy,[72,73] hyperkinetic states including aortic insufficiency, anemia, and hypovolemia,[73,74] and mitral valve prolapse.[75–78] SAM has also been found in the absence of detectable heart disease.[67,74,79]

The two-dimensional echocardiographic description of systolic anterior motion of the mitral valve in hypertrophic cardiomyopathy is discussed at length in Chapter

10. Here we review only the salient features of SAM in hypertrophic cardiomyopathy. Henry et al[80] were among the first to describe SAM of the anterior mitral leaflet into the left ventricular outflow tract. SAM was defined as a systolic anterior motion of the body of the anterior mitral leaflet, a motion involving convex bowing of the leaflet body toward the ventricular septum. More recently, however, others have emphasized other possible mechanisms for the production of SAM in hypertrophic cardiomyopathy. Rodger[81] described SAM as a complex of echoes from the chordae tendineae, papillary muscle, and anterior mitral leaflet, with the latter structure being the farthest from, and not impinging upon, the septum. In addition, Tajik and coworkers,[82] using wide-angle two-dimensional echocardiography, noted the site of obstruction in hypertrophic cardiomyopathy as occurring at various levels within the left ventricular outflow tract. Three sites of obstruction have been recognized: (1) high, caused by apposition of the ventricular septum and anterior mitral leaflet; (2) upper third of outflow tract, caused by apposition of the septum and the mitral chordal junction—i.e., the distal free edge of the anterior mitral leaflet and the proximal chordae tendineae, and (3) midventricular, caused by apposition of the ventricular septum and papillary muscles (see Chapter 10).

Recently, Shah and associates,[83] using apical four-chamber views, noted abnormal mitral valve coaptation only in those patients with hypertrophic cardiomyopathy and left ventricular outflow gradients. They proposed that the presence of "residual" anterior leaflet (that portion protruding into the left ventricular outflow tract) was necessary for developing SAM. Various etiologies may therefore exist for the systolic anterior motion of the mitral valve in hypertrophic obstructive cardiomyopathy.

A form of SAM known as chordal SAM, or "mitral chordal buckling,"[78] has been described in normals and in patients with mitral valve prolapse. This form of SAM generally appears on M-mode as an abrupt angular motion of the mitral apparatus in early systole which returns to the C-D line in mid- to late-systole. The mitral D-E excursion is greater than normal; the left ventricular ejection fraction may be increased while the ventricular septal and free wall thicknesses are normal. In the patients with mitral valve prolapse, early systolic SAM may be followed by late systolic prolapse (Figure 4-23). Two-dimensional echocardiography reveals early- to midsystolic angulation of the mitral leaflet–chordal junction, giving rise to the appearance of "buckling" or kinking of that structure. The body of the anterior mitral leaflet moves normally—i.e., not toward the septum during systole (Figure 4-24). Mitral chordal buckling can be visualized either in the parasternal long- or short-axis view or in the apical four-chamber view; the parasternal long-axis view appears to be the best for imaging this phenomenon. This form of SAM has not been associated with left ventricular outflow tract obstruction in normals or in patients with mitral valve prolapse.

DILATED CARDIOMYOPATHY

The mitral valve in dilated cardiomyopathy generally demonstrates decreased leaflet excursion reflecting diminished transvalvular flow and an increase in the distance between the E point of the anterior mitral leaflet and the left ventricular septum (Figure 4-6). Mitral regurgitation may occur in patients with dilated cardiomyopathy or patients with a dilated left ventricle of other etiology. One of the mechanisms, i.e., papillary muscle dysfunction (Figure 4-25), has been described earlier in this chapter. It has also been suggested that dilatation of the mitral valve ring may play

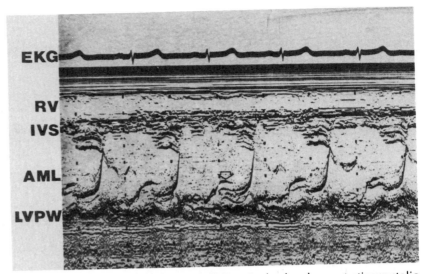

Figure 4-23. M-mode echocardiogram at the level of the mitral valve demonstrating systolic anterior motion (SAM) beginning abruptly early in systole followed by short systolic mitral valve prolapse. IVS denotes interventricular septum; LVPW, left ventricular posterior wall. (From Gardin JM, Talano JV, Stephanides L, Systolic anterior motion in the absence of asymmetric septal hypertrophy: A buckling phenomenon of the chordae tendineae. Circulation 63:181–188, 1981. With permission.)

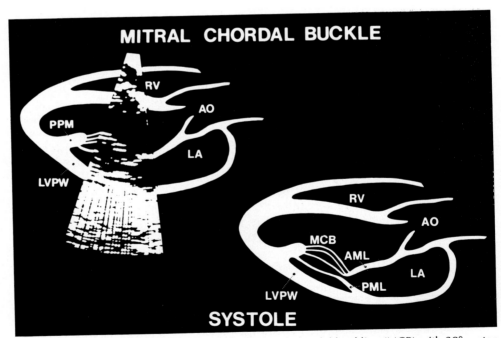

Figure 4-24. Diagrammatic long-axis views of mitral chordal buckling (MCB) with 30° sector scan interposed in drawing on left. Note the angulation toward the septum of the mitral chordae, or leaflet-chordal position. The body of the anterior mitral leaflet moves normally during systole—i.e., not toward the septum. PPM denotes posterior papillary muscle. (From Gardin JM, Talano JV, Stephanides L, et al: Systolic anterior motion in the absence of asymmetric septal hypertrophy: A buckling phenomenon of the chordae tendineae. Circulation 63:181–188, 1981. With permission.)

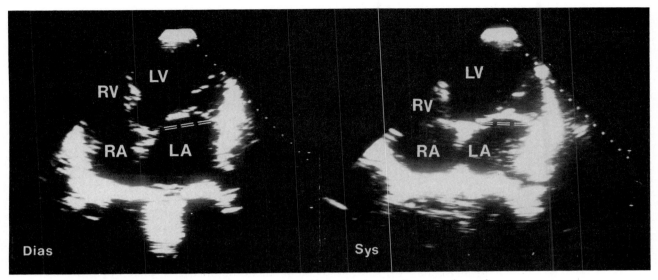

Figure 4-25. Apical four-chamber frames from a patient with congestive cardiomyopathy and papillary muscle dysfunction. The mitral leaflet excursion is markedly diminished during diastole, and leaflet coaptation is abnormally displaced into the left ventricle in systole.

an important role in the genesis of mitral regurgitation.[84] One report has noted that dilatation of the mitral annulus can occur in patients with dilated cardiomyopathy; however, this dilatation is not proportional to left ventricular dilatation.[85] Mitral regurgitation in left ventricular dilatation may therefore be due to other mechanisms, such as loss of sphincteric action of the annulus or malalignment of the papillary muscles, independent of mitral annulus dilatation.[86]

MYXOMA AND VEGETATIONS

The two-dimensional echocardiographic findings of mitral valve vegetations and of left myxoma are discussed in detail in Chapter 12.

CONGENITAL MITRAL VALVE DISORDERS

Congenital mitral stenosis, parachute mitral valve, cleft mitral leaflet, and other congenital conditions involving the mitral valve are described in Chapter 13.

MITRAL VALVE PROLAPSE

Mitral valve prolapse has been identified as a clinical syndrome with various electrocardiographic, echocardiographic, auscultatory, and skeletal muscle abnormalities. The anatomic features include large, redundant scalloped and thickened valves associated with myxomatous changes of the mitral–chordal structures and annular dilatation. Myxomatous changes cause a loss of collagenous support, allowing for leaflet stretching and systolic prolapse into the left atrium. It is not known whether the myxomatous changes are due to an as yet unidentified local factor or to a primary defect in mucopolysaccharide metabolism.[88] Primary and secondary forms of mitral prolapse have been identified by Jeresaty[87] and Barlow and Pocock.[88] Primary mitral valve prolapse includes a spectrum which ranges from mild prolapse of one leaflet without clinical symptoms to severe prolapse of one or two leaflets with severe mitral regurgitation and multiple cardiovascular symptoms.[89,90] Secondary mitral prolapse can result from any abnormality which affects the normal mitral–chordal apparatus, i.e., myocarditis, rheumatic, primary cardiomyopathy, or endocarditis.

Mitral tissue within the left atrium during systole is the hallmark of the disease. Diagnostic techniques such as angiography, M-mode echocardiography, and now two-dimensional echocardiography, which allows for imaging of the mitral leaflets during the cardiac cycle, are most helpful in establishing the diagnosis. However, the "gold standard" among diagnostic techniques is yet to be defined. The incidence of mitral valve prolapse in the general population has been reported as varying from 5 to 28 percent depending on the diagnostic criteria and the age and sex of the population.[91–93] The ability of echocardiography to image the mitral valve and define location of the leaflets during systole might suggest that this method is the procedure of choice. However, experience with M-mode echocardiography has identified some limitations of the technique. Jeresaty[87] preferred that the systolic nonejection click and late systolic murmur on auscultation serve as the standard. However, he himself admits that up to 17 percent of mitral valve prolapses are silent in auscultation. Several investigators have proposed left ventricular cineangiography as the diagnostic standard. However, the normal mitral valve has variable patterns on cineangiography with the most common projection, the right anterior oblique view, obscuring the anterior mitral leaflet during systole.[87] There is also considerable interobserver variability in the angiographic diagnosis of mitral valve prolapse, making this a poor "gold standard."[94]

Problems with M-Mode Echocardiography

Shah and Gramiak[95] described two patterns—a posterior midsystolic buckling of the mitral valve and a posterior hammocking displacement of the mitral valve—as the M-mode echocardiographic hallmarks of mitral valve prolapse. Others subsequently have described similar M-mode echocardiographic features that are considered relatively specific for mitral prolapse.[96,97] However, variations in technique provided many false-positive and false-negative studies in these patients. It became apparent that transducer position and angulation were critical in the M-mode diagnosis of mitral prolapse. Markiewicz et al[91] nicely demonstrated that if the transducer is positioned high on the chest wall and angled caudad (inferiorly), it might be directed in a plane posterior to the closure point of the mitral valve; the mitral leaflets move perpendicular to the M-mode beam, away from the transducer, providing a false-positive dipping of the mitral valve. Conversely, if the transducer is placed too low on the chest wall and pointed cephalad (superiorly), the posterior mitral leaflets may not be visualized and anterior mitral leaflet prolapse may be masked, producing a false-negative study.

The sensitivity of M-mode echocardiography ranges from 50 to 82 percent when left ventricular angiography is used as a standard.[91,98,99] This limitation may result from a transducer position too low on the chest wall, or if the major portion of the prolapsed leaflet is superiorly, rather than posteriorly, directed. Given the limitation of the "ice-pick" view of M-mode echocardiography, mitral valve prolapse can more accurately be diagnosed by two-dimensional echocardiography.

Two-Dimensional Echocardiographic Findings

The advent of two-dimensional echocardiography provides the clinician with a better tool for the diagnosis of mitral valve prolapse. The spatial orientation of the mitral valve is better imaged by the two-dimensional technique. Cardiac landmarks can be identified and more precise measurements of mitral valve motion can be made. Mitral coaptation patterns can be better identified, standardized, and classified. Sahn and coworkers,[100] using two-dimensional echocardiography, studied mitral coaptation in mitral valve prolapse and found that the prolapsing motion of the leaflets is superiorly as well as posteriorly directed. M-mode echocardiographic patterns of midsystolic prolapse and holosystolic prolapse could be clearly identified in the same patient by differences in beam angulation. The multiple lines seen on M-mode echocardiograms were found to be due to simultaneous intersection of different portions of the prolapsed mitral valve by the ultrasound beam. False-negative M-mode echocardiographic studies for mitral prolapse could easily be identified by the demonstration of superior prolapsed motion of the body of the posterior mitral leaflet on two-dimensional echocardiography. Thus, the two-dimensional technique appears more accurate in diagnosing and differentiating the various types of mitral valve prolapse.

Gilbert et al[101] used two-dimensional echocardiography to study characteristic patterns of mitral valve coaptation in patients with angiographically proved mitral valve prolapse. In normal subjects without mitral prolapse, on cardiac catheterization no superior movement (prolapse) of the leaflets occurred above the plane of the mitral annulus (Figure 4-26). In patients with angiographically proved mitral valve prolapse, the most important two-dimensional echocardiographic finding was superior motion of either the anterior, the posterior, or both mitral leaflets during systole above the plane of the mitral annulus. The majority of patients (68 percent) demonstrated both anterior and posterior mitral leaflet prolapse, several (30 percent) had isolated posterior leaflet prolapse, and a rare patient had isolated anterior leaflet prolapse (2 percent). Two-dimensional echocardiography was more sensitive than angiography in identifying isolated anterior mitral leaflet prolapse. Left ventricular angiography was more likely to miss anterior leaflet prolapse because the anterior leaflet was superimposed on a ventricular silhouette opacified by the contrast.

More recently, the apical four-chamber view has been reported to increase sensitivity of the two-dimensional echocardiographic diagnosis of mitral valve prolapse. In the four-chamber view, the mitral annulus is horizontal and perpendicular to the interventricular septum. Therefore, the motion of the leaflets and the point of coaptation can be clearly analyzed in relation to the mitral annulus. Using the apical four-chamber view, Naito et al[102] demonstrated that the majority of mitral prolapse patients had both anterior and posterior mitral prolapse. The parasternal long-axis view demonstrated mitral prolapse in only half of these patients. Posterior leaflet prolapse was also more commonly seen in the apical four-chamber view than in the long-axis view.

Using two-dimensional echocardiography, four patterns of systolic mitral coaptation can be identified using the parasternal long-axis view. The superior border of

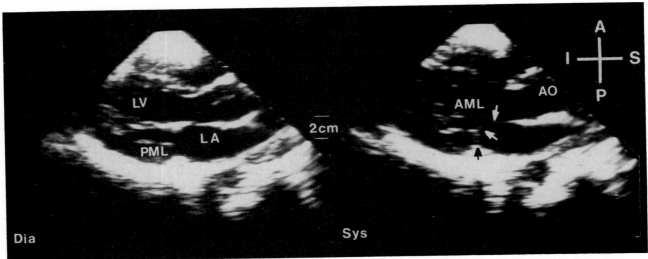

Figure 4-26. Two-dimensional long-axis view of the left ventricle in normal (Type I) subject. Note coaptation of the normal mitral valve (oblique arrow) well within the left ventricular cavity. The superior portion of the left ventricle is defined as an area caudad to an imaginary annular line drawn from the hinge point of the anterior mitral leaflet and posterior aortic wall (vertical white arrow) to the atrioventricular sulcus (vertical black arrow).

the left ventricular cavity is defined by two-dimensional echocardiography as an area caudad (inferior) to an imaginary line (i line) drawn from the hinge point of the anterior mitral leaflet and posterior aortic wall to the atrioventricular sulcus. In normals (Type 1), systolic coaptation of the mitral leaflets occurs within the cavity and the leaflets remain there throughout systole (Figure 4-26). In one form of mitral prolapse (Type 2), mitral coaptation occurs well within the left ventricle. However, in late systole the anterior mitral leaflet, which is larger than normal, bows toward the left atrium superior (cephalad) to the atrioventricular junction (i line), overshooting the posterior leaflets (Figure 4-27). There is excessive coaptation of the anterior and posterior mitral leaflets and a decreased (more acute) angle between the atrial surface of the anterior mitral leaflet and the posterior aortic wall. Superior arching of the anterior mitral leaflet is above the i line, evidence considered positive for mitral prolapse (Figure 4-28). In another pattern (Type 3), the anterior and posterior mitral leaflets coapt either caudad to or at the i line (Figure 4-29). During late systole, however, the posterior mitral leaflet moves cephalad to the atrioventricular junction and prolapses into the left atrium. There is unusual systolic curling of the posterior mitral annulus on the adjacent myocardium. The posterior leaflet predominantly prolapses superiorly and posteriorly. In a fourth pattern (Type 4), there is mitral coaptation within the left ventricular cavity or at the i line (Figure 4-30). In late systole both the anterior and posterior leaflets arch superiorly (cephalad) into the left atrium. The most frequent patterns in our experience have been Types 3 and 4. Type 2 is infrequently seen in mitral valve prolapse.

The apical four-chamber view (Figure 4-31) is particularly useful in defining the mitral annulus, since it moves perpendicular to the ultrasound beam. It is especially helpful in detecting mitral valve prolapse because the systolic arching into the left atrium is easily observed.[103] A foreshortened apical four-chamber view can yield a false-positive diagnosis of anterior mitral prolapse.

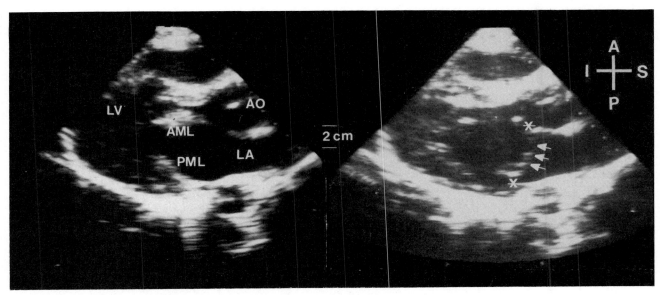

Figure 4-27. Two-dimensional long-axis view of the left ventricle in Type 2 mitral coaptation. Note the unusually large anterior mitral leaflet that bows toward the left atrium superior to the atrioventricular sulcus and overshoots the posterior mitral leaflet. The asterisks define the anterior and posterior borders of the mitral valve annulus. The arrows indicate the prolapsing anterior mitral valve leaflet.

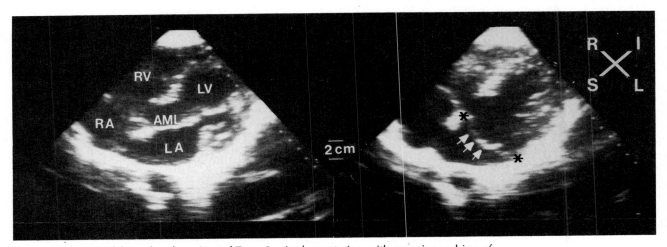

Figure 4-28. Apical four-chamber view of Type 2 mitral coaptation with superior arching of the anterior mitral leaflet above the atrioventricular sulcus. The asterisks define the anterior and posterior borders of the mitral valve annulus. The arrows indicate the prolapsing mitral valve.

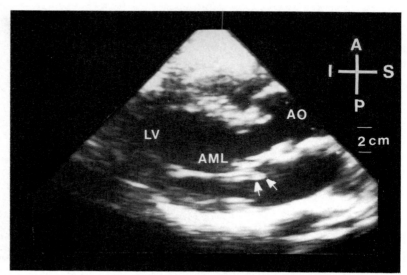

Figure 4-29. Parasternal long-axis view of Type 3 mitral coaptation. Note that in late systole only the posterior mitral leaflet (arrows) moves cephalad to the atrioventricular junction and prolapses into the left atrium.

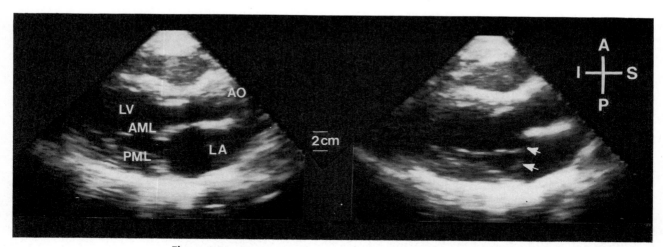

Figure 4-30. Long-axis parasternal view of the left ventricle in Type 4 mitral coaptation. Note how in late systole both the anterior and posterior mitral leaflets (arrows) arch superiorly into the left atrium.

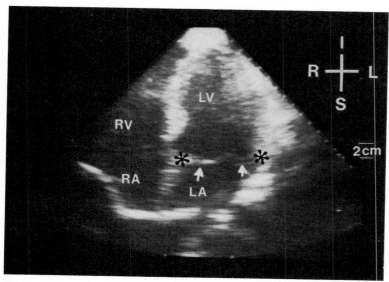

Figure 4-31. Apical four-chamber view in Type 4 mitral coaptation. Both the anterior and posterior mitral leaflets (arrows) arch superiorly into the left atrium during systole above the atrioventricular sulcus.

REFERENCES

1. Ormiston JA, Shah PM, Tei C, et al: Size and motion of the mitral valve annulus in man. I. A two-dimensional echocardiographic method and findings in normal subjects. Circulation 64:113–120, 1981

2. Edler I, Gustafson A: Ultrasound cardiogram in mitral stenosis. Acta Med Scand 169:85–90, 1957

3. Nichol PM, Gilbert BW, Kisslo JA: Two-dimensional echocardiographic assessment of mitral stenosis. Circulation 55:120–128, 1977

4. Wann LS, Weyman AE, Feigenbaum H, et al: Determination of mitral valve area by cross-sectional echocardiography. Ann Intern Med 88:337–341, 1978

5. Feigenbaum H: Echocardiography (ed 3). Philadelphia, Lea & Febiger, 1981, pp 239–267

6. Cope GD, Kisslo JA, Johnson ML, et al: A reassessment of the echocardiogram in mitral stenosis. Circulation 52:664–670, 1975

7. Levisman JA, Abassi AS, Pearce ML: Posterior mitral leaflet motion of mitral stenosis. Circulation 51:511–514, 1975

8. Shiu MF, Jenkins BS, Webb-Peploe MM: Echocardiographic analysis of posterior mitral leaflet movement in mitral-stenosis. Br Heart J 40:372–376, 1978

9. Fisher ML, Parisi AF, Plotnick GD, et al: Assessment of severe mitral stenosis by echocardiographic leaflet separation. Arch Intern Med 139:402–406, 1979

10. Beasley B, Kerber R: Does mitral prolapse occur in mitral stenosis? Echocardiographic–angiographic observations. Chest 80:56–60, 1981

11. Henry WL, Griffith JM, Michaelis LL, et al: Measurement of mitral orifice area in patients with mitral valve disease by real-time two-dimensional echocardiography. Circulation 51:827–831, 1975

12. Gorlin R, Gorlin SG: Hydraulic formula for calculation of the area of the stenotic mitral valve, other cardiac valves, and central circulatory shunts. Am Heart J 41:1–29, 1951

13. Henry WL, Kastl DJ: Echocardiographic evaluation of patients with mitral stenosis. Am J Med 62:813–818, 1977

14. Martin RP, Rakowski H, Kleiman JH, et al: Reliability and reproducibility of two-dimensional echocardiographic measurement of the stenotic mitral valve orifice area. Am J Cardiol 43:560–568, 1979

15. Chandraratna PAN, Aronow WS, Lurie M: Cross-sectional echocardiographic observations on the

mechanism of preservation of the opening snap in calcific mitral stenosis. Chest 78:822–825, 1980

16. Segal BL, Likoff W, Kingsley B: Echocardiography: clinical application in mitral regurgitation. Am J Cardiol 19:50, 1967

17. Burgess J, Clark R, Kamigaki M, et al: Echocardiographic findings in different types of mitral regurgitation. Circulation 48:97–106, 1973

18. Patton R, Dragatakis L, Marpole D, et al: The posterior left atrial echocardiogram of mitral regurgitation. Circulation 57:1134–1139, 1978

19. Wann LS, Feigenbaum H, Weyman AE, et al: Cross-sectional echocardiographic detection of rheumatic mitral regurgitation. Am J Cardiol 41:1258–1263, 1978

20. Mintz GS, Kotler MN, Segal BL, et al: Two-dimensional echocardiographic evaluation of patients with mitral insufficiency. Am J Cardiol 44:670–678, 1979

21. Kotler MN, Mintz GS, Parry WR, et al: M-mode and two-dimensional echocardiography in mitral and aortic regurgitation: Pre- and postoperative evaluation of volume overload of the left ventricle. Am J Cardiol 46:1144–1152, 1980

22. Lewis BS, Colsen PR, Rosenfeld T, et al: An unusual case of mitral valve aneurysm: two-dimensional echocardiographic and cineangiocardiographic features. Am J Cardiol 49:1293–1296, 1982

23. Gehl LG, Mintz GS, Kotler MN, et al: Left atrial volume overload in mitral regurgitation: a two-dimensional echocardiographic study. Am J Cardiol 49:33–38, 1982

24. Burch GE, DePasquale NP, Phillips JH: Clinical manifestations of papillary muscle dysfunction. Arch Intern Med 112:112–117, 1963

25. Phillips JH, Burch GE, DePasquale NP: The syndrome of papillary muscle dysfunction. Ann Intern Med 59:508–520, 1963

26. Tallury VK, DePasquale NP, Burch GE: The echocardiogram in papillary muscle dysfunction. Am Heart J 83:12–18, 1972

27. Millward DK, McLaurin LP, Craige E: Echocardiographic studies of the mitral valve in patients with congestive cardiomyopathy and mitral regurgitation. Am Heart J 85:413–421, 1973

28. Ogawa S, Hubbard FE, Mardelli TJ, et al: Cross-sectional echocardiographic spectrum of papillary muscle dysfunction. Am Heart J 97:312–321, 1979

29. Godley RW, Wann L, Rodgers EW, et al: Incomplete mitral leaflet closure in patients with papillary muscle dysfunction. Circulation 63:565–571, 1981

30. Mirro MJ, Rodgers EW, Weyman AE, et al: Angular displacement of the papillary muscles during the cardiac cycle. Circulation 60:327–333, 1979

31. Erbel R, Schwezer P, Bardos P, et al: Two-dimensional echocardiographic diagnosis of papillary muscle rupture. Chest 79:595–598, 1981

32. Sweatman T, Selzer A, Kamagaki M: Echocardiographic diagnosis of mitral regurgitation due to ruptured chordae tendineae. Circulation 47:580–586, 1972

33. DeMaria AM, King JF, Bogren HG, et al: The variable spectrum of echocardiographic manifestations of the mitral valve prolapse syndrome. Circulation 50:33–41, 1974

34. Meyer JF, Frank MJ, Goldberg S, et al: Systolic mitral flutter, an echocardiographic clue to the diagnosis of ruptured chordae tendineae. Am Heart J 93:3–9, 1977

35. Burgess J, Clark R, Kamagaki M, et al: Echocardiographic findings in different types of mitral regurgitation. Circulation 48:77–106, 1973

36. Duchak JM, Chang S, Feigenbaum H: Echocardiographic features of torn chordae tendineae (Abstract). Am J Cardiol 29:260, 1972

37. Mintz GS, Kotler MN, Segal BL, et al: Two-dimensional echocardiographic recognition of ruptured chordae tendineae. Circulation 57:244–250, 1978

38. Child JS, Skorton DJ, Taylor RD, et al: M-mode and cross-sectional echocardiographic features of flail posterior mitral leaflets. Am J Cardiol 44:1303–1390, 1979

39. Nishimura T, Takahashi M, Osakada G, et al: Two-dimensional echocardiographic findings in ruptured chordae tendineae of the mitral valve. J Cardiogr 8:589, 1978

40. Ogawa S, Mardelli TJ, Hubbard FE: The role of cross-sectional echocardiography in the diagnosis of flail mitral leaflet. Clin Cardiol 1:85–90, 1978

41. Mintz GS, Kotler MN, Parry WR, et al: Statistical comparison of M-mode and two-dimensional echocardiographic diagnosis of flail mitral leaflets. Am J Cardiol 45:253–259, 1980

42. Howard PF, Cabizuca SV, Desser KB, et al: The echocardiographic diagnosis of calcified mitral annulus. Am J Med Sci 273:267–271, 1977

43. Gabor GE, Mohr BD, Goel PC, et al: Echocardiographic and clinical spectrum of mitral annular calcification. Am J Cardiol 38:836–841, 1976

44. Curati WL, Petitclerc R, Winsberg F: Ultrasonic features of mitral annulus calcification. A report of 21 cases. Radiology 122:215–217, 1977

45. Dashkoff N, Karacuschansky M, Come PC, et al: Echocardiographic features of mitral annulus calcification. Am Heart J 94:585–592, 1977

46. D'Cruz I, Cohen HC, Prabhu R, et al: Clinical manifestations of mitral annulus calcification with emphasis on its echocardiographic features. Am Heart J 94:367–377, 1977

47. Schott CR, Kotler MN, Parry WR, et al: Mitral annular calcification. Clinical and echocardiographic correlations. Arch Intern Med 137:1143–1150, 1977

48. D'Cruz I, Panetta F, Cohen H, et al: Submitral calcification or sclerosis in elderly patients: M-mode and two-dimensional echocardiography in "mitral annulus calcification." Am J Cardiol 44:31–38, 1979

49. Kronzon I, Mitchell J, Shapiro J, et al: Two-dimensional echocardiography in mitral annulus calcification. AJR 134:355–358, 1980

50. Meltzer RS, Martin RP, Robbins BS, et al: Mitral annular calcification: clinical and echocardiographic features. Acta Cardiol 35:189–202, 1980

51. Arvan SB, Weisman JS: The calcified mitral annulus: clinical and echocardiographic features. Practical Cardiol 4:104–127, 1978

52. Feigenbaum H: Echocardiography (ed 3). Philadelphia, Lea & Febiger, 1981, pp 315–318

53. Roberts WC, Perloff JK: Mitral valvular disease: a clinicopathologic survey of the conditions causing the mitral valve to function abnormally. Ann Intern Med 77:939–975, 1971

54. Korn D, DeSanctis RW, Sell S: Massive calcification of the mitral annulus, a clinicopathological study of fourteen cases. N Engl J Med 267:900–909, 1962

55. Hirschfeld DS, Emilson BB: Echocardiogram in calcified mitral annulus. Am J Cardiol 36:354–356, 1975

56. Hammer WJ, Roberts WC, DeLeon AC: "Mitral stenosis" secondary to combined massive mitral annular calcific deposits and small hypertrophied left ventricles. Am J Med 64:371–376, 1978

57. Hakki AH, Iskandrian AS: Obstruction to left ventricular inflow secondary to combined mitral annular calcification and hypertrophic subaortic stenosis. Cathet Cardiovasc Diagn 6:191–196, 1980

58. Osterberger LE, Goldstein S, Khaja F, et al: Functional mitral stenosis in patients with massive mitral annular calcification. Circulation 64:472–476, 1981

59. Ramirez J, Flowers NC: Severe mitral stenosis secondary to massive calcification of the mitral annulus with unusual echocardiographic manifestations. Clin Cardiol 3:284–287, 1980

60. Shah PM, Gramiak R, Kramer DH: Ultrasound localization of left ventricular outflow obstruction and hypertrophic obstructive cardiomyopathy. Circulation 40:3–11, 1979

61. Popp RL, Harrison DC: Ultrasound in the diagnosis and evaluation of therapy of idiopathic hypertrophic subaortic stenosis. Circulation 40:905–914, 1969

62. Shah PM, Gramiak R, Adelman AG, et al: Role of echocardiography in diagnostic and hemodynamic assessment of hypertrophic subaortic stenosis. Circulation 44:891–898, 1971

63. Henry WL, Clark CE, Glancy DL, et al: Echocardiographic measurement of left ventricular outflow gradient in idiopathic hypertrophic subaortic stenosis. N Engl J Med 288:989–993, 1973

64. Pridie RB, Oakley CM: Mechanism of mitral regurgitation in hypertrophic obstructive cardiomyopathy. Br Heart J 32:203–208, 1970

65. Mintz GS, Kotler MN, Segal BL, et al: Systolic anterior motion of the mitral valve in the absence of asymmetric septal hypertrophy. Circulation 57:256–263, 1976

66. Crawford MH, Groves BM, Horowitz LD: Dynamic left ventricular outflow tract obstruction and systolic anterior motion of the mitral valve in the absence of asymmetric septal hypertrophy. Am J Med 65:703–708, 1978

67. Cooperberg P, Hazell S, Ashmore GP: Parachute accessory anterior mitral valve leaflet causing left ventricular outflow tract obstruction. Report of a case with emphasis on the echocardiographic findings. Circulation 53:908–911, 1976

68. Boughner DR, Rakowski H, Wigle ED: Mitral valve systolic anterior motion in the absence of hypertrophic cardiomyopathy (Abstract). Circulation 58(Suppl II):235, 1978

69. Davis RH, Feigenbaum H, Chang S, et al: Echocardiographic manifestations of discrete subaortic stenosis. Am J Cardiol 33:277–280, 1974

70. Nanda NC, Gramiak R, Manning JA, et al: Echocardiographic features of subpulmonic obstruction in dextro-transposition of the great vessels. Circulation 51:515–521, 1975

71. Goodman DJ, Rossen RM, Popp RL: Echocardiographic pseudo-idiopathic hypertrophic subaortic stenosis. Chest 66:573–574, 1974

72. Maron BJ, Gottdiener JS, Roberts WC, et al: Left ventricular outflow tract obstruction due to systolic anterior motion of the anterior mitral leaflet in patients with concentric left ventricular hypertrophy. Circulation 57:527–533, 1978

73. Come PC, Bulkley BH, Goodman ZB, et al: Hypercontractile cardiac states simulating hypertrophic cardiomyopathy. Circulation 55:901–908, 1977

74. Bulkley BH, Fortuin NJ: Systolic anterior motion of the mitral valve without asymmetric septal hypertrophy. Chest 69:694–696, 1976

75. Terasawa Y, Tanaka M, Niita K, et al: Production mechanism of systolic click in mid-systolic–late systolic murmur syndrome. J Cardiogr 6:593, 1976

76. Feigenbaum H: Echocardiography (ed 2). Philadelphia, Lea & Febiger, 1976, p 122

77. Sahn DJ, Allen HD, Goldberg SJ, et al: Mitral valve prolapse in children. A problem defined by real-time cross-sectional echocardiography. Circulation 53:651–657, 1976

78. Gardin JM, Talano JV, Stephanides L, et al: Systolic anterior motion in the absence of asymmetric septal hypertrophy: A buckling phenomenon of the chordae tendineae. Circulation 63:181–188, 1981

79. Lombardi A, Nanda N, Gramiak R: Significance of abnormal mitral systolic anterior movements (Abstract). First Meeting of the World Federation for Ultrasound in Medicine and Biology, 1976

80. Henry WL, Clark CE, Griffith J, et al: Mechanism of left ventricular outflow obstruction in patients with obstructive asymmetric septal hypertrophy (idiopathic hypertrophic subaortic stenosis). Am J Cardiol 35:337–345, 1975

81. Rodger JC: Motion of mitral apparatus in hypertrophic cardiomyopathy with obstruction. Br Heart J 38:732–737, 1976

82. Tajik AJ, Seward JB, Hagler DJ: Detailed analysis of hypertrophic obstructive cardiomyopathy by wide-angle two-dimensional sector echocardiography (Abstract). Am J Cardiol 43:348, 1979

83. Shah PM, Taylor RD, Wong M: Abnormal mitral valve coaptation in hypertropic obstructive cardiomyopathy: Proposed role in systolic anterior motion of mitral valve. Am J Cardiol 48:258–262, 1981

84. Flint A: A Practical Treatise on the Diagnosis, Pathogenesis and Treatment of Diseases of the Heart. Philadelphia, Henry C Lea, 1870, p 134

85. Bulkley BH, Roberts WC: Dilatation of the mitral annulus. A rare cause of mitral regurgitation. Am J Med 59:457–463, 1975

86. Chandraratna PAN, Aronow WS: Mitral valve ring in normal vs. dilated left ventricle: cross-sectional echocardiographic study. Chest 79:151–154, 1981

87. Jeresaty RM: Mitral Valve Prolapse. New York, Raven Press, 1979

88. Barlow JB, Pocock WA: Mitral valve prolapse, the specific billowing mitral leaflet syndrome, or an insignificant non-ejection systolic click. Am Heart J 97:277–285, 1979

89. Read RC, Thai AP: Surgical experience with symptomatic myxomatous valvular transformation (the floppy valve syndrome). Surgery 59:173–182, 1966

90. Read RC, Thai AP, Wendy VE: Symptomatic valvular myxomatous transformation (the floppy valve syndrome): a possible forme fruste of the Marfan syndrome. Circulation 32:897–910, 1965

91. Markiewicz W, Stoner J, London E, et al: Mitral valve prolapse in one hundred presumably healthy young females. Circulation 53:464–473, 1976

92. Procacci PM, Savran SV, Schreiter SL, et al: Prevalence of clinical mitral valve prolapse in 1169 young women. N Engl J Med 294:1086–1088, 1976

93. Gardin JM, Henry WL, Savage DD, et al: Echocardiographic evaluation of an older population without clinically apparent heart disease (Abstract). Am J Cardiol 41:377, 1978

94. DeMaria AN, Neumann A, Lee G, et al: Echocardiographic identification of the mitral valve prolapse syndrome. Am J Med 62:819–829, 1977

95. Shah PM, Gramiak R: Echocardiographic recognition of mitral valve prolapse (Abstract). Circulation 42(SupplIII):III-45, 1970

96. Dillon JC, Haine CL, Chang S, et al: Use of echocardiography in patients with prolapsed mitral valve. Circulation 43:503–507, 1971

97. Kerber RE, Isaeff DM, Hancock EW: Echocardiographic patterns in patients with the syndrome of systolic click and late systolic murmur. N Engl J Med 284:691–3, 1971

98. Malcolm AD, Boughner DR, Kostuk WJ, et al: Clinical features and investigative findings in presence of mitral leaflet prolapse. Study of 85 consecutive patients. Br Heart J 38:244–256, 1976

99. Boughner DR: Correlation of echocardiographic and angiographic abnormalities in mitral valve prolapse. Ultrasound Med Biol 1:55–62, 1975

100. Sahn DJ, Allen HD, Goldberg SJ, Friedman WF: Mitral valve prolapse in children. A problem defined by real-time cross-sectional echocardiography. Circulation 53:651–657, 1976

101. Gilbert BW, Schatz RA, VonRamm OT, et al: Mitral valve prolapse. Two-dimensional echocardiographic and angiographic correlation. Circulation 54:716–723, 1976

102. Naito M, Morganroth J, Mardelli TJ, et al: Apical cross sectional echocardiography: the standard for diagnosis of mitral valve prolapse (Abstract). Circulation 59,60(Suppl II):II-154, 1979

CHAPTER **5**

Diseases of the Aortic Valve and Aorta

James V. Talano

— AORTIC VALVE

Normal Aortic Valve

The aortic valve can be best examined by two-dimensional echocardiography from the parasternal long-axis and short-axis views (see Chapter 3). In long axis, the aorta, aortic valve, left atrium, and left ventricular outflow tract can be imaged. The normal aortic valve is imaged during systole as two parallel echoes near the aortic wall (Figure 5-1). During diastole the aortic cusps close and are imaged as a dominant single echo in the middle of the aorta. The bodies of the cusps are only occasionally visualized, unless they are thickened.

To obtain a short-axis view of the aorta and aortic valve, the transducer is rotated 90° from the parasternal long axis. The aortic valve is seen within the center of the image with the tricuspid valve to the left of the image (anatomic right), the pulmonic valve is seen superior and to the right, and the left atrium is just posterior to the aorta. With careful 5° to 10° cephalad or caudad angulation of the transducer, the three cusps of the aortic valve can usually be imaged (Figure 5-2). In diastole the three cusps form an inverted "Mercedes Benz sign." With slight (5° to 10°) counterclockwise rotation of the transducer, all three cusps, i.e., right, left, and non-coronary, can usually be imaged. During systole the three cusps usually open up to the aortic wall and become indistinguishable from the aortic wall echoes. In conditions in which forward stroke volume is diminished, the aortic valve orifice changes from a circular to a triangular configuration during systole, allowing visualization of all three cusps.

The Bicuspid Aortic Valve

The bicuspid aortic valve is a common congenital lesion that is usually underdiagnosed in the general population.[1] The risks of this lesion include aortic valvular regurgitation,[1–3] progressive valvular stenosis,[2–5] and vegetative endocarditis.[2–7]

The M-mode echocardiographic description of the bicuspid aortic valve has been that of an eccentrically located cusp—i.e., one that is closer to one or the other wall of the aorta. An eccentricity index has been developed for the M-mode diagnosis[8,9]; however, this index has been plagued by many false-positive and false-negative

103

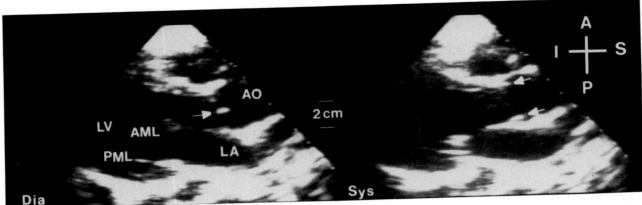

Figure 5-1. Parasternal long-axis view of normal aortic valve. Note the dominant single echo of the aortic cusps (arrow) in diastole. During systole the aortic cusps are seen as two parallel echoes near the aortic wall (parallel arrows). LA denotes left atrium; LV, left ventricle; AO, aorta; AML, anterior mitral leaflet; PML, posterior mitral leaflet.

results.[9] Two-dimensional echocardiography provides a better method for assessing the spatial relationships of the aortic cusps and thus has become more useful in diagnosis (Figures 5-3A, B, C). The most common characteristics of the bicuspid aortic valve on two-dimensional echocardiography are (1) visualization of only two aortic cusps in short axis, (2) irregularity or folding over of cusp margins, (3) abnormal location of commissural insertion, and (4) marked asymmetry of valve closure.[10]

In the short-axis view shown in Figure 5-3B, only two aortic cusps can be identified during valve opening and closing. In diastole the cusp margins of the bicuspid valve

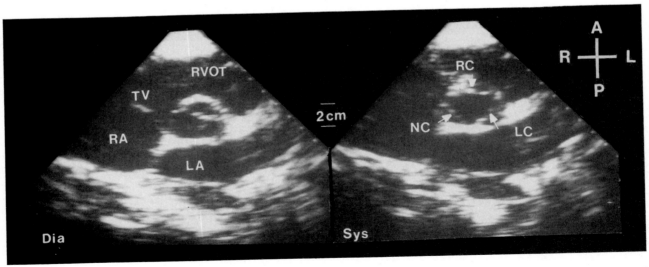

Figure 5-2. Parasternal short-axis view of normal aortic valve. In diastole the three cusps of the aortic valve are seen to form an inverted "Mercedes Benz sign." During systole all cusps of the aortic valve can usually be imaged. RC denotes right coronary cusp, LC, left coronary cusp; NC, noncoronary cusp; RVOT, right ventricular outflow tract; TV, tricuspid valve; RA, right atrium.

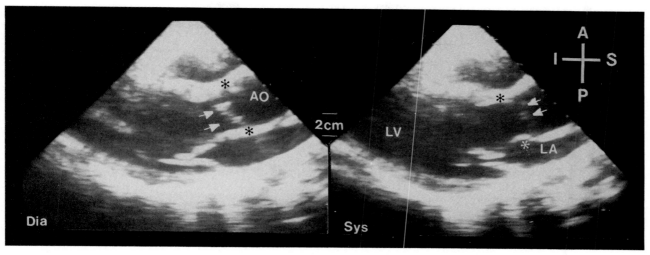

Figure 5-3A. Parasternal long-axis view of a congenital bicuspid aortic valve. The anterior and posterior aortic ring margins are marked by asterisks. Note doming of the aortic valve superiorly (cephalad) during systole (arrows). During diastole the bicuspid aortic valve will frequently prolapse inferiorly (caudad) in the left ventricular outflow tract (arrows).

can be folded over and appear redundant, often forming a sigmoid pattern.[10] The bicuspid valve often has commissures which insert eccentrically into the aorta.

In the parasternal long-axis views of Figures 5-3A and C, systolic doming of the aortic valve is seen. Doming of the aortic valve is not necessarily characteristic of the bicuspid valve but is seen with an abnormally thickened tricuspid aortic valve. Whether in a bicuspid or abnormal tricuspid aortic valve, however, in the experiences of Fowles et al[10] the presence of systolic doming was always correlated with the highest peak systolic gradient. These workers further found that systolic doming was correctly identified by two-dimensional echocardiography in patients in whom it had also been shown by angiography.

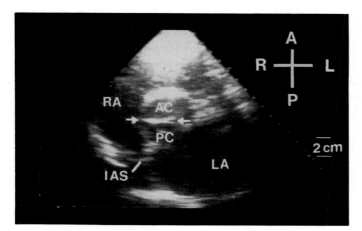

Figure 5-3B. Parasternal short-axis view of a congenital bicuspid aortic valve in diastole. Note that the closure line of the aortic valve in diastole may be single and at times "S" shaped or sigmoid (arrows). AC denotes anterior cusp; PC, posterior cusp; IAS, interatrial septum.

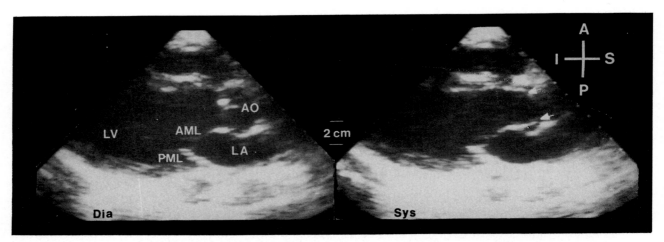

Figure 5-3C. Parasternal long-axis view of a congenital bicuspid aortic valve. Note systolic doming superiorly (cephalad) of the bicuspid valve (arrows).

Aortic Stenosis

Aortic stenosis is of several etiologies, but the most frequent cause in a child or adult is congenital.[2,3,11] Aortic stenosis and regurgitation are progressive valvular lesions that affect the adult, usually after age 30.[6] Unicuspid aortic stenosis is generally a disease of infants and children, but it has also been reported in adults.[11] Rheumatic valvular disease often affects both the aortic and mitral valves, and occasionally the tricuspid valve; thus, isolated aortic valvular disease is uncommon in rheumatic heart disease. For purposes of clarity aortic stenosis is discussed according to the level and type of obstruction (see Table 5-1).

Congenital Aortic Stenosis

Congenital aortic stenosis in young adults is characterized by little, if any, thickening or calcium in the valve. The M-mode echocardiogram can therefore be unusual and, at times, confusing, depending on where the "ice-pick" M-mode beam intersects the aortic valve. The congenitally stenotic aortic valve domes cephalad during systole. If the M-mode beam were to transect the valve near its attachment to the aortic valve ring, the aortic cusp echoes during systole would appear normal and any judgment of severity of aortic obstruction would be erroneous.

Two-dimensional echocardiography provides an important tool in the qualitative assessment of congenital aortic stenosis. In diastole the congenitally stenotic valve demonstrates multiple echoes from a thickened valve cusp (Figure 5-4). During systole the valve is domed, with a limited orifice at its apex. It is this doming of the valve that is the most important two-dimensional criterion for the qualitative diagnosis of aortic valve stenosis (Figures 5-5 and 5-6A, B, C, D).[12,13]

Echocardiography can also provide quantitative assessment of the severity of aortic valve stenosis. M-mode echocardiography has been utilized to quantify peak left ventricular systolic pressure (LVSP) by assuming that peak systolic circumferential wall stress is constant.[14,15] From measurements of left ventricular systolic internal dimension (LVS) and posterior wall thickness ($LVPW_S$), peak left ventricular systolic pressure can be estimated. By subtracting brachial artery systolic pressure (BAP) from

Table 5-1

Aortic Stenosis

Valvular aortic stenosis
 Congenital valvular stenosis
 Rheumatic valvular stenosis
Discrete subaortic stenosis
 Membranous type
 Tubular (tunnel) or fibromuscular type
Idiopathic hypertrophic subaortic stenosis
Supravalvular aortic stenosis
 Membranous type
 Tubular or fibromuscular type
Hypoplastic aorta and aortic atresia

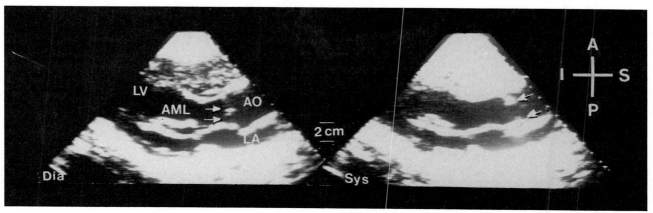

Figure 5-4. Parasternal long-axis view of congenital aortic stenosis. Note multiple echoes from the thickened valve during diastole (arrows). During systole the thickened cusps are seen to dome and the aortic cusp separation (arrows) is slightly reduced (1.4 cm).

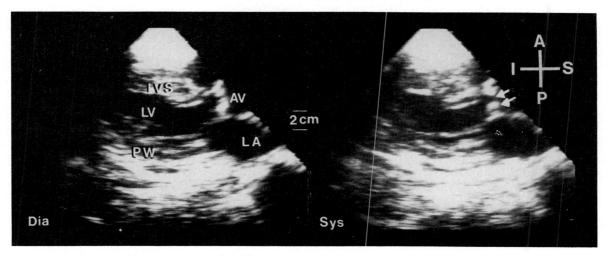

Figure 5-5. Parasternal long-axis view of mild aortic stenosis. Note marked thickening of the aortic cusps during diastole. The aortic cusp separation during systole is reduced (1.2 cm). Note mild concentric hypertrophy of the septum (IVS) and left ventricular posterior wall (PW). AV denotes aortic valve.

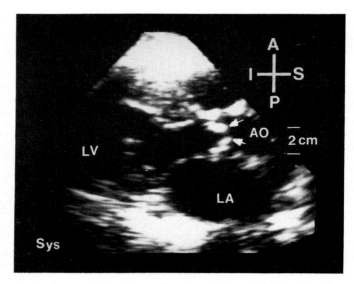

Figure 5-6A. Parasternal long-axis view of moderate aortic stenosis in systole (aortic valve gradient 35 mm Hg). Note marked thickening of the aortic valve cusp and reduced aortic cusp separation (1.0 cm). There is also left atrial enlargement.

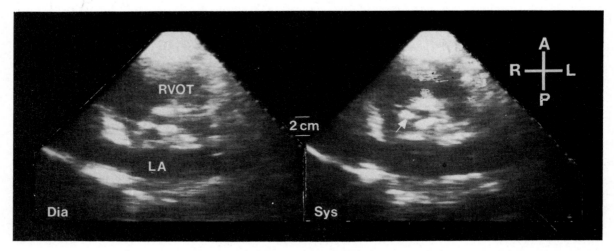

Figure 5-6B. Parasternal short-axis view of moderate aortic stenosis in diastole and systole. Note the thickened cusp and the reduced aortic cusp separation in systole (arrow).

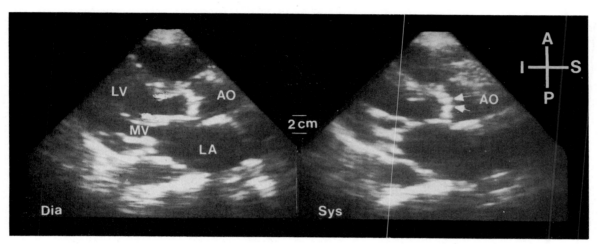

Figure 5-6C. Parasternal long-axis view in severe aortic stenosis (aortic valve gradient 75 mm Hg). Note minimal aortic cusp separation in systole (arrows). MV denotes mitral valve.

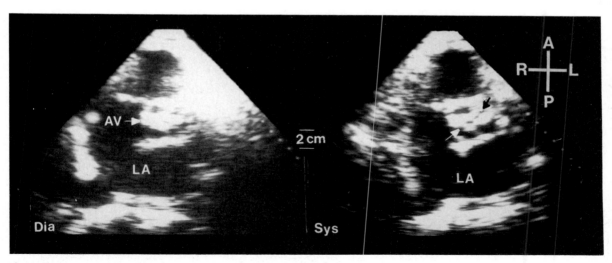

Figure 5-6D. Parasternal short-axis view in same patient as Figure 5-6C with severe aortic stenosis. Note minimal aortic cusp separation during systole (arrows).

left ventricular systolic pressure, the estimated aortic valve systolic pressure gradient can be derived. The formula[14] is as follows:

$$LVSP \text{ (mm Hg)} = \frac{225 \times LVPW_s}{LVS}$$

$$\text{Aortic valve gradient (mm Hg)} = LVSP - BAP$$

This method has been useful in children and young adults who fulfill several prerequisites: (1) aortic valvular insufficiency is trivial, (2) there is no left ventricular failure, and (3) there has been no previous aortic valvuloplasty.[14]

Two-dimensional echocardiography was utilized by Weyman et al[12,13] to estimate the severity of congenital aortic stenosis by noting the maximum aortic leaflet separation in the parasternal long-axis views. In the absence of left ventricular failure, maximum aortic cusp separation (MACS) should have a direct relationship to the severity of aortic stenosis. In normal subjects, the MACS should be nearly equal to the aortic annulus diameter. In aortic stenosis, the ratio of MACS to aortic annulus diameter (AOD) should be markedly reduced (Figure 5-7). In one study, when the MACS to AOD ratio was less than 80 percent, the aortic valve gradient was greater than 20 mm Hg.[10] This ratio is helpful in evaluating congenital aortic stenosis when the cusps are pliable and the orifice is circular. In calcific aortic stenosis, however, the orifice becomes more ellipsoid or oval and the ratio of MACS to AOD is less reliable.

The parasternal short-axis view theoretically should provide a more accurate assessment of the true aortic valve orifice size and shape. During examination in short axis, however, the plane of the valve changes in relation to the transducer. If the transducer beam transects the aortic cusps near their attachments to the annulus, an exaggerated orifice size is obtained. If, on the other hand, the aortic leaflets are transected near the tip of the dome, the true narrowed aortic valve orifice can be measured[13] (Figure 5-6D).

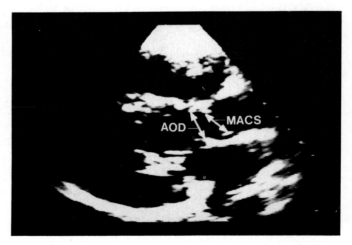

Figure 5-7. Parasternal long-axis view of aortic valve shown to measure maximal aortic cusp separation (MACS) and aortic annulus diameter (AOD) in estimating the severity of aortic stenosis.

Rheumatic Aortic Stenosis

Rheumatic valvular stenosis is difficult to distinguish echocardiographically from congenital stenosis. Nevertheless, frequently three aortic cusps with fusion of the commissures are visualized in the short-axis view. Once thickening and calcium distort the valve, however, it is unlikely that two-dimensional imaging can distinguish between the two types of stenosis.

Discrete Subaortic Stenosis

Discrete subaortic stenosis is of two anatomic types: (1) membranous and (2) diffuse fibromuscular. M-mode echocardiography has been quite useful in differentiating discrete subvalvular from valvular aortic stenosis. In subaortic stenosis the aortic valve shows early- or midsystolic notching with partial closure, followed by coarse fluttering or high-frequency vibration of the cusps (Figure 5-8). Anomalous linear echoes below the aortic valve are occasionally identified.[16–21] In one series aortic valve abnormalities were noted in only half of the patients with subaortic stenosis.[16]

Two-dimensional echocardiography has been more helpful than M-mode in identifying the level of obstruction in discrete subaortic stenosis.[18,22–24] The narrow

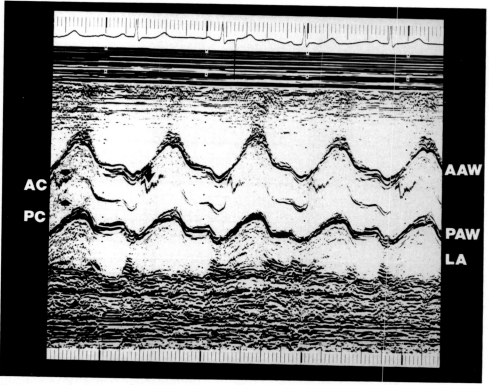

Figure 5-8. M-mode echocardiogram taken at the aorta in a patient with discrete subaortic stenosis. Note early systolic notching, persistent closure, and fluttering of the anterior and posterior aortic cusps (AC and PC). AAW denotes anterior aortic wall; PAW, posterior aortic wall.

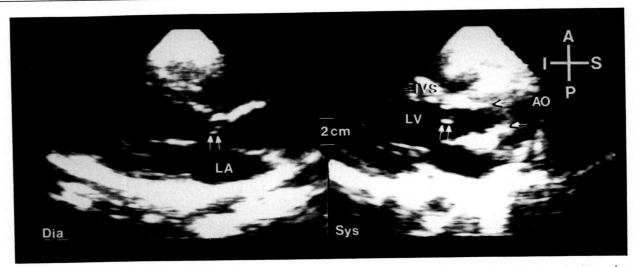

Figure 5-9A. Parasternal long-axis view of congenital discrete subaortic stenosis. Note the discrete linear membrane just below the aortic valve in diastole and systole (vertical arrows). Note also that the discrete membrane interferes with the complete opening of the anterior aortic cusp (top horizontal arrow).

subaortic obstruction can be visualized and the difference between the membranous and diffuse fibromuscular type can be made (Figure 5-9A). In the fibromuscular type, the obstruction is caused by excessive tissue protruding from the junction between the anterior mitral leaflet and the posterior aortic wall. Tissue also protrudes from the interventricular septum, forming a ringlike subaortic obstruction (Figure 5-9B). The entire subvalvular membrane, including its attachment to the walls of the left

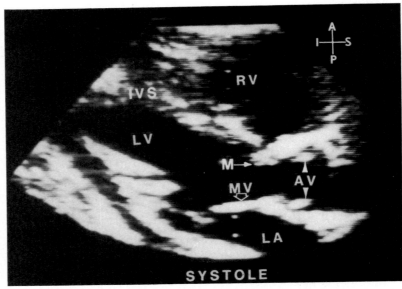

Figure 5-9B. Parasternal long-axis view, discrete membranous subvalvular aortic stenosis. The left ventricular outflow tract is narrowed by the linear echo produced by the membrane (M) beneath the septum.

ventricular outflow tract (Figure 5-9B), can be visualized by two-dimensional echocardiography. Thus the distinction among membranous, fibromuscular, and the more severe tunnel-like subaortic obstruction can be made. In one series two-dimensional echocardiography was found more sensitive than angiography in recognizing and characterizing the morphology of the obstructing subaortic lesion.[18]

Idiopathic Hypertrophic Subaortic Stenosis

Idiopathic hypertrophic subaortic stenosis (IHSS) is discussed in detail in Chapter 10.

Supravalvular Aortic Stenosis

Supravalvular aortic stenosis can be of the membranous or the fibromuscular type. M-mode echocardiography has limited utility in assessing supravalvular aortic stenosis. Slow-speed scanning of the ascending aorta will usually show a normal aortic valve with a narrowed aortic annulus. As the transducer is angulated cephalad, the ascending aorta diminishes in size; thereafter, more cephalad angulation shows a normal ascending aorta. Frequent misangulation of the M-mode beam outside the aorta can give a distorted picture and may mimic supra-aortic stenosis.

Two-dimensional echocardiography provides a more useful tool because of the improved spatial orientation in distinguishing the ascending aorta from the aortic valve and annulus.[25–27] The supravalvular narrowing becomes apparent with cephalad angulation of the transducer from the standard parasternal long-axis view (Figure 5-10). Occasionally, moving the transducer up one intercostal space will allow better imaging of the ascending aorta.

Further examples of the congenital form of aortic stenosis can be found in Chapter 13.

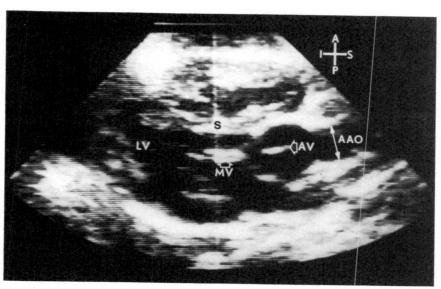

Figure 5-10. Parasternal long-axis view, supravalvular aortic stenosis. The aortic valve (AV) is normal. There is diffuse narrowing of the ascending aorta (AAO) just above the aortic sinus. S denotes interventricular septum.

Hypoplastic Aorta and Aortic Atresia

The more extreme forms of aortic obstruction are hypoplastic aorta and aortic atresia. In these cases two-dimensional echocardiography is far superior to M-mode in distinguishing the size of the aorta. The aortic root is extremely narrowed, and usually an aortic valve cannot be seen in the hypoplastic aorta. In aortic atresia there is hypoplasia of the left ventricle, which is therefore not imaged well.[27]

Aortic Regurgitation

Aortic Valve Prolapse

Prolapse of the aortic valve (Figure 5-11) has recently been described.[28-31] The echocardiographic hallmarks are (1) abnormal diastolic echoes protruding into the left ventricular outflow tract, (2) location of abnormal echoes anterior to the mitral leaflets in diastole, (3) extra left ventricular echoes in the aorta during systole, and (4) diastolic high-frequency fluttering of one or more aortic cusps.[28]

In addition, these patients frequently have a flail or absent aortic cusp, with fluctuation in one or another coronary cusp. The condition is frequently associated with vegetative endocarditis, but other causes include nonvegetative myxomatous changes of the aortic valve[29] and trauma to the aorta. Prolapse of the aortic valve is, however, difficult to distinguish from a vegetation attached to an aortic cusp in the left ventricular outflow tract. Unlike mitral valve prolapse, aortic prolapse commonly is associated with disruption or fenestration of one or more of the aortic cusps.

Flail Aortic Leaflet

Flail aortic leaflet may appear the same anatomically and echocardiographically as aortic valve prolapse. With a flail aortic cusp, diastolic fluttering of echoes can be seen in the left ventricular outflow tract independent of, and anterior to, the anterior mitral leaflet.[33-36] During systole the flail cusp can be seen in the aorta.

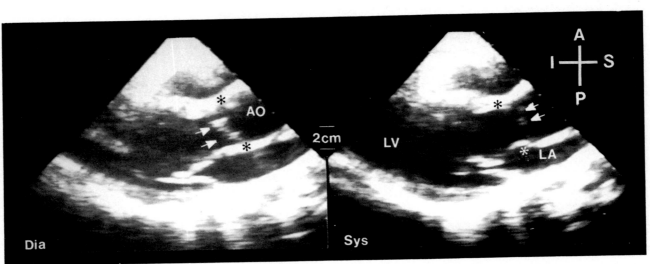

Figure 5-11. Parasternal long-axis view of aortic valve prolapse. Note how in diastole the aortic valve prolapses into the left ventricular outflow tract (arrows). During systole the aortic valve domes superiorly (arrows).

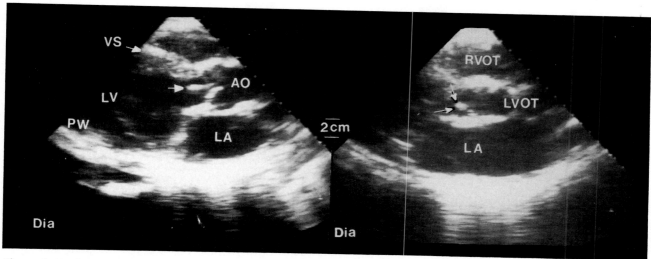

Figure 5-12. Parasternal long-axis view of aortic valve in diastole (left) and short axis-view in diastole (right) of a flail aortic leaflet from aortic valve endocarditis. Note the diastolic echoes (arrow, left), which represent the flail aortic leaflet and vegetation in the left ventricular outflow tract (arrows, right). VS denotes interventricular septum.

Since flail aortic cusps are frequently associated with vegetations, the two may be indistinguishable by two-dimensional echocardiography.[37] The flail cusp and the vegetation are frequently found together in the left ventricular outflow tract (Figure 5-12).

Occasionally a flail aortic cusp occurs in patients with myxomatous changes of the aortic valve. In the myxomatous aortic valve, a ruptured or fenestrated cusp may be present without vegetations.[30,31,33] Abnormal echoes in the left ventricular outflow tract in diastole can also be caused by a ruptured chordae tendineae to the mitral valve. In one reported case, abnormal echoes in the outflow tract were caused by swollen and confluent chordae tendineae disrupted from the anterolateral papillary muscle.[34]

Aortic Regurgitation

The M-mode evaluation can provide direct and indirect clues as to the presence of aortic regurgitation. The direct M-mode findings are those of aortic valve prolapse or flail or fenestrated aortic leaflet; bicuspid aortic valve (see preceding discussion); aortic dissection; sinus of Valsalva rupture; ascending aortic root dilatation; or aortic valve vegetation. The most frequent clues, however, are the indirect findings, which include diastolic fluttering of the anterior and posterior mitral leaflets; diastolic fluttering of the ventricular septum; left ventricular volume overload; and exaggerated septal excursion with midsystolic notching. With severe aortic regurgitation presystolic closure of the mitral valve can be recorded.

Two-dimensional echocardiography can be helpful in differentiating the etiology. However, the direct features of aortic regurgitation are seen only when a flail or prolapsed aortic cusp is present.[38] In congenital aortic stenosis the aortic valve domes cephalad during systole. If regurgitation is present, there is inversion of the aortic cusps into the left ventricular outflow tract during diastole.

Persistent separation of the aortic cusps during diastole (Figure 5-13A) may be a useful sign in aortic regurgitation.[39,40] When the aortic valve was viewed echocardiographically in parasternal long and short axis, persistent diastolic aortic cusp separation of greater than 2 mm was associated in all patients with aortic regurgitation that had been revealed by aortic root angiography (Figures 5-13B, C). This finding appears to be characteristic of chronic aortic regurgitation in which the thickened aortic cusps can be distinguished in diastole. The finding, however, requires careful application of technique in evaluating the aortic cusps. The aortic valve normally moves in and out of the plane of imaging during the cardiac cycle; consequently, to demonstrate this finding, it is important to image the aortic cusps in long and short axis.

The effects of the regurgitant jet on the mitral valve serve as the M-mode marker of this lesion. These oscillations are of such high frequency that at times they are difficult to detect by two-dimensional echocardiography. Diastolic fluttering of the interventricular septum may also occur if the regurgitant aortic jet is directed toward the left side of the septum. This fluttering is due to regurgitation through or near the posterior or noncoronary cusp of the aortic valve.[41] Occasionally diastolic fluttering of the left ventricular free wall may also be detected.

Distortion of the anterior mitral leaflet by the regurgitant jet can alter the E point, or opening of the mitral valve. Incomplete reopening of a portion of the mitral valve occurs in early diastole, resulting in multiple echoes of the anterior mitral leaflet on two-dimensional echocardiography. Severe aortic regurgitation distorts a portion of the mitral valve in diastole where the regurgitant jet impinges on the anterior leaflet (Figure 5-14). In patients with severe aortic regurgitation and elevated end-diastolic pressures, early closure of the mitral valve occurs prior to the onset of ventricular systole.[42]

Attempts to judge the severity of chronic aortic regurgitation have been made by estimates of left ventricular volume from M-mode echocardiographic measurement. These, however, have not been successful.[43] Henry and coworkers[44] have used left ventricular systolic dimensions in aortic regurgitation to predict surgical outcome in patients undergoing aortic valve replacement for chronic aortic regurgitation. In patients in whom the end-systolic dimension was 5.5 cm or greater, the results of valve replacement were poor. This implies that once myocardial slippage occurs to beyond a defined cavity size, surgical improvement is unlikely.

Quantitative estimates of severity of aortic regurgitation have been obtained with pulsed Doppler echocardiography. Ciobanu et al[45] have used Doppler echocardiography to study 27 patients with aortic regurgitation documented by aortography. Doppler echocardiography was utilized to estimate the degree of aortic regurgitation by assessing the distribution of disturbed diastolic flow in the left ventricular outflow tract and body. A disturbed diastolic flow pattern was found in the left ventricular outflow tract in all but one patient—a sensitivity of 96 percent. A significant correlation (r = 0.88) was found between the Doppler and angiographic estimates. However, several factors appear to influence Doppler estimation of aortic regurgitation; they are (1) the direction of the regurgitant jet, i.e., toward the anterior mitral leaflet or toward the septum; (2) interference with mitral valve flow, especially in mitral stenosis; (3) low cardiac output, which influences the degree of regurgitation. (Further evaluations of Doppler echocardiography are presented in Chapter 15.)

Quantitative assessment of aortic regurgitation has also been attempted with radionuclide angiography. By calculating the difference between counts at end-diastole

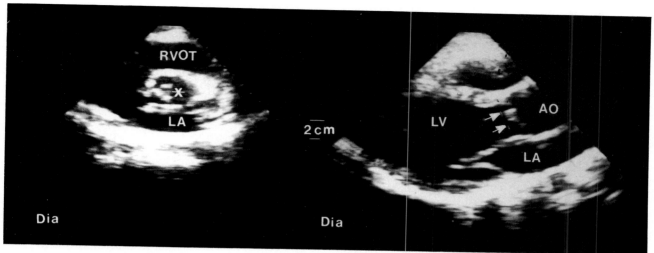

Figure 5-13A. Parasternal short-axis view in diastole (left) and long-axis view in diastole (right) in aortic regurgitation due to a congenitally bicuspid aortic valve. Note persistent diastolic separation of the aortic cusps in short axis (asterisk) and in long axis (arrows).

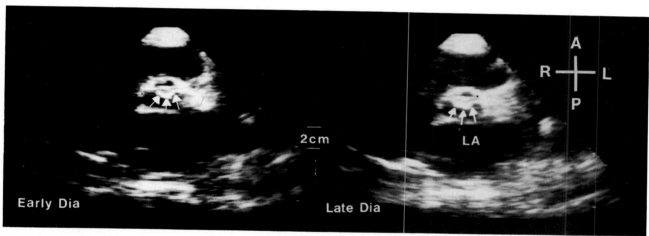

Figure 5-13B. Parasternal short-axis view in aortic regurgitation from a bicuspid aortic valve. Note persistent separation of the aortic cusps in early and late diastole.

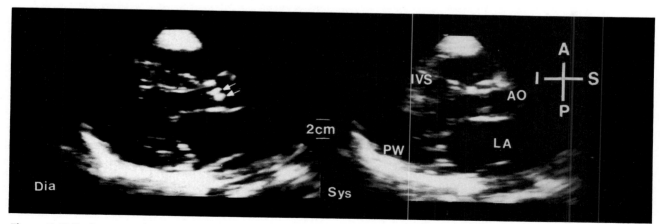

Figure 5-13C. Parasternal long-axis view in rheumatic aortic regurgitation. Note persistent separation of the thickened aortic cusps in diastole (arrows).

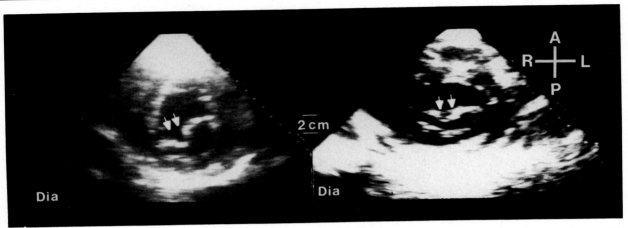

Figure 5-14. Parasternal short-axis view in diastole of the mitral valve in two patients with aortic regurgitation. Note distortion of the medial portion of the anterior mitral leaflet by the regurgitant jet (arrows, left) and of the midportion of the leaflet (arrows, right).

and end-systole in the left ventricle and right ventricle, the regurgitant volume of the left ventricle can be estimated. A correlation coefficient (r = 0.81) has been found.[45] (See also Chapter 17.)

--- **AORTA**

Method of Evaluation

The parasternal long axis is the best position from which to evaluate the ascending aorta. It is also helpful at times to move the transducer one interspace higher from the standard position to better evaluate the second portion of the ascending aorta (Figure 5-15). The transverse aortic arch is better evaluated from the suprasternal

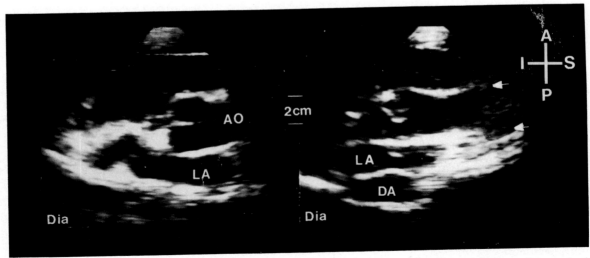

Figure 5-15. Parasternal long-axis view of the normal ascending aorta from the standard interspace (left) and from one interspace above (right). Arrows on the right point to the anterior and posterior walls of the ascending aorta. DA denotes descending aorta.

notch position. From this view the brachiocephalic, left carotid, and left subclavian arteries can be seen originating from the transverse aortic arch. Although the initial portion of the descending aorta can be seen in the suprasternal notch view, it is sometimes better evaluated from the parasternal position. In the parasternal long-axis view, the descending aorta appears as a circular, echo-free structure posterior to the left ventricle and left atrial wall (Figure 5-16A). With slight clockwise rotation of the transducer, the examining plane becomes parallel to the long axis of the descending aorta (Figure 5-16B). Aneurysms of the descending thoracic aorta can be imaged from this position.

Aortic Root Dilatation (Marfan's Syndrome)

Two-dimensional echocardiography has been helpful in detecting both dilatation of the ascending aorta and aortic aneurysm.[47–49] M-mode echocardiography is adequate for measuring transverse aortic root diameter: the normal aortic root diameter should not exceed 4.0 cm at the level of the aortic valve. With Marfan's syndrome

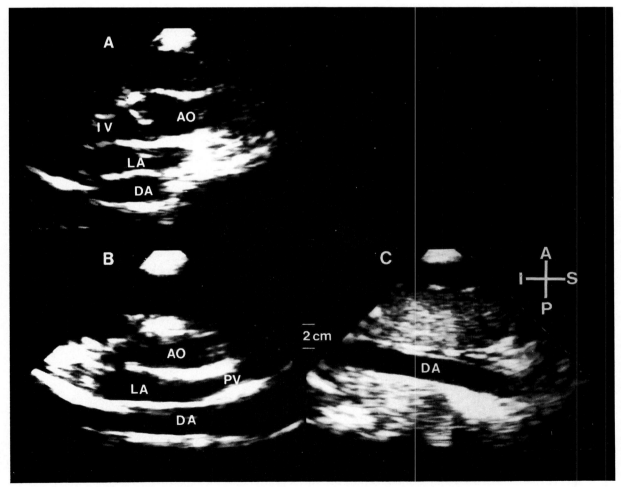

Figure 5-16. A: Normal descending aorta seen from the parasternal long-axis position. B: Oblique view. C: Subxiphoid view. PV denotes pulmonary vein seen entering the left atrium.

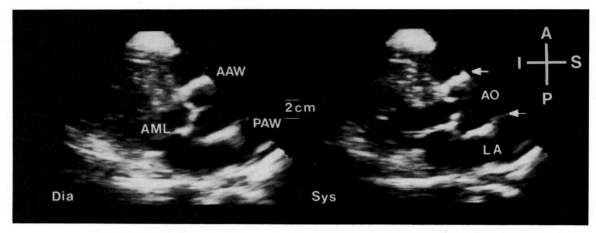

Figure 5-17. Parasternal long-axis view of aortic root dilatation in Marfan's syndrome. Note the annulo-aortic ectasia. The aortic root measures 4.2 cm.

(Figure 5-17) there is annulo-aortic ectasia, with dilatation of the aortic annulus as well as the ascending aorta.[50,51] Occasionally with dilatation of the ascending aorta to the right of the sternum, the aortic root diameter measured at the aortic valve in the standard left parasternal position may be normal. With the transducer held perpendicular to the chest wall in the right parasternal position, aortic root dilatation can be better assessed.[47]

Occasionally, aortic valve notching in early systole has been identified in patients with aortic root dilatation similar to that seen with subaortic stenosis.[48–50] The explanation given is that the dilated aortic root produces eddy-current beyond the aortic annulus that partially precloses the valve in early systole (Figure 5-18).

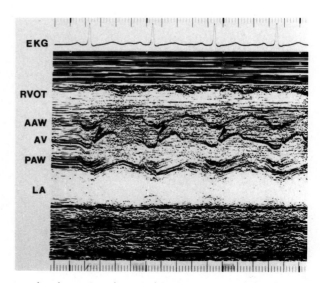

Figure 5-18. M-mode echocardiogram of early aortic valve notching in a patient with a dilated aorta. Note that the valve reopens in systole after early notching.

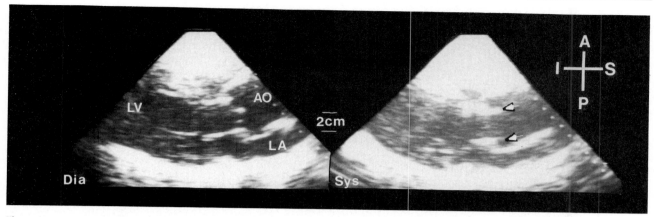

Figure 5-19. Parasternal long-axis view of a patient with aortic root aneurysm. The aorta measures 5.8 cm in diameter. Aortic cusps in systole (arrows) are maximally separated and do not touch the aortic walls during systole.

Ascending Aortic Aneurysm

Aortic aneurysms can be of several types: congenital, dissecting, or traumatic. Congenital aneurysms are seen in children and usually involve the arch or the descending aorta. Aortic dissections may also be of congenital origin but are frequently associated with Marfan's syndrome and cystic medial degeneration. Traumatic aneurysm is usually the result of blunt chest trauma and may involve the ascending, transverse, or descending aorta (Figures 5-19 and 5-20).

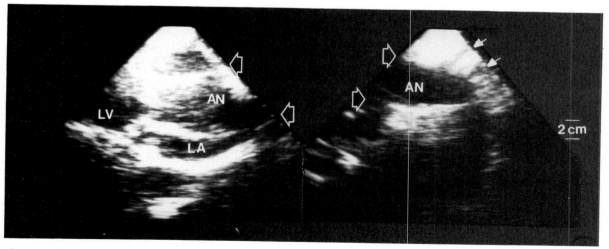

Figure 5-20. Ascending and transverse aortic aneurysms (AN) in the parasternal long-axis (left) and suprasternal (right) views. Note the left common carotid and left subclavian arteries as they originate from the transverse aorta (small arrows). The open arrows mark the margins of the dilated aorta.

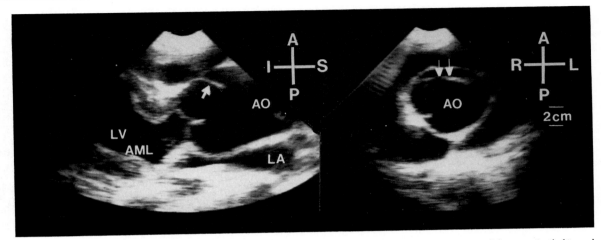

Figure 5-21. Aortic root dissection in Marfan's syndrome in parasternal long-axis (left) and short-axis (right) views. Note the intimal flap in the ascending aorta (single arrow) and the false lumen (double arrows) of the dissection.

Aortic Dissection

In aortic dissection there are duplication of echoes from the aortic wall and aortic root dilatation. The inner echoes represent the confines of the true lumen, whereas the outer echoes represent the confines of the false lumen.[52–55] Whether the reduplicated echoes occur anteriorly or posteriorly depends on the position and extent of the aortic dissection. If the dissection is circumscribed around the entire aortic root, reduplicated echoes will be seen anteriorly and posteriorly[54] (Figure 5-21). Occasionally other conditions mimic aortic dissection, e.g., abscess in the interventricular septum, dilatation of the sinus of Valsalva, false dissecting hematoma, and severe aortic root sclerosis.

Two-dimensional echocardiography has been useful in detecting aortic dissection[56–59] and in preventing false-positive M-mode diagnosis.[59] In a study by DeMaria and associates[58] measurement of the aortic root diameter in patients with aortic aneurysm was more accurate with two-dimensional than with M-mode echocardiography when compared with angiography. The site and nature of the aneurysm is more accurately defined by two-dimensional than by M-mode echocardiography.[56] Thus, two-dimensional echocardiography is generally reliable for detecting and localizing aneurysm of the ascending aorta. It has been very helpful in screening patients with suspected aortic dissection.

Descending Aortic Aneurysm

Two-dimensional echocardiography has been shown to be of value in evaluating aneurysms of the descending thoracic aorta[58] (Figure 5-22). In normal persons the descending aorta is seen as a circular structure in the posterior atrioventricular groove from the standard parasternal long-axis view (see Figure 5-16A). When the left atrium enlarges, the descending aorta is displaced several centimeters superior to the atrioventricular groove. In patients with left ventricular hypertrophy, it is displaced inferiorly behind the left ventricular posterior wall in diastole. In normal subjects the

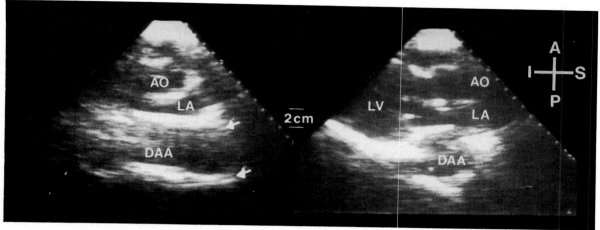

Figure 5-22. Descending thoracic aortic aneurysm (DAA) in parasternal oblique (left) and long-axis (right) views. Note that the descending aortic aneurysm enlarges posterior to the left atrium and inferior to the left ventricle. The aortic aneurysm measures 5.1 cm.

descending aorta measures 10 ± 1.4 mm/M² in diastole. In patients with ischemic heart disease, hypertension, and aortic valve disease, the descending aorta is larger. Descending aortic aneurysm can be seen posterior to the heart in the parasternal long-axis view in Figure 5-22. Occasionally in Type II aortic dissection, the false lumen can be differentiated from the true lumen. In thoracic and abdominal aortic aneurysms, the size of the aorta can be determined and the diagnosis can be made more accurately by ultrasound than by plain radiography.[60]

Sinus of Valsalva Aneurysm

Sinus of Valsalva aneurysms have different and variable echocardiographic features, depending on their location, whether intact or ruptured, and into what structure the rupture occurs. The aneurysm can present as a group of echoes in the left ventricular outflow tract in diastole, moving back into the aorta with systole.[61–63] The aneurysm behaves similarly to a flail or prolapsing aortic cusp; but, unlike the cusp, the walls of the aneurysm are thicker and better defined (Figure 5-23). The sinus of Valsalva aneurysm may dissect into the septum, left ventricle, right ventricle or right atrium.[63] On two-dimensional echocardiography the sinus of Valsalva aneurysm may be seen to protrude into the coronary sinus. If it ruptures into the right side of the heart, a communication can be seen from the coronary sinus to the right side of the heart.[64]

Calcification of Sinotubular Junction

The embryonic tube that forms the ascending aorta joins with the sinus of Valsalva at the sinotubular junction. In the elderly this point becomes prominent and eventually may calcify (Figures 5-24 A and B). On M-mode echocardiograms calcification of the sinotubular junction can be mistaken for aortic dissection or a calcified aortic valve. There is no known clinical complication of this entity.

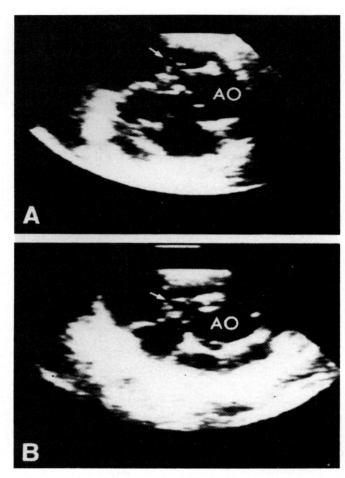

Figure 5-23. Parasternal long-axis (A) and short-axis (B) views in a patient with a ruptured right sinus of Valsalva aneurysm. The ruptured aneurysm is indicated by the arrow. (From Weyman AE: Clinical Application of Cross-Sectional Echocardiography. Philadelphia, Lea & Febiger, 1982. With permission.)

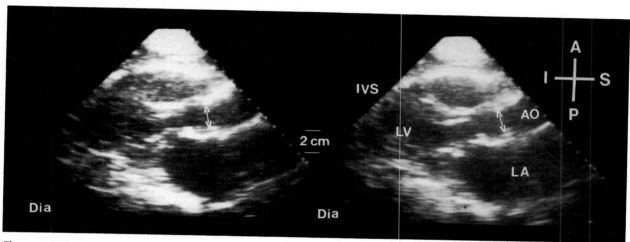

Figure 5-24A. Parasternal long-axis views in diastole of calcification of the sinotubular junction above the aortic valve (arrow). Note left atrial enlargement.

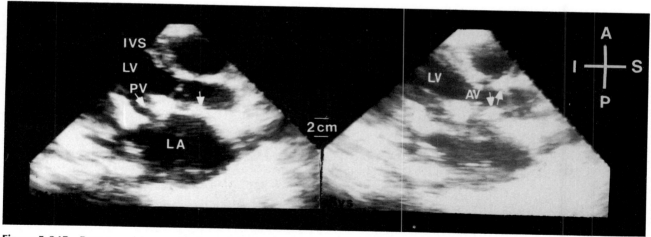

Figure 5-24B. Parasternal long-axis view of the ascending aorta in a patient with a porcine mitral valve (PV). Note heavy calcification of the sinotubular junction (arrows).

REFERENCES

1. Osler W: The biscuspid condition of the aortic valves. Trans Assoc Am Physicians 2:185–192, 1886
2. Roberts WC: The congenitally bicuspid aortic valve. A study of 85 autopsy cases. Am J Cardiol 26:72–83, 1970
3. Fenoglio JJ Jr, McAllister HA Jr, DeCastro CM, et al: Congenital bicuspid aortic valve after age 20. Am J Cardiol 39:164–169, 1977
4. Smith DE, Matthews MB: Aortic valvular stenosis with coarctation of the aorta. With special reference to the development of aortic stenosis upon congenital bicuspid valves. Br Heart J 17:198–206, 1955
5. Bacon APC, Matthews MB: Congenital bicuspid aortic valves and the aetiology of isolated aortic valvular stenosis. Q J Med 28:545–560, 1959
6. Stein PD, Sabbah HN, Pitha JV: Continuing disease process of calcific aortic stenosis. Role of microthrombi and turbulent flow. Am J Cardiol 39:159–163, 1977
7. Schlant RC: Calcific aortic stenosis. Am J Cardiol 27:581–583, 1971
8. Nanda NC, Gramiak R, Manning J, et al: Echocardiographic recognition of the congenital bicuspid aortic valve. Circulation 49:870–875, 1974
9. Radford DJ, Bloom KR, Izukawa T, et al: Echocardiographic assessment of bicuspid aortic valves. Angiographic and pathologic correlates. Circulation 53:80–85, 1976
10. Fowles RE, Martin RP, Abrams JM, et al: Two-dimensional echocardiographic features of bicuspid aortic valve. Chest 75:434–440, 1979
11. Falcone MW, Roberts WC, Morrow AG, et al: Congenital aortic stenosis resulting from a unicommissural valve: Clinical and anatomic features in twenty-one adult patients. Circulation 44:272–280, 1971
12. Weyman AE, Feigenbaum H, Dillon JC, et al: Cross-sectional echocardiography in assessing the severity of valvular aortic stenosis. Circulation 52:828–834, 1975
13. Weyman AE, Feigenbaum H, Hurwitz RA, et al: Cross-sectional echocardiographic assessment of the severity of aortic stenosis in children. Circulation 55:773–778, 1977
14. Schwartz A, Vignola PA, Walker HJ, et al: Echocardiographic estimation of aortic-valve gradient in aortic stenosis. Ann Intern Med 89:329–335, 1978
15. Aziz KU, van Grondelle A, Paul MH, et al: Echocardiographic assessment of the relation between left ventricular wall and cavity dimensions and peak systolic pressure in children with aortic stenosis. Am J Cardiol 40:775–780, 1977
16. Berry TE, Aziz KU, Paul MH: Echocardiographic assessment of discrete subaortic stenosis in childhood. Am J Cardiol 43:957–961, 1979
17. Chandraratna PAN, Cohen LS: Pre- and postoperative echocardiographic features of discrete subaortic stenosis. Cardiology 61:181–188, 1976
18. Wilcox WD, Seward JB, Hagler DJ, et al: Discrete subaortic stenosis: Two-dimensional echocardiographic features with angiographic and surgical correlation. Mayo Clin Proc 55:425–433, 1980
19. Popp RL, Silverman JL, French JW, et al: Echocardiographic findings in discrete subvalvular aortic stenosis. Circulation 49:226–231, 1974
20. Davis RH, Feigenbaum H, Chang S, et al: Echocardiographic manifestations of discrete subaortic stenosis. Am J Cardiol 33:277–280, 1974
21. Popp RL, Silverman JF, French JW, et al: Echocardiographic findings in discrete subvalvular aortic stenosis. Circulation 49:226–231, 1974
22. Chang S: Localization of left ventricular outflow obstruction by cross-sectional echocardiography. Am J Med 60:33–38, 1976
23. Weyman AE, Feigenbaum H, Hurwitz RA, et al: Cross-sectional echocardiography in evaluating patients with discrete subaortic stenosis. Am J Cardiol 37:358–365, 1976
24. Reichek N, Devereux RB, Perloff JK, et al: Echocardiographic assessment of left ventricular outflow obstruction. Cardiovasc Clin 9 (No. 2):85–96, 1978
25. Williams DE, Sahn DJ, Friedman WF: Cross-sectional echocardiographic localization of sites of left ventricular outflow tract obstruction. Am J Cardiol 37:250–255, 1976
26. Ali N, Sheckh M, Mehratra P, et al: Echocardiographic diagnosis of supravalvular aortic stenosis. South Med J 70:759–764, 1977
27. Weyman AE, Caldwell RL, Hurwitz RA, et al: Cross-sectional echocardiographic characterization of aortic obstruction. I. Supravalvular aortic stenosis and aortic hypoplasia. Circulation 57:491, 1978

28. El Shahawy M, Graybeal R, Pepine CJ, et al: Diagnosis of aortic valvular prolapse. Chest 69:411–413, 1976

29. Chandraratna PAN, Samet P, Robinson MJ, et al: Echocardiography of the floppy aortic valve. Circulation 52:959–962, 1975

30. Chandraratna PAN, Robinson MJ, Byrd C, et al: Significance of abnormal echoes in left ventricular outflow tract. Br Heart J 39:381–389, 1977

31. Estevez CN, Dillon JC, Walker PD, et al: Echocardiographic manifestations of aortic cusp rupture in a case of myxomatous degeneration of the aortic valve. Chest 69:685–687, 1976

32. Wray TM: Echocardiographic manifestations of flail aortic valve leaflets in bacterial endocarditis. Circulation 51:832–835, 1975

33. Whipple RL III, Morris DC, Felner JM, et al: Echocardiographic manifestations of flail aortic valve leaflets. JCU 5:417, 1977

34. Van Leeuwen K, Fast JH, Deppenbroek JHM, et al: Abnormal echoes in the left ventricular outflow tract caused by ruptured chordae tendineae of the mitral valve. Chest 81:1, 1982

35. Srivastava TN, Flowers NC: Echocardiographic features of flail aortic valve. Chest 73:90, 1978

36. Shiu MF, Coltart DJ, Braimbridge MV: Echocardiographic findings in prolapsed cusp with vegetation. Br Heart J 41:118, 1979

37. Mardelli TJ, Morganroth J, Naito M, et al: Cross-sectional echocardiographic identification of aortic valve prolapse (Abstract). Circulation 60 (Suppl. II):797, 1979

38. Fujioka T, Ueda K, Ohkawa S, et al: A clinicopathological study of aortic regurgitation with septal fluttering on echocardiogram. J Cardiogr 8:697, 1978

39. Koda J, Nakamura K, Atsuchi Y, et al: Diastolic aortic cusp separation in aortic regurgitation. J Cardiogr 7:163, 1977

40. D'Cruz I, Cohen HC, Prabhu R, et al: Flutter of left ventricular structures in patients with aortic regurgitation, with special reference to patients with associated mitral stenosis. Am Heart J 9:684, 1976

41. Nakao S, Tanaka H, Tahara M, et al: An experimental study on the mechanism of echocardiographic findings in aortic regurgitation: with special reference to the direction of regurgitant jet (Abstract). Circulation 60 (Suppl. II):798, 1979

42. Ambrose JA, Meller J, Teichholz LE, et al: Premature closure of the mitral valve: echocardiographic clue for the diagnosis of aortic dissection. Chest 73:121, 1978

43. Abdulla AM, Frank MJ, Canedo MI, et al: Limitations of echocardiography in the assessment of left ventricular size and function in aortic regurgitation. Circulation 61:148, 1980

44. Henry WL, Bonow RO, Borer JS, et al: Observations on the optimum time for operative intervention for aortic regurgitation. I. Evaluation of the results of aortic valve replacement in symptomatic patients. Circulation 61:471–483, 1980

45. Ciobanu M, Abbasi AS, Allen M, et al: Pulsed Doppler echocardiography in the diagnosis and estimation of severity of aortic insufficiency. Am J Cardiol 49:339–343, 1982

46. Manyari DE, Nolewajka AJ, Kostuk WJ: Quantitative assessment of aortic valvular insufficiency by radionuclide angiography. Chest 81:170–176, 1982

47. D'Cruz IA, Jain DP, Hirsch L, et al: Echocardiographic diagnosis of dilatation of the ascending aorta using right parasternal scanning. Radiology 129:465–469, 1978

48. Atsuchi Y, Nagai Y, Komatsu Y, et al: Echocardiographic manifestations of annulo-aortic ectasia: its "paradoxical" motion of the aorta and premature systolic closure of the aortic valve. Am Heart J 93:428, 1977

49. Tanaka K, Yoshikawa J, Kato H, et al: Echocardiographic assessment of cardiac abnormalities in Marfan's syndrome. Cardiovasc Sound Bull 5:437–442, 1975

50. Atsuchi Y, Nagai Y, Komatsu Y, et al: Echocardiographic manifestations of annulo-aortic ectasia. Cardiovasc Sound Bull 5:653–664, 1975

51. Koiwaya Y, Tomoike H, Tanaka S, et al: UCG findings in annulo-aortic ectasia: comparison with operative findings in two cases. Cardiovasc Sound Bull 5:667–671, 1975

52. Millward DK, Robinson NJ, Craige E: Dissecting aortic aneurysm diagnosed by echocardiography in a patient with rupture of the aneurysm into the right atrium. Am J Cardiol 30:427–432, 1972

53. Moothart RW, Spangler RD, Blount SG Jr: Echocardiography in aortic root dissection and dilatation. Am J Cardiol 36:11–17, 1975

54. Nanda NC, Gramiak R, Shah PM: Diagnosis of aortic root dissection by echocardiography. Circulation 48:506–511, 1973

55. Kasper W, Meinertz T, Kersting F, et al: Diagnosis of dissecting aortic aneurysm with suprasternal echocardiography. Am J Cardiol 42:291–299, 1978

56. Krueger SR, Wilson CS, Weaver WF, et al: Aortic root dissection: Echocardiographic demonstration of torn intimal flap. JCU 4:35–39, 1976

57. Matsumoto M, Matsuo H, Ohara T, et al: Use of kymo-two-dimensional echoaortocardiography for the diagnosis of aortic root dissection and mycotic aneurysm of the aortic root. Ultrasound Med Biol 3:153, 1977

58. DeMaria AN, Bommer W, Neumann A, et al: Identification and localization of aneurysms of the ascending aorta by cross-sectional echocardiography. Circulation 59:755, 1979

59. Matsumoto M, Matsuo H, Ohara T, et al: A two-dimensional echoaortocardiographic approach to dissecting aneurysms of the aorta to prevent false-positive diagnoses. Radiology 127:491, 1978

60. Mintz GS, Kotler MN, Segal BL, et al: Two-dimensional echocardiographic recognition of the descending thoracic aorta. Am J Cardiol 44:232–238, 1979

61. Rothbaum DA, Dillon JC, Chang S, et al: Echocardiographic manifestation of right sinus of Valsalva aneurysm. Circulation 49:768–774, 1974

62. Matsumoto M, Matsuo H, Beppu S, et al: Echocardiographic diagnosis of ruptured aneurysm of sinus of Valsalva: report of two cases. Circulation 53:382–388, 1976

63. DeSa'Neto A, Padnick MB, Desser KB, et al: Right sinus of Valsalva–right atrial fistula secondary to nonpenetrating chest trauma: a case report with description of noninvasive diagnostic features. Circulation 60:205–212, 1979

64. Nishimura K, Hibi N, Kato T, et al: High-speed ultrasonocardiotomography: echographic manifestation of right sinus of Valsalva aneurysm ruptured into the right ventricle. J Cardiogr 6:149–155, 1976

Diseases of the Right Ventricle, Right Atrium, and the Tricuspid and Pulmonic Valves

P. A. N. Chandraratna

The right atrium has received less echocardographic attention and investigative effort than has the normal and abnormal left atrium. Similarly, although a great deal has been written about the determination of left ventricular volumes, ejection fraction, and left ventricular wall motion by two-dimensional echocardiography, relatively little attention has been paid to ascertaining right ventricular function by echocardiography. Despite this lack of focus, determining right ventricular anatomy and function is important in detecting intrinsic right ventricular dysfunction as well as right ventricular hypertrophy and failure secondary to left ventricular failure or mitral valve disease.

RIGHT VENTRICLE

The right ventricular cavity can be divided into a posteriorly and inferiorly positioned right ventricular inflow tract, which contains the tricuspid valve (see Figures 2-2A, B), and an anteriorly and superiorly positioned right ventricular outflow tract, from which the pulmonary artery originates (see Figures 2-3C, D). The wall of the inflow tract is heavily trabeculated, whereas the outflow tract (also called the infundibulum) is sparsely trabeculated. These two tracts are separated by prominent muscular bands called the parietal band, the crista supraventricularis, the septal band, and the moderator band, which form an almost circular orifice that in the normal heart is widely patent. In conditions producing right ventricular hypertrophy, these bands may be markedly thickened. A prominent, hypertrophied moderator band may be mistaken for a right ventricular mass by the uninitiated observer. An example of a prominent moderator band is shown in Figure 6-1.

Because of its irregular shape and its relatively inaccessible intrathoracic position, the right ventricle is difficult to image reliably by M-mode echocardiography. On the other hand, two-dimensional echocardiography is particularly useful in studying the right ventricle because it uses several acoustic windows. With two-dimensional echocardiography the right ventricle can be imaged in the parasternal long- and short-axis views, in the apical four-chamber view, and from the subcostal position.[1-3]

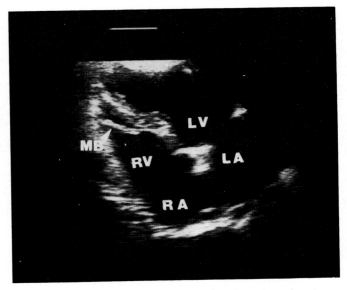

Figure 6-1. Two-dimensional echocardiogram in the apical four-chamber view showing a prominent moderator band (MB). LV denotes left ventricle; RV, right ventricle; RA, right atrium; LA, left atrium.

The ability to visualize the right ventricle from different positions is a distinct advantage because of its irregular shape which makes evaluation of the right ventricle from a single position inadequate. A long-axis view of the right ventricular inflow tract may be obtained by placing the transducer in the parasternal long-axis plane of the left ventricle and rotating the transducer slightly clockwise while tilting it inferomedially[2] (see Figure 2-2D). An excellent image of the right atrium, tricuspid valve, and right ventricle may be obtained from this view. A long-axis view of the right ventricular outflow tract can be recorded by further clockwise rotation and superior tilting of the transducer (see Figure 2-1E). The long-axis views of the right ventricular inflow and outflow tracts are useful in evaluating right atrial and right ventricular enlargement, detecting mass lesions in the right heart, evaluating tricuspid valve abnormalities, and detecting pulmonic valve pathology. Parasternal short-axis views at various levels may also be utilized to image the right atrium, right ventricle, tricuspid valve, right ventricular outflow tract, pulmonary artery, and pulmonic valve (Figures 2-3D, 2-4B, 6-2, and 6-3). Subcostal views are helpful in studying the inferior vena cava, right atrium, interatrial septum, right ventricle, right ventricular outflow tract, and pulmonic valve (see Figure 2-9B).

Right ventricular dilatation may occur (1) in right ventricular volume overload, such as with atrial septal defect or tricuspid regurgitation; (2) in right ventricular pressure overload with failure; (3) in right ventricular infarction; and (4) in dilated cardiomyopathies, involving both left ventricle and right ventricle, or selectively involving the right ventricle. Right ventricular hypertrophy may occur as a consequence of valvular or infundibular pulmonary stenosis, primary or secondary pulmonary hypertension, or in association with hypertrophic cardiomyopathy. Two-dimensional echocardiography is superior to M-mode echocardiography in the detection of right ventricular dilatation. In many instances the cause of right ven-

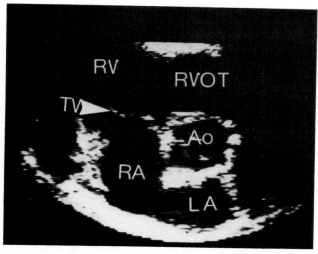

Figure 6-2. Parasternal short-axis view at the level of the aortic root demonstrates a dilated right ventricle and right ventricular outflow tract (RVOT) in a patient with right ventricular infarction. TV denotes tricuspid valve; AO, aortic valve.

tricular dilatation (such as atrial septal defect or tricuspid regurgitation) may be evident from the two-dimensional study. Right ventricular hypertrophy may also be diagnosed by two-dimensional echocardiography. A short-axis view at the level of the aortic root and a short-axis view at the level of the left ventricular papillary muscles from a patient with right ventricular dilatation due to right ventricular infarction are depicted in Figures 6-2 and 6-3, respectively. An apical four-chamber view from a patient with marked dilatation of the right ventricle and right atrium due to an atrial septal defect is presented in Figure 6-4.

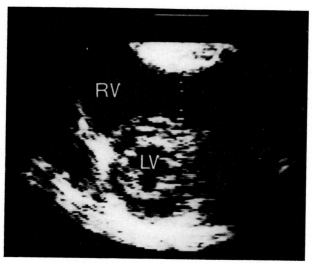

Figure 6-3. Parasternal short-axis view at the level of the left ventricular papillary muscles in a patient with right ventricular infarction, showing a dilated right ventricular cavity.

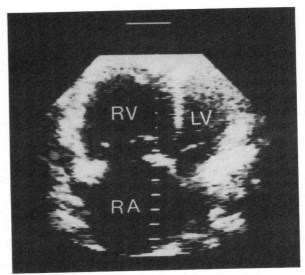

Figure 6-4. Apical four-chamber view from a patient with marked dilatation of the right ventricle and right atrium due to an atrial septal defect. Note that the left ventricle is considerably smaller than the right ventricular cavity.

Right Ventricular Volume and Function

Bommer and associates[4] performed two-dimensional echocardiography on right heart casts obtained at autopsy, noting a good correlation between ultrasound and actual cast dimensions. Echocardiographic dimensions of the long and short axes of the right atrium and right ventricle from right heart casts correlated closely with the volume of these structures as determined by water displacement. In addition, these investigators measured the right atrial and right ventricular long and short axes in the apical four-chamber view in a group of normal patients and in a group of patients with right ventricular volume overload. The mean values for right atrial short-axis and long-axis measurements were significantly higher in the right ventricular volume overload group. The right ventricular area and short-axis dimensions were also greater than normal in the volume overload group (see p. 181).

Using Simpson's rule, Ninomiya and associates[5] correlated right ventricular volumes and ejection fractions determined from two-dimensional echocardiography with those estimated from cineangiography and found an excellent correlation between them, although the correlation between the two methods for right ventricular volume was less striking. Right ventricular volumes calculated from echocardiography were consistently smaller than those estimated from angiography.

Right Ventricular Volume Overload

Dilatation of the right ventricle and paradoxical motion of the interventricular septum are the echocardiographic hallmarks of right ventricular volume overload. The cause of the paradoxical septal motion has been the subject of much debate and has only recently been elucidated.[6–9] Investigations using two-dimensional echocardiography suggest that paradoxical septal motion is the result of an abnormal configuration of the interventricular septum during diastole. Patients with right ventricular volume overload have marked dilatation of the right ventricle with conse-

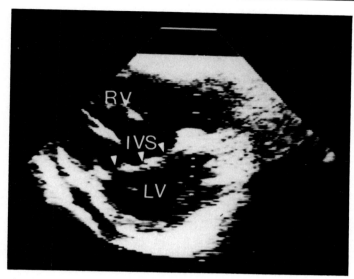

Figure 6-5. Parasternal short-axis diastolic frame of the left and right ventricle in a patient with right ventricular pressure and volume overload. The right ventricle is markedly dilated and is larger than the left ventricle; the interventricular septum bulges (IVS) into the left ventricle.

quent indentation of the interventricular septum toward the left ventricle in diastole. During ventricular systole the indentation is corrected and the septum moves toward the right ventricle, i.e., anteriorly in a paradoxical manner.

Figure 6-5 shows a diastolic frame of a short-axis view of the left and right ventricles in a patient with right ventricular volume and pressure overload. The right ventricle is markedly dilated and is larger than the left ventricle; the interventricular septum

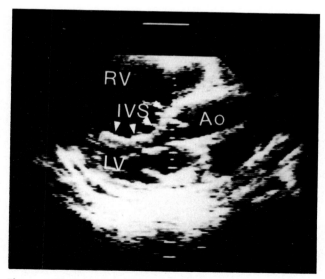

Figure 6-6. Parasternal long-axis view in diastole from the same patient described in Figure 6-5 shows a markedly dilated right ventricle with bulging of the interventricular septum into a much smaller left ventricle. Note that the interventricular septum is concave anteriorly (arrows). AO denotes aorta.

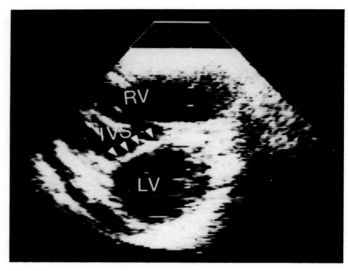

Figure 6-7. Parasternal short-axis view in systole from the patient described in Figures 6-5 and 6-6. Note that the septum has moved anteriorly toward the right ventricular cavity.

bulges into the left ventricle. The parasternal long-axis view (Figure 6-6) on the same patient also illustrates the markedly dilated right ventricle with bulging of the interventricular septum into a much smaller left ventricle in diastole. In systole the interventricular septum (Figures 6-7 and 6-8) moves anteriorly toward the right ventricular cavity, resulting in paradoxical motion of the septum. It should be emphasized that although motion of the interventricular septum is paradoxical, it moves toward the center of the larger cardiac chamber during systole. There is no intrinsic abnormality of the ventricular septum—e.g., in degree of systolic thickening—in

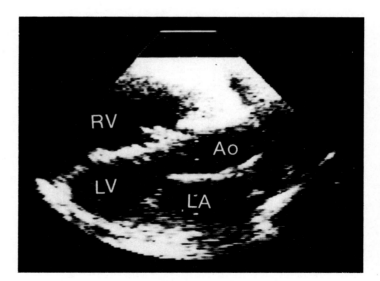

Figure 6-8. Parasternal long-axis view in systole from the patient described in Figures 6-5, 6-6, and 6-7. Note the anterior paradoxical motion of the interventricular septum toward the right ventricle.

right ventricular volume overload. Although two-dimensional echocardiography is probably more sensitive than M-mode in diagnosing right ventricular dilatation, the two techniques may be equally sensitive in detecting paradoxical septal motion.

Right Ventricular Hypertrophy

A small right ventricular cavity and a thickened right ventricular free wall are found in right ventricular hypertrophy. An example of severe right ventricular hypertrophy in a patient with hypertrophic cardiomyopathy is given in Figure 6-9. This patient was found to have an aortic subvalvular gradient. Right ventricular hypertrophy more commonly occurs secondary to pulmonary hypertension or right ventricular outflow tract obstruction caused by congenital valvular or subvalvular pulmonic stenosis. In such cases severe septal hypertrophy may be seen even in the absence of left ventricular disease. Dilatation of the right ventricle usually does not occur except with severe elevation of right ventricular pressure. When right ventricular failure or tricuspid regurgitation occurs, right ventricular dilatation takes place; in some patients both right ventricular dilatation and paradoxical septal motion may be seen.

Intrinsic Disease of the Right Ventricular Muscle

Dilatation of the right ventricle due to intrinsic disease of the right ventricular muscle may occur in patients with right ventricular infarction, Uhl's anomaly, and primary right ventricular cardiomyopathy. We have performed two-dimensional echocardiograms on a few patients with right ventricular infarction. These patients had right ventricular dilatation with a marked decrease in right ventricular wall motion (see Figure 6-3). A similar appearance may be noted in primary right ventricular cardiomyopathy, which has been found to be associated with recurrent ventricular tachycardia.

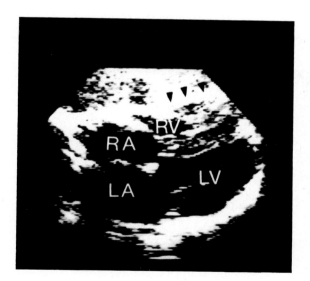

Figure 6-9. Subcostal four-chamber view from a patient with hypertrophic cardiomyopathy. Note the marked thickening of the right ventricular anterior wall (arrows) and the small right ventricular cavity. The arrows point to the anterior surface of the right ventricle.

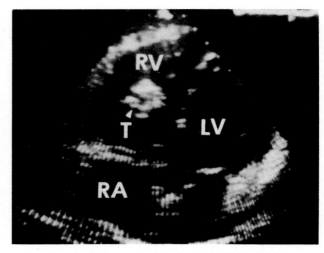

Figure 6-10. Apical four-chamber view demonstrating a myxoma in the right ventricle. Note the dense mass present in the right ventricular cavity. T denotes tumor. (From Chandraratna PAN, Aronow W, Wong D: Echocardiography of intracardiac and extracardiac tumors. Semin Ultrasound 2:143–148, 1981. With permission.)

Right Ventricular Masses

Although M-mode echocardiography is a useful method for diagnosing right ventricular masses, two-dimensional echocardiography provides more information regarding the size, attachment, and motion of such mass lesions. Furthermore, small masses which may be missed by the M-mode technique may sometimes be detected by the two-dimensional method. An echocardiogram from a patient with a right ventricular myxoma is shown in Figure 6-10.[10] Other mass lesions, such as right ventricular thrombi, may also be detected by this technique. A pacemaker or balloon-type catheter in the right ventricle (Figure 6-11) may produce a cluster of echoes which could be confused with a right ventricular mass. However, a right ventricular

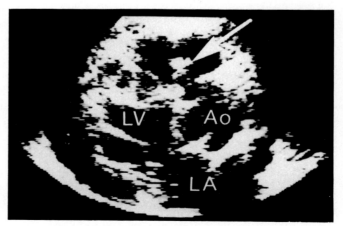

Figure 6-11. Parasternal long-axis view showing a Swan-Ganz catheter (white arrow) in the right ventricular cavity. This dense echo could be mistaken for a right ventricular mass. Ao denotes aortic root.

catheter can be distinguished from a tumor because it produces a dense linear echo which may be seen to traverse the right atrium, the right ventricle, and (in the case of a balloon catheter) the pulmonary artery. A prominent moderator band in a patient with severe right ventricular hypertrophy may produce a dense echo within the right ventricle that may be misinterpreted as a cardiac mass.

RIGHT ATRIUM

The right atrium consists of a posterior smooth-walled portion that receives the superior and inferior venae cavae and an anterior thin-walled trabeculated section. These sections are separated by a ridge of muscle called the crista terminalis. The right atrial appendage is a superior triangular extension of the right atrium. The anterior rim of the ostium to the inferior vena cava has a fold of tissue called the eustachian valve. When very large, this valve has numerous perforations which form a lacelike structure known as the Chiari network. The posteromedial wall of the right atrium is the interatrial septum, the central portion of which is thin and depressed and is known as the fossa ovalis. The right atrium can be visualized from either the apical or the subcostal four-chamber view, the parasternal long-axis view of the right ventricular inflow tract, or the parasternal short-axis view.

The right atrial appendage is usually visualized in the apical four-chamber view as a rounded structure moving to and fro on the lateral border of the right atrium near the atrioventricular junction. It could be misinterpreted as a right atrial mass or tricuspid valve vegetation, especially if the echo beam is slightly off-axis (Figure 6-12).

The distal part of the inferior vena cava and its entrance into the right atrium can be visualized by placing the transducer in the subcostal position. The entrance of the hepatic vein into the inferior vena cava can also be delineated. Extension of a renal tumor into the inferior vena cava and right atrium can be detected by this technique.

Chiari Network

The two-dimensional echocardiographic appearance of the Chiari network has been recently described.[11] This appears as a rapidly moving, long thin echo located in the right atrium which moves in a lateral-to-medial direction across the atrium; it also exhibits a whiplike motion toward and away from the tricuspid valve ring

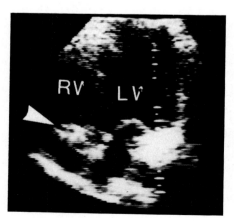

Figure 6-12. A slightly off-axis apical four-chamber view shows a dense oval atrial appendage (white arrow). This atrial appendage could be mistaken for a right atrial mass, especially since the appendage demonstrates vigorous motion during the cardiac cycle.

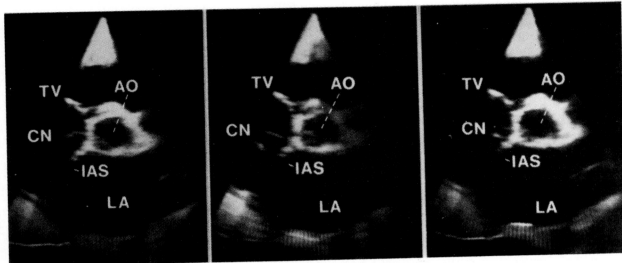

Figure 6-13. Parasternal short-axis view at the level of the aorta. Three stop-frames demonstrate the whiplike mobility of the Chiari network (CN) as well as its separation from the tricuspid valve and interatrial septum (IAS). (From Werner JA, Cheitlin MD, Gross BW, et al: Echocardiographic appearance of the Chiari network: Differentiation from right-heart pathology. Circulation 63:1104–1109, 1981. By permission of the American Heart Association, Inc.)

(Figure 6-13). The most striking motion of this structure is its movement toward the tricuspid valve in early diastole, and its largest excursion is toward the reopening tricuspid leaflets during the atrial systole.[11] The structure moves in and out of the scan plane and appears fixed at the junction of the inferior vena cava and the right atrium. Werner and associates[11] found evidence of a Chiari network in 1.5 percent of patients studied in their echocardiography laboratory. The echocardiographic appearance of the Chiari network may be confused with other echo targets, such as right heart vegetations, ruptured tricuspid valve chordae tendineae, right atrial thrombus, and right heart tumor.

Atrial Septal Configuration

The configuration of the atrial septum may provide useful clues to the relative pressures in the left atrium and right atrium. When the left atrial pressure is elevated (as in mitral stenosis) with normal or mild elevation of right atrial pressure, the interatrial septum bulges toward the right atrium.[12,13] Conversely, when the right atrial pressure is markedly elevated with normal left atrial pressure, the septum bulges convexly into the left atrium. A detailed and elegant analysis of the motion of the atrial septum in normal and diseased hearts was made by Tei and associates.[14,15] They placed the two-dimensional transducer in the third and fourth interspaces at the right sternal border and angulated it posteromedially and superiorly so that the right atrium, interatrial septum, and left atrium were recorded. An M-mode echocardiogram of the interatrial septum was obtained by passing a cursor through the midportion of the septum. They noted that the septum was normally convex toward the right atrium in mid- and late-ventricular systole and in early-ventricular diastole; it was flat or convex toward the left atrium in mid- and end-diastole and in early systole.

Tei and coworkers[14,15] identified abnormalities of atrial septal motion in various disease states. In patients with mitral stenosis the septum bulged toward the right atrium both in systole and in diastole, whereas with acute mitral regurgitation the septum was markedly convex toward the right atrium in end-systole and slightly convex toward the left atrium in diastole, resulting in an accentuated motion of the interatrial septum during the cardiac cycle. Patients with chronic mitral regurgitation had moderate convexity of the septum toward the right atrium in systole; the septum was flat or slightly convex toward the right atrium in diastole. In tricuspid regurgitation the septum was more convex toward the left atrium, or less convex toward the right atrium, in systole than in diastole. Using an animal model these workers demonstrated that the change in configuration of the atrial septum was related to the interatrial pressure gradient during the cardiac cycle.

Atrial Septal Defect

As stated earlier, the atrial septum can be visualized from several transducer positions. Hence, atrial septal defects can be readily detected.[12,13] However, since drop-out of echoes from the region of the fossa ovalis—a particularly thin area of the atrial septum—is a common phenomenon, a great deal of attention should be paid to proper gain settings. The atrial septum should be imaged from several different transducer positions to avoid a misdiagnosis of atrial septal defect. The subcostal view is probably the best projection for diagnosis of atrial septal defect, since the ultrasound beam is perpendicular to the atrial septum in this view.

Echocardiographic contrast studies are of value in confirming the presence of an atrial septal defect. Injection of saline or indocyanine green into a peripheral vein will result in the appearance of microbubbles in the right atrium. If there is a left-to-right shunt at the atrial level, shunting of blood that does not contain microbubbles from the left atrium to the right atrium will result in a negative contrast effect, as shown in Figure 6-14. Since some patients with atrial septal defects who have predominant left-to-right shunts may also have a small right-to-left shunt, micro-

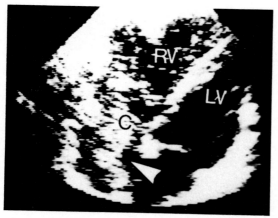

Figure 6-14. Apical four-chamber view recorded during injection of saline into a peripheral vein. Note the dilated right ventricle. A contrast effect (C) is seen in the right atrium and right ventricle and an absence of contrast—i.e., a "negative contrast effect" (white arrow)—is seen due to shunting of non-contrast-containing blood from the left atrium into the right atrium through an atrial septal defect.

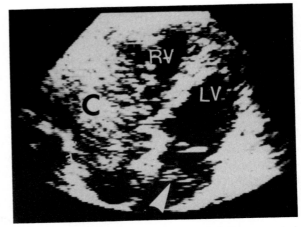

Figure 6-15. Apical four-chamber view from a patient with an atrial septal defect recorded during saline injection into a peripheral vein. Note that the contrast effect (C) is seen in both the right atrium and the right ventricle as well as in the left atrium (white arrow), indicating that there is a small right-to-left shunt. This patient was found to have an atrial septal defect with predominant left-to-right shunt at cardiac catheterization.

bubbles may be seen to cross the atrial septal defect from the right to the left atrium, as shown in Figure 6-15.

Right Atrial Masses

Masses such as right atrial thrombi and right atrial tumors can be reliably diagnosed by two-dimensional echocardiography. This technique is probably superior to M-mode echocardiography in the detection of small right atrial tumors. An example of a right atrial tumor is shown in Figure 6-16.

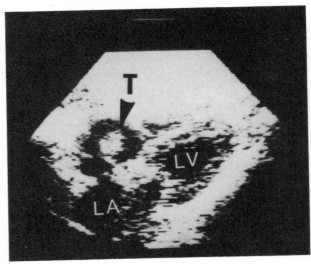

Figure 6-16. Subcostal four-chamber view from a patient with a right atrial myxoma. Note the dense oval echo in the right atrium indicated by a black arrow (T), which represents the myxoma.

TRISCUSPID VALVE

Several two-dimensional echocardiographic projections may be used to visualize the tricuspid valve. Portions of the tricuspid valve may be seen in the parasternal long-axis view, but the tricuspid leaflets are better visualized by rotating the transducer slightly clockwise and angulating it inferomedially so that the right ventricular long-axis view is obtained (see Figures 2-2C, D, and E). A parasternal short-axis view at the level of the aortic root enables excellent visualization of the tricuspid leaflets, as does the apical or subcostal four-chamber view. The normal tricuspid valve has three leaflets which coapt in systole and open widely in diastole. The tricuspid leaflets are attached more caudally than the mitral leaflets; this difference is helpful in distinguishing the two atrioventricular valves. The leaflets are attached to the tricuspid annulus, which can be imaged from the apical four-chamber view and the right ventricular long-axis view. This technique is thus useful in detecting a dilated tricuspid annulus and tricuspid valve prolapse.

Abnormal thickening of the tricuspid valve may be detected by two-dimensional echocardiography. Rheumatic tricuspid valve stenosis is characterized by thickening of the leaflets with restricted leaflet motion and doming of the leaflets in early diastole.[16] Three patients with proved rheumatic tricuspid stenosis have been studied in our laboratory. Although these preliminary observations suggest that tricuspid stenosis may be detected by two-dimensional echocardiography, further studies on a larger number of patients are required to assess the sensitivity and specificity of this technique in detecting tricuspid stenosis. Carcinoid infiltration of the tricuspid valve may also result in marked thickening and restriction of mobility of the valve leaflets[17] (Figure 6-17).

Two-dimensional echocardiography is probably more sensitive than M-mode echocardiography in the detection of tricuspid valve prolapse. In this condition, the leaflets are seen to protrude superior to the tricuspid annulus into the right atrium[18] (Figure 6-18). The apical and subcostal four-chamber views have been found to be particularly useful in making the diagnosis, since the attachment of leaflets to the tricuspid

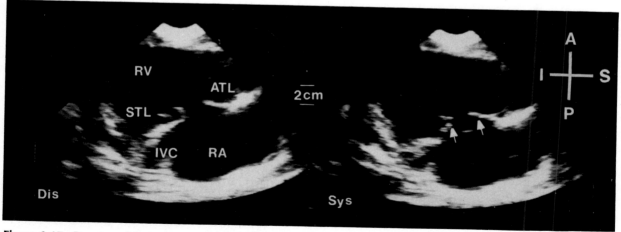

Figure 6-17. Parasternal long-axis view of the tricuspid valve in acquired tricuspid stenosis due to carcinoid infiltration. Note thickening of the anterior tricuspid leaflet (ATL) and septal tricuspid leaflet (STL). The leaflets fail to coapt during systole (arrows), causing severe tricuspid regurgitation. There are right atrial, right ventricular, and inferior vena cava (IVC) enlargement.

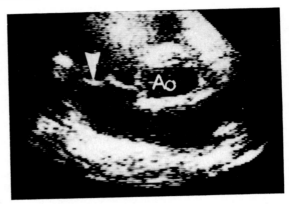

Figure 6-18. Two-dimensional echocardiogram in a modified parasternal short-axis view demonstrating tricuspid valve prolapse.

annulus can be nicely visualized.[19] These patients usually have associated mitral valve prolapse[20] (see Chapter 4).

Ebstein's Anomaly

Two-dimensional echocardiography is very useful in the diagnosis of Ebstein's anomaly of the tricuspid valve.[21] Once the tricuspid annulus is identified, the displacement of one or more of the tricuspid leaflets toward the right ventricular apex can be readily discerned (Figure 6-19). The right atrium is usually markedly dilated and associated abnormalities such as atrial septal defect can be detected. Occasionally, when the displaced tricuspid leaflets are quite small, echocardiographic identification of these rudimentary structures may be difficult.

Tricuspid Valve Vegetations

Two-dimensional echocardiography is superior to M-mode echocardiography in identifying right heart vegetations. A tricuspid valve vegetation appears as a discrete mass attached to the valve; the mass usually moves in a chaotic fashion during the

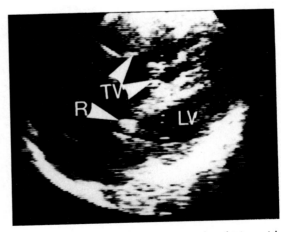

Figure 6-19. Apical four-chamber view from a patient with Ebstein's anomaly of tricuspid valve. Note the displacement of the tricuspid leaflets (TV) into the right ventricular cavity. The level of the tricuspid valve annulus (R) is shown.

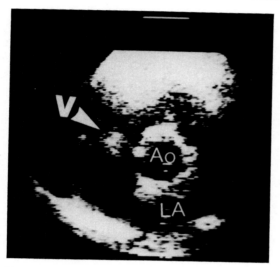

Figure 6-20. Parasternal short-axis view at the level of the aortic root (Ao). Note the dense rounded mass of echoes on the tricuspid valve (arrow) due to a vegetation (V) on the valve.

cardiac cycle (Figure 6-20). The size, attachment, and motion of the vegetation on the tricuspid valve can be accurately assessed by two-dimensional echocardiography. Small vegetations that may not be identified by M-mode echocardiography can be detected by the two-dimensional technique. Furthermore, changes in the size of the vegetation that may result from embolization or, occasionally, following bacteriologic cure can be assessed by the two-dimensional technique.

Tricuspid Regurgitation

Two-dimensional echocardiography has been established as a reliable method for diagnosing tricuspid regurgitation,[22] which is especially important in patients who are scheduled to undergo mitral valve replacement. If significant tricuspid regurgitation is not surgically corrected, such as with tricuspid annuloplasty, considerable difficulty may be encountered in weaning the patient off cardiopulmonary bypass.

Right ventricular dilatation with paradoxical septal motion and right atrial dilatation may be noted on the echocardiogram when significant tricuspid regurgitation is present. The definitive method of diagnosing tricuspid regurgitation is by contrast echocardiography.[22,23] Saline or indocyanine green is injected into an arm vein while the two-dimensional echocardiogram is being recorded. In normal subjects, microcavitations seen in the right atrium rapidly pass into the right ventricle and subsequently clear in a few seconds. When tricuspid regurgitation is present, to-and-fro motion of the microbubbles between the right ventricle and the right atrium is noted, and the contrast effect lasts for a long time (Figure 6-21). Because prolonged persistence of microcavitations in the right heart chambers may also be noted in patients with severe right ventricular dysfunction, identification of microbubbles during systole in the inferior vena cava or hepatic veins after an arm vein injection is crucial to the diagnosis of tricuspid regurgitation (Figure 6-22). The inferior vena cava, hepatic vein, and right atrium are identified by placing the transducer in the subcostal position. By placing an M-mode cursor over the hepatic veins, the appearance of microcavitations can be timed to the QRS complex. Microcavitations seen only after the QRS complex are highly suggestive of tricuspid regurgitation:

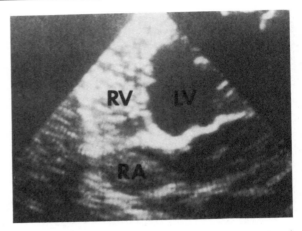

Figure 6-21. Apical four-chamber view recorded during an injection of saline into a peripheral vein, showing a contrast effect in the right atrium and right ventricle. Microcavitations were seen to move back and forth between the right atrium and right ventricle, indicating the presence of tricuspid regurgitation.

contrast appears in the hepatic veins middle and late systole and may spill over into diastole.[22] In the presence of severe right ventricular hypertrophy, a strong right atrial contraction may cause contrast to appear in the inferior vena cava during presystole, corresponding to the "a" wave on the right atrial pressure recording.

Patients with tricuspid regurgitation have larger inferior vena caval (IVC) dimensions than do normal subjects.[22] Because of the overlap between groups, however, the IVC dimension alone is not helpful in making the diagnosis of tricuspid regurgitation. In one study[22] tricuspid regurgitation was present in all patients with an

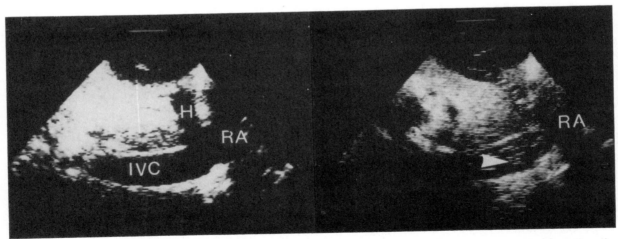

Figure 6-22. Two-dimensional echocardiogram of the inferior vena cava and hepatic vein (H) obtained by placement of the transducer in the subcostal position in a patient with tricuspid regurgitation. A: The inferior vena cava, hepatic vein, and right atrium prior to the peripheral intravenous injection of saline. B: The echocardiogram obtained during the injection of saline into the arm vein. Note the appearance of microcavitations (arrow) in the inferior vena cava and also in the hepatic vein.

IVC dimension (at the onset of QRS complex or at the maximum "v" pulsation) of greater than 24 mm and absent in all patients with an IVC dimension of less than 16 mm. Mintz and associates[24] studied the cyclical variation of IVC size and observed a small presystolic a wave and a systolic v wave affecting IVC dimension. The normal a wave was less than 125 percent and the normal v wave less than 140 percent of end-diastolic IVC dimension. The IVC size correlated with right atrial pressure; a large a wave was indicative of a high right ventricular end-diastolic pressure; a large v wave signified tricuspid insufficiency; lack of respiratory variation in IVC size indicated severe right ventricular dysfunction.

PULMONIC VALVE

The pulmonic valve is best visualized in the parasternal short-axis view at the level of the aortic root. The right atrium, septal tricuspid leaflet, right ventricle, right ventricular outflow tract, pulmonic valve, and main pulmonary artery can be seen in this view (see Figure 2-3D). The right ventricular outflow tract and pulmonic valve may also be imaged from the subcostal view. In many instances only one cusp of the pulmonic valve is visualized. When the pulmonary artery is dilated or in children, however, two of the three cusps may be seen. The cusps of the pulmonic valve open widely in systole and coapt in diastole. In patients with congenital valvular pulmonary stenosis, cusp excursion is diminished and doming of the pulmonic valve in systole is noted (Figure 6-23).

Abnormal echoes within the pulmonic valve cusps may be produced by several conditions. A right ventricular tumor or pulmonic valve vegetation may protrude through the pulmonic valve in systole and give rise to a mass of echoes within the valve. These echoes may disappear in diastole as the tumor or vegetation flops back during right ventricular relaxation. A Swan-Ganz catheter in the pulmonary artery may give rise to a band of echoes within the pulmonic valve that persists in both systole and diastole. Vegetations on the pulmonic valve usually produce a cluster

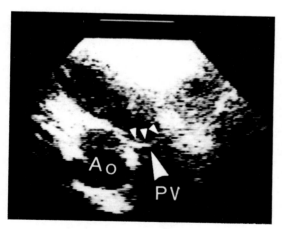

Figure 6-23. Parasternal short-axis view at the level of the aortic valve (Ao) which has been blown up to show the pulmonic valve (multiple small arrows). There is doming of the pulmonic valve (PV) toward the pulmonary artery during systole with diminished cusp excursion, indicating the presence of valvular pulmonic stenosis.

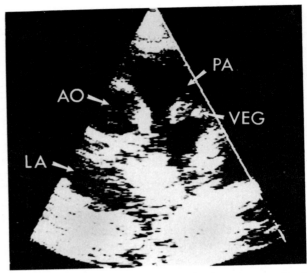

Figure 6-24. Parasternal short-axis view of the pulmonic valve. Vegetation in a young patient with a patent ductus arteriosus. PA denotes pulmonary artery. (From Bianchi HE, Gardin JM, Dixon GH, et al: Pulmonic valve vegetation associated with patent ductus arteriosus. J Ultrasound Med 1:261–263, 1982. With permission.)

of echoes within the valve which demonstrate irregular chaotic motion quite different from that seen with a Swan-Ganz catheter.[25] We have observed one patient with vegetations on the pulmonic valve (Figure 6-24).

The main pulmonary artery and its bifurcation into the right and left pulmonary artery branches may be seen in the short-axis view. Dilatation of the pulmonary artery may be noted in patients with severe pulmonary hypertension. The characteristic M-mode echocardiographic features described for pulmonary hypertension—namely, diminished diastolic a wave, midsystolic notching, and prolonged preejection period with shortened ejection time, cannot be detected by the two-dimensional technique because of its slower sampling rate.[26] Two-dimensional echocardiography has not proved as useful as the M-mode technique in the diagnosis of pulmonary hypertension.

The right pulmonary artery may also be imaged from the suprasternal notch. The diagnosis of branch pulmonary artery stenosis by suprasternal placement of the transducer has been reported.[27] Furthermore, patent ductus arteriosus generally appears as a curvilinear superior, rightward extension of the main pulmonary artery that becomes confluent with the descending aorta posteriorly. Two-dimensional echocardiography has been shown to be useful in imaging and estimating the size of the patent ductus arteriosus in infants and children.[28]

REFERENCES

1. Silverman NH, Schiller NB: Apex echocardiography. A two-dimensional technique for evaluating congenital heart disease. Circulation 57:503–511, 1978
2. Tajik A, Seward J, Hagler D, et al: Two-dimensional real-time ultrasonic imaging of the heart and great vessels. Mayo Clin Proc 53:271–303, 1978

3. Popp RL, Fowles R, Coltart DJ, et al: Cardiac anatomy viewed systematically with two dimensional echocardiography. Chest 75:579–585, 1979
4. Bommer W, Weinert L, Neumann A, et al: Determination of right atrial and right ventricular size by two-dimensional echocardiography. Circulation 60:91–100, 1979
5. Ninomiya K, Duncan WJ, Cook DH, et al: Right ventricular ejection fraction and volumes after Mustard repair: Correlation of two-dimensional echocardiograms and cineangiograms. Am J Cardiol 48:317–324, 1981
6. Weyman AE, Wann LS, Feigenbaum H, et al: Mechanism of abnormal septal motion in patients with right ventricular volume overload: A cross-sectional echocardiographic study. Circulation 54:179–186, 1976
7. Fukui Y, Kato T, Hibi N, et al: Clinical study of atrial septal defect by means of ultrasono-cardiotomography: with special reference to the backward deviation of interventricular septum. J Cardiogr 6:519–526, 1976
8. Tomoda H: Real-time, two-dimensional echocardiographic assessment of interventricular septal performance. J Cardiogr 6:527–534, 1976
9. Kabasawa T, Ohno M, Kamei K, et al: Study of volume and/or pressure overload by real time, two-dimensional echocardiography: Motion of the interventricular septum and motion and shape of the left ventricular cavity. J Cardiogr 8:55–66, 1978
10. Chandraratna PAN, Aronow W, Wong D: Echocardiography of intracardiac and extracardiac tumors. Semin Ultrasound 2:143–148, 1981
11. Werner JA, Cheitlin MD, Gross BW, et al: Echocardiographic appearance of the Chiari Network: Differentiation from right-heart pathology. Circulation 63:1104–1109, 1981
12. Dillon JC, Weyman AE, Feigenbaum H, et al: Cross-sectional echocardiographic examination of the interatrial septum. Circulation 55:115–120, 1977
13. Bierman FZ, Williams RG: Subxyphoid two-dimensional imaging of the interatrial septum in infants and neonates with congenital heart disease. Circulation 60:80–90, 1979
14. Tei C, Tanaka H, Kashina T, et al: Real-time cross-sectional echocardiographic evaluation of the interatrial septum by right atrium—interatrial septum—left atrium direction of ultrasound beam. Circulation 60:539–546, 1979
15. Tei C, Tanaka H, Kashima T, et al: Echocardiographic analysis of interatrial septum. Am J Cardiol 44:472–477, 1979
16. Feigenbaum H: Echocardiography (ed 3). Philadelphia, Lea & Febiger, 1981, p 286
17. Reid CL, Chandraratna PAN, Kawanishi DT, et al: Echocardiographic features of carcinoid heart disease. Am Heart J (in press)
18. Morganroth J, Jones RH, Chen C, et al: Two-dimensional echocardiography in mitral, aortic and tricuspid valve prolapse. Am J Cardiol 46:1164–1177, 1980
19. Inoue D. Katsuma H, Watanabe T, et al: Tricuspid valve prolapse detected by subxyphoid two-dimensional echocardiography. J Cardiogr 9:387–393, 1979
20. Werner JA, Schiller NB, Prasquier R: Occurrence and significance of echocardiographically demonstrated tricuspid valve prolapse. Am Heart J 96:180–186, 1978
21. Ports TA, Silverman NH, Schiller NB: Two-dimensional echocardiographic assessment of Ebstein's anomaly. Circulation 58:336–343, 1978
22. Meltzer R, van Hoogenhuyze D, Serruys P, et al: Diagnosis of tricuspid regurgitation by contrast echocardiography. Circulation 63:1093–1099, 1981
23. Wise N, Myers S, Fraker T, et al: Contrast M-mode ultrasonography of the inferior vena cava. Circulation 63:1100–1103, 1981
24. Mintz GS, Kottler MN, Parry WR, et al: Real-time inferior vena caval ultrasonography: Normal and abnormal findings and its use in assessing right heart function. Circulation 64:1018–1025, 1981
25. Brachi HE, Gardin JM, Dixon GH, et al: Pulmonic valve vegetation associated with patent ductus arteriosis. J Ultrasound Med 1:261–263, 1982
26. Feigenbaum H: Echocardiography (ed 3). Philadelphia, Lea & Febiger, 1981, pp 213–216
27. Tinker DD, Nanda NC, Harris JP, et al: Two-dimensional echocardiographic identification of pulmonary artery branch stenosis. Am J Cardiol 50:814–820, 1982
28. Sahn DJ, Allen HD: Real-time, cross-sectional echocardiographic imaging and measurement of the patent ductus arteriosus in infants and children. Circulation 58:343–354, 1978

CHAPTER 7

Prosthetic Heart Valves

David J. Mehlman

M-MODE ECHOCARDIOGRAPHY

Prosthetic heart valves are subject to many complications, including mechanical malfunction and disruption, infection, thrombosis, and regurgitation. M-mode echocardiography with or without phonocardiography has proved to be a useful non-invasive method to gauge prosthetic valve function. The M-mode echocardiogram, when properly obtained, permits easy determination of prosthetic valve motion and allows for rapid comparison with the electrocardiogram and phonocardiogram.[1] In a retrospective study of patients with surgically proved prosthetic valve malfunction, 70 percent of the patients had a preoperative M-mode echocardiogram or phonocardiogram demonstrating an abnormality in prosthesis function.[2]

There are several problems, however, that the M-mode echocardiographer encounters when evaluating a patient with suspected prosthetic valve malfunction. Since patients with left ventricular dysfunction and prosthetic valve malfunction may have similar symptoms and signs, it is important that left ventricular size and wall motion be fully evaluated. The narrow field of examination provided by M-mode echocardiography, though, is inadequate to permit complete evaluation of left ventricular wall motion (particularly the apical and lateral myocardial segments). Likewise, the narrow imaging field sometimes does not permit adequate examination of the cardiac prosthesis itself. For example, prosthetic valves are best examined when the ultrasound beam is parallel to the predominant axis of prosthesis motion. Thus, with certain mechanical prostheses such as the mitral ball-in-cage and disc-in-cage types, proper examination requires that the transducer be placed at the left ventricular apex. From this position, however, the examiner may have difficulty locating the prosthesis or aligning the ultrasound beam with the axis of prosthesis motion. This is a particular problem in patients with multiple prostheses since each prosthesis must be located, identified, and evaluated separately. Prosthetic valves are composed of very refractile metals and synthetics that often produce numerous extraneous echoes. With M-mode echocardiography, it is difficult to distinguish reverberations from pathological causes of extraneous echoes, such as vegetations or thrombi.

149

TWO-DIMENSIONAL ECHOCARDIOGRAPHY

By providing improved spatial orientation, two-dimensional echocardiography aids in the evaluation of mechanical and tissue prosthetic cardiac valves in each of these situations. First, its wider field of examination permits imaging of the prosthesis from a known vantage point. Second, its wide field of examination enables spatial relationships of the prosthesis to the surrounding heart tissue to be understood. This permits identification of prosthesis valve location and analysis of left ventricular wall motion and may help distinguish artifact from pathologic echoes.

Since the two-dimensional imaging of each prosthesis is related directly to the valve's structure, knowledge of the structure and pattern of motion of each prosthetic valve type will enable the echocardiographer to interpret the image more easily. Each of the commercially available prostheses has a circular sewing ring by which it is attached to the valve annulus. The sewing ring also serves as the physical support for those parts of the prosthesis whose motion allows blood to pass through the prosthesis orifice.

In the case of mechanical prostheses, the mobile portion of the valve may be a ball or a disc. In either case a device is needed to limit ball or disc motion. In the ball-in-cage valve a tall cage limits the excursion of the ball (Figure 7-1a). Several types of disc valves have been in use. If the disc moves parallel to the sewing ring, a flattened cage restricts disc motion (Figure 7-1b). In other disc valves the disc tilts like a one-way swinging door (Figure 7-1c). Another type of tilting disc valve has two hemicircular discs that pivot along a diameter of the sewing ring (Figure 7-1d). In tilting disc valves the device which restricts disc motion is incorporated into or near the sewing ring. The sewing ring of the bioprosthetic or heterograft valve (Figure

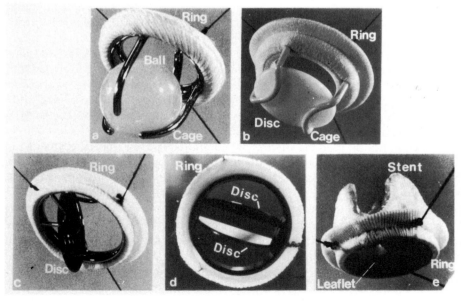

Figure 7-1. Prosthetic valve types. a: Ball-in-cage (Smeloff Cutter; Cutter Biomedical, San Diego, CA). b: Disc-in-cage (Beall Model 104; Surgitool, Pittsburgh, PA). c: Tilting disc (Bjork-Shiley; Shiley Laboratories, Irvine, CA). d: Double tilting disc (St. Jude Medical; St. Paul, MN). e: Bioprosthesis (Edwards xenograft; Edwards Laboratory, Santa Ana, CA).

7-1e) supports a three-part stent that, in turn, supports three valve leaflets fashioned from porcine aortic or bovine pericardial tissue. The stent is large and quite refractile. Each of these mechanical and bioprosthetic heart valves will be discussed in more detail.

Ball-in-Cage Echogram

The two dimensional echogram of the ball-in-cage valve in the atrioventricular position is most easily obtained from the cardiac apex in a modified apical four-chamber or long-axis view. From this position, the sewing ring, ball, and cage can each be identified (Figure 7-2). Ball excursion can be measured directly from the two-dimensional image or from a derived M-mode echocardiogram. With the onset of diastole the ball moves from the sewing ring to the apex of the cage. It may "bounce" on striking the cage apex. With the onset of systole the ball returns to the

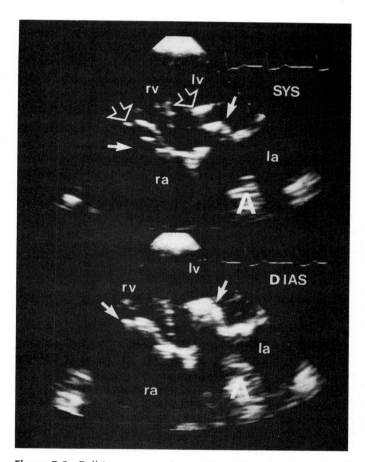

Figure 7-2. Ball-in-cage prostheses (Starr-Edwards; Edwards Laboratory, Santa Ana, CA) in the mitral and tricuspid positions imaged in the apical four-chamber view in systole and diastole. During systole the balls (solid arrows) of the tricuspid and mitral valves are seated in their respective sewing rings, permitting imaging of the prostheses' cages (open arrows). During diastole the ball and cage echoes merge. Note the artifact (A) within the left atrium (1a) that moves concordantly with mitral ball motion. This is a "reverbation" echo from the ball. Label rv indicates right ventricle; ra, right atrium; lv, left ventricle.

sewing ring. Exaggerated rocking of the cage or sewing ring suggests sewing ring (valve) dehiscence. Increased echoes surround the sewing ring and cage apex owing to their highly refractile metal content. As a result, it is frequently difficult to judge whether small clots or vegetations are present. Ball-in-cage valves in the atrioventricular position can also be examined from the parasternal position, but interpretation of the images is difficult since the predominant ball motion is often not parallel to the ultrasound beam.

It is also difficult to obtain two-dimensional images of ball-in-cage valves in the aortic position. When examined with the transducer at the apical, suprasternal, or supraclavicular positions, the cage tends to be lost in the aortic root echoes. Even if the cage cannot be imaged, however, the two-dimensional technique is useful in determining the proper transducer position from which to obtain an appropriate derived M-mode echocardiogram of the aortic ball-in-cage valve. When an M-mode transducer is used alone, it is frequently difficult to obtain an echogram of an aortic prosthesis from the apical or supraclavicular positions.

Disc-in-Cage Echogram

Although the disc-in-cage valve is no longer being implanted, many patients remain with these valves in the mitral position. Like the ball-in-cage prosthesis, this valve is easily imaged with the two-dimensional technique from the apical position (Figure 7-3). The sewing ring, disc and cage can be identified. The motion of the disc is similar to that of the ball described previously. As the disc is much smaller than the ball, its image is smaller as well. The cage of the disc-in-cage valve is also flattened, so that the cage is relatively close to the sewing ring.

As the disc opens and closes the prosthesis orifice, the plane of the disc remains

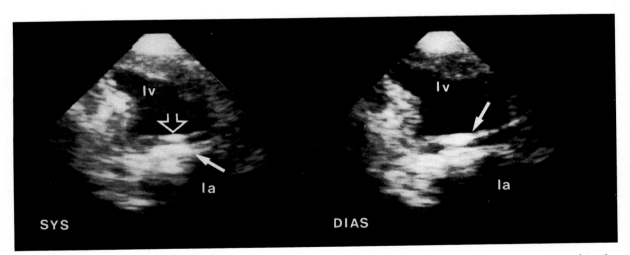

Figure 7-3. Disc-in-cage prosthesis (Beall Model 104) in the mitral position imaged in the apical long-axis view in systole and diastole. During systole the disc (solid arrow) seats on the sewing ring, permitting the cage to be imaged (open arrow). Artifactual echoes (side lobes) appear on either side of the cage. During diastole the disc moves towards the cage, causing the cage echo to become very refractile. The side lobe artifact increases as well. As the disc moves to the cage, the sewing ring image is noted. Reverberations from the sewing ring are noted within the left atrium.

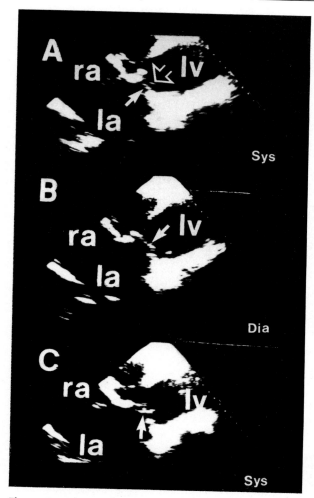

Figure 7-4. Disc-in-cage prosthesis (Beall Model 104) in the mitral position imaged in the apical four-chamber view. In A (systole), the disc (solid arrow) is seated on the sewing ring. The cage (open arrow) is imaged as a fine line. In B (diastole), the disc has moved to the cage. Another systolic frame is shown in C. In this frame, however, the disc (arrow), instead of moving parallel to the disc and sewing ring planes, is seen to be "cocked," with the disc forming a 45° angle with the plane of the sewing ring. This is an example of intermittent disc cocking due to severe disc variance, confirmed at surgery. The solid arrow indicating the disc is drawn perpendicular to the disc.

nearly parallel to the planes of the sewing ring and cage apex. Disc variance (excessive wearing of the disc so that the disc becomes smaller than normal and grooved) may be diagnosed if disc motion is not parallel to the sewing ring (Figure 7-4).

Tilting Disc Echogram

Tilting disc prostheses, mainly the Bjork-Shiley and Lillehei-Kaster valves, are widely used in both aortic and atrioventricular positions. Depending on how the prosthesis is oriented at the time of surgery, meaningful two-dimensional echocar-

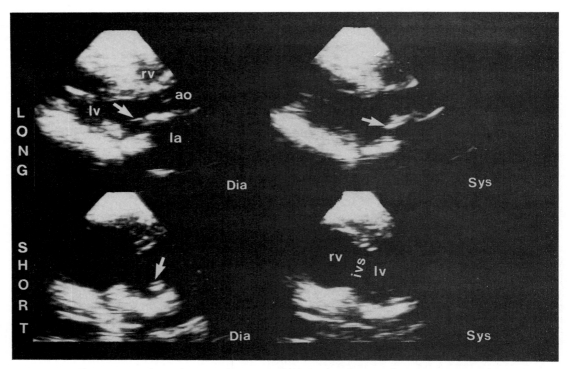

Figure 7-5. Tilting disc prosthesis (Bjork-Shiley) in the mitral position imaged from the parasternal position. In the parasternal long-axis view (top panels), the disc swings open toward the ventricular apex (arrow) during diastole. During systole, the disc (arrow) is seen in the same plane as the sewing ring. In a parasternal short-axis view just below the mitral annulus as the disc opens (diastole) and moves toward the ventricular apex, the disc image (arrow) appears within the left ventricle. No prosthesis is noted during systole. Label ivs indicates interventricular septum; ao, aorta.

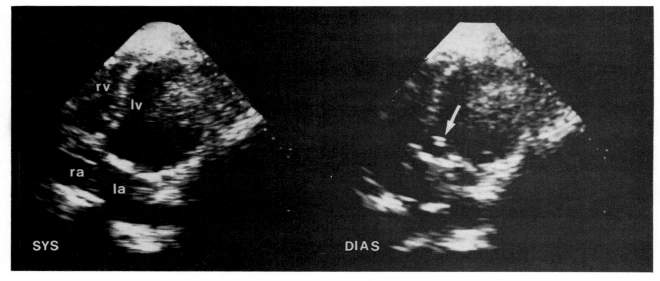

Figure 7-6. Tilting disc prosthesis (Bjork-Shiley) in the mitral position imaged in the apical four-chamber view. During systole the disc and sewing ring echoes merge. During diastole the disc (arrow) swings toward the ventricular apex. The disc excursion is approximately 1 cm. Lung tissue obscures much of the lateral and apical left ventricular wall segments.

diograms may or may not be obtained from the parasternal position (Figure 7-5). In almost all patients this type of prosthesis can be imaged from the ventricular apex (Figure 7-6). The sewing ring is well demonstrated, though only portions of the disc are usually visualized. When open (during systole in the aortic position, during diastole in the mitral position), the disc echo separates from the sewing ring echo. When closed, the disc echo either merges with the sewing ring echo or is seen within the plane of the sewing ring. Of major interest is the motion of the disc and the maximum distance between sewing ring and disc during valve opening (disc excursion). The distance can be measured directly from the two-dimensional echogram (Figure 7-7) or from an M-mode echocardiogram derived from a cursor directed through the disc echo.

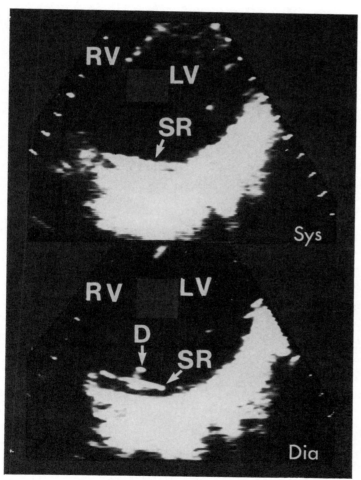

Figure 7-7. Mitral tilting disc prosthesis (Bjork-Shiley) imaged from the apical position. The left ventricle and a small portion of the right ventricle are seen; the atria are truncated in order to view the prosthesis. During systole the disc image is overshadowed by the sewing ring (SR) and not seen. During diastole the disc (D) separates from the sewing ring and moves toward the ventricular apex. The maximal disc excursion (distance from disc to sewing ring) is less than 0.5 cm, suggestive of prosthesis thrombosis, which was confirmed at surgery.

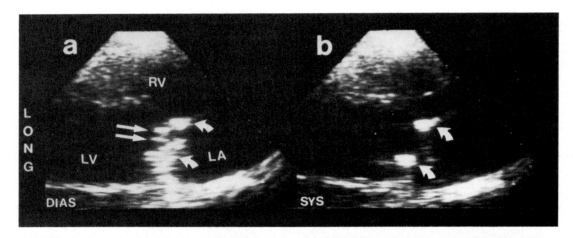

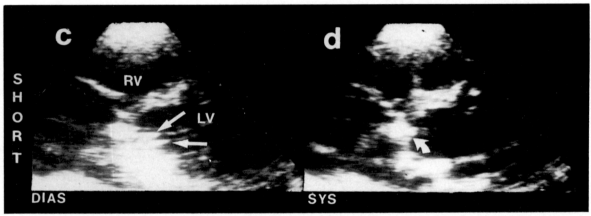

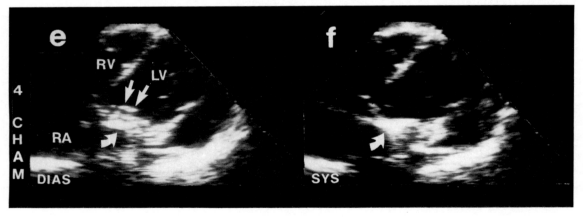

Figure 7-8. Double tilting disc prosthesis (St. Jude Medical) in the mitral position imaged in the parasternal long-axis (a, b), parasternal short-axis (c, d), and apical four-chamber (e, f) views. The curved arrows indicate the sewing ring, the straight arrows indicate the hemicircular discs. During diastole the discs are parallel to one another and perpendicular to the plane of the sewing ring. During systole the discs are not seen well as they merge into the sewing ring plane. Note that in panel e, the two discs appear as a single structure owing to limitations in lateral resolution.

Double Tilting Disc Echogram

The St. Jude prosthesis, composed of two hemicircular tilting discs, produces a unique echocardiogram. When the valve is open, the two discs are perpendicular to the plane of the sewing ring.[3] This can be demonstrated by two-dimensional echocardiograms obtained with the transducer in the apical or left parasternal position (Figure 7-8). The ability to obtain an echogram from a particular position depends upon the orientation of the valve when implanted.[4-6] Thrombosis within 30 days of implantation of the St. Jude mitral valve in the mitral position has been reported.[7]

Bioprosthetic Valve Echogram

Because bioprostheses are composed of three valve leaflets suspended on a stent, the two-dimensional echocardiogram is similar to that obtained from the native aortic valve, regardless of the annulus position in which the bioprosthesis is placed. Useful ultrasound images are obtained from both parasternal long-axis (Figure 7-9) and

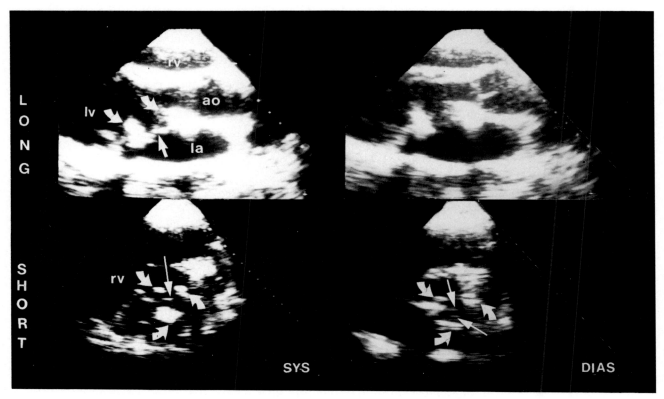

Figure 7-9. Bioprosthesis (Hancock heterograft) in the mitral position imaged in the parasternal long-axis (top panels) and parasternal short-axis (bottom panels) views. The curved arrows indicate the stent; the straight arrows indicate the leaflets. In the long-axis views only two of the three parts of the stent are imaged at a time. In the parasternal short-axis view all three parts of the stent can be imaged at once. In the short-axis view during diastole, the leaflets are seen separated. During systole only the single leaflet coaptation point is seen. The leaflets lie in the plane of the sewing ring on the long-axis view.

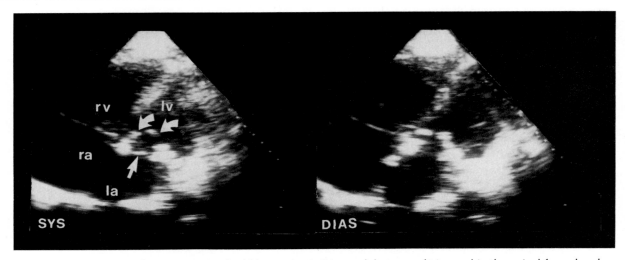

Figure 7-10. A mitral bioprosthesis (Hancock heterograft) imaged in the apical four-chamber view. The curved arrows indicate the stent within the left ventricle, the straight arrow points to the heterograft leaflets. During systole the leaflets are within the sewing ring plane.

apical four-chamber (Figure 7-10) views. The two-dimensional echocardiogram shows the leaflets separated from one another when the valve is open, and the leaflets together when the valve is closed. The three components of the stent and sewing ring are also visualized, though leaflets and stent may be seen best with differing reject and coarse gain settings.[8–10] The leaflets of the normal bioprosthesis are imaged as fine lines. Thickening or calcification of the leaflets causes the leaflets to appear as dense echoes (Figure 7-11). Likewise, flail leaflets may be seen prolapsing into the left atrium[8] in patients with mitral bioprostheses. Exaggerated rocking motion of the entire bioprosthesis suggests valve dehiscence, especially if the sewing ring is seen separated from the valve annulus.[9,11] Minor degrees of prosthesis tilting are common during examination. As the prosthesis tilts, portions of the stent may enter the imaging field transiently, mimicking a vegetation or mass.

Advantages of Two-Dimensional Echocardiography

Two-dimensional echocardiography permits routine imaging of cardiac prostheses from the most useful angle, generally that angle which demonstrates full disc or ball excursion. With M-mode echocardiography, optimal imaging of disc or ball excursion frequently requires an apical transducer position from which it is sometimes difficult to adequately image the prosthesis. For example, in the critically ill patient with prosthesis malfunction shown in Figure 7-7 the disc valve could not be located with M-mode echocardiography alone. Using the two-dimensional technique the prosthesis was located by virtue of its known spatial relationships to the left ventricular walls. Once located, the limitation in disc motion could be observed on the two-dimensional echocardiogram or on a derived M-mode tracing utilizing an adjustable cursor.

The patient whose cardiac prostheses are imaged in Figure 7-2 demonstrates another advantage of two-dimensional echocardiography. With ball-in-cage valves present in both atrioventricular positions, it was easy for the examiner to find a prosthetic valve image with the M-mode technique. It was quite difficult, though,

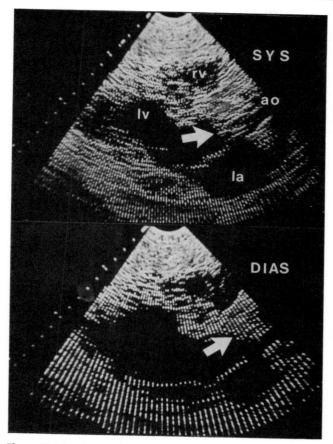

Figure 7-11. Bioprosthesis (Hancock heterograft) in the aortic position (parasternal long-axis view). Dense echoes (arrows) are seen in the aortic root between the stents, suggestive of calcified leaflets. Note that the mitral valve is closed during diastole: This patient had severe aortic insufficiency with early mitral valve closure. At surgery the heterograft leaflets were calcified and immobile; one leaflet had a large perforation.

for the examiner to be certain which valve was being imaged. Again, the spatial relationships of the cardiac structures provided by two-dimensional imaging make the differentiation of the two prostheses simple.

In another example, a patient with three cardiac prostheses (tilting disc aortic prosthesis, tilting disc tricuspid prosthesis, and ball-in-cage mitral prosthesis) had congestive heart failure. Using the M-mode technique from the apical position, only the mitral prosthesis could be adequately imaged. Two-dimensional echocardiography permitted imaging of all three prostheses from the apical position (Figure 7-12). The immobility of the disc of the tricuspid tilting disc valve was apparent from the two-dimensional echocardiogram, as was the normal motion of the other two prostheses.

Left ventricular dysfunction may clinically mimic prosthetic valve dysfunction. In the patient with suspected prosthesis dysfunction, therefore, it is important to examine left ventricular function. Two-dimensional is superior to M-mode echocardiography in the evaluation of left ventricular wall motion, particularly in patients with segmental myocardial disease involving the lateral and apical left ventricular walls.

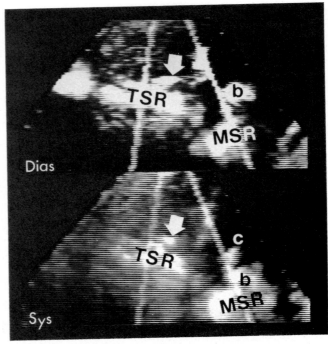

Figure 7-12. Tilting disc prosthesis (Lillehei-Kaster) in the tricuspid position and ball-in-cage prosthesis (Starr-Edwards) in the mitral position (apical four-chamber view). This patient, who also had a Bjork-Shiley aortic valve, had heart failure. With M-mode echocardiography it was not possible to locate each prosthesis. With the two-dimensional technique each pros-thesis could be located and identified. The tricuspid prosthesis sewing ring (TSR) and mitral prosthesis sewing ring (MSR) are indicated. In diastole the ball (b) of the ball-in-cage mitral valve is at the apex of its cage. In systole, the ball returns to its sewing ring seat and the cage (c) is seen. The arrow indicates the disc of the tricuspid prosthesis. Note that in both systole and diastole the disc maintains the same relationship to the tricuspid sewing ring—i.e., the disc is immobile. This echocardiogram shows abnormalities seen with a thrombosed prosthesis partially open. The findings were confirmed at surgery.

Artifacts and Other Confusing Echoes

Periprosthetic valve masses, such as vegetations or thrombi, may occur and in some cases be confused with echoes arising from the prosthesis.[12] There are several technical factors to be considered, however, including damping, side-lobe artifacts, and reverberations.[13] (See Chapter 1.) As prosthetic valves are strong reflectors of ultrasound, their components often appear bright and fuzzy when ultrasonograph instrument settings optimal for viewing surrounding cardiac structures are used. These prominent echoes can be mistaken for small thrombi or vegetations. It is thus necessary to view prostheses with varying reject and gain settings in order to eliminate some of these potentially confusing echoes.

Side-lobe artifacts, principally a problem with phased-array equipment, are fre-quently noted when prosthetic valves are examined. As demonstrated in Figure 7-3, these echoes are seen at the same depth as the structure with which they are associated, and the side lobes move with the structure. They are most prominent if they are not superimposed by more dominant, real echoes.

Reverberations, another source of artifact, are usually (but unfortunately, not al-ways) recorded behind the true cardiac echogram. They are particularly prominent when mechanical (ball-in-cage or disc) prostheses are imaged. The reverberations

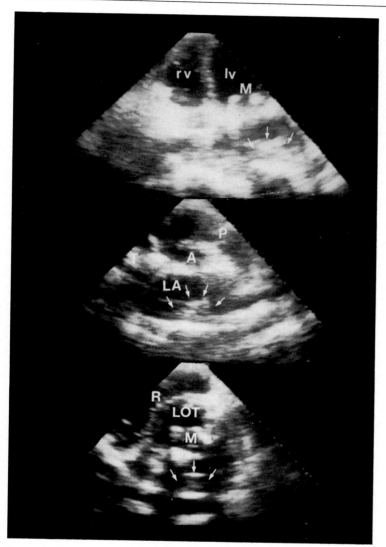

Figure 7-13. Mitral (M) and tricuspid bioprostheses (Hancock heterograft) in the mitral and tricuspid positions with a left atrial mass, presumably thrombus. The mass (arrows), is seen in three different views (top, apical four-chamber; middle, parasternal short-axis at level of aortic (A) annulus; bottom, parasternal short-axis at level of mitral prosthesis). LOT denotes left ventricular outflow tract; R, right ventricle; P, pulmonic valve.

are often large (see Figure 7-2) and move in the same direction as the major echo, although the amplitude of motion may differ.

Refractile prosthesis, side lobe artifact, and reverberation must all be considered in the differential diagnosis when prostheses are examined, as their presence may suggest (or hide) the presence of a thrombus or vegetation. In this regard two-dimensional echocardiography may be advantageous, as it permits examination of the cardiac structures and prosthesis from different angles. For example, if a thrombus is present, its echo image will be seen in the same anatomic area of the heart from any angle (Figure 7-13). If the echoes are related to artifact, the apparent cardiac location of the echoes will change as the structures are imaged from differing chest wall locations.

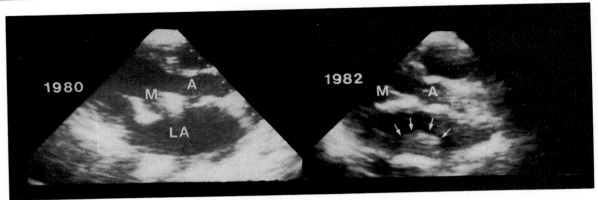

Figure 7-14. Mitral bioprosthesis (Hancock heterograft) imaged in a parasternal long-axis view. The aortic valve (A), mitral prosthesis (M), and left atrium are seen on the left. The image on the right was taken approximately 18 months later. The echo plane is similar; aorta and mitral prosthesis are again seen. Within the left atrium, a mass, presumably clot (small arrows), has appeared.

A small paraprosthetic thrombus or vegetation not affecting disc, ball or leaflet motion is likely to be overlooked, as the increased echoes from the sewing ring or stent are difficult to separate from small masses. Large thrombi or vegetations, however, should be echocardiographically apparent. A previous echocardiogram showing the same prosthesis without the echoes thought to represent the mass, makes the apparent mass even more likely to be real (Figure 7-14). Consequently, baseline postoperative two-dimensional echocardiograms can be helpful in the management of the patient with a prosthetic heart valve.

SUMMARY

Two-dimensional echocardiography has been demonstrated to be useful in the evaluation of porcine heterograft valves, adding important information to the M-mode study. Whether the same is true of mechanical prostheses is at present uncertain. In a study of 36 consecutive patients with prosthesis malfunction confirmed by visual inspection at surgery or at postmortem examination, two-dimensional echocardiography alone recognized dysfunction in only 6 of 23 abnormal mechanical prostheses and in only 2 of 4 abnormal tissue prostheses.[14] Two-dimensional and M-mode echocardiography appear to be complementary procedures in the evaluation of cardiac prostheses, as the two-dimensional technique permits determination of the optimal transducer angle for the M-mode study and also permits evaluation of left ventricular wall motion. The M-mode format, however, permits easy evaluation of the phonocardiogram, which is a useful tool in the assessment of mechanical valves. In addition, measurements of leaflet motion or "poppet" motion are also easier from an M-mode echocardiogram.

REFERENCES

1. Mehlman DJ: Ultrasonic visualization of prosthetic heart valves. Semin Ultrasound 2:134–142, 1981
2. Cunha CLP, Giuliani ER, Callahan JA, et al: Echophonocardiographic findings in patients with prosthetic valve malfunction. Mayo Clin Proc 55:231–242, 1980

3. Tri TB, Schatz RA, Watson TD, et al: Echocardiographic evaluation of the St. Jude Medical prosthetic valve. Chest 80:278–284, 1981

4. Feldman HJ, Gray RJ, Chaux A, et al: Noninvasive in vivo and in vitro study of the St. Jude mitral valve prosthesis. Evaluation using two-dimensional and M-mode echocardiography, phonocardiography and cinefluoroscopy. Am J Cardiol 49:1101–1109, 1982

5. Tri TB, Schatz RA, Watson TD, et al: Echocardiographic evaluation of the St. Jude medical prosthetic valve. Chest 80:278–283, 1981

6. DePace NL, Kotler MN, Mintz GS, et al: Echocardiographic and phonocardiographic assessment of the St. Jude cardiac valve prosthesis. Chest 80:272–277, 1981

7. Commerford PJ, Lloyd EA, De Nobrega JA: Thrombosis of St. Jude medical cardiac valve in the mitral position. Chest 80:326–327, 1981

8. Alam M, Madrazo AC, Magilligan DJ, et al: M-mode and two-dimensional echocardiographic features of porcine valve dysfunction. Am J Cardiol 43:502–509, 1979

9. Schapira JN, Martin RP, Fowles RE, et al: Two-dimensional echocardiographic assessment of patients with bioprosthetic valves. Am J Cardiol 43:510–519, 1979

10. Martin RP, French JW, Popp RL: Clinical utility of two-dimensional echocardiography in patients with bioprosthetic valves, in Vogel JHK (ed): Current Concepts in Clinical Cardiology. Basel, Karger, 1980. Adv Cardiol 27:294–304, 1980

11. Mehta A, Kessler KM, Tamer D, et al: Two-dimensional echographic observations in major detachment of a prosthetic aortic valve. Chest 101:231–233, 1981

12. Mikell FL, Asinger RW, Rourke T, et al: Two-dimensional echocardiographic demonstration of left atrial thrombi in patients with prosthetic mitral valves. Circulation 60:183–190, 1979

13. Gilbert BW, Rakowski H: 2-D echo and LA thrombi. Circulation 61:667–668, 1980

14. Miller FA, Tajik AJ, Seward JB, et al: Prosthetic valve dysfunction: two-dimensional echocardiographic assessment. Circulation 64(Suppl IV):315, 1981

CHAPTER 8

Ventricular Volume and Function

Edward D. Folland and Alfred F. Parisi

Ventricular function can be described in terms of global *pump performance* and *regional muscle function*. The two are obviously related, as pump performance is the end-product of regional function; nevertheless, it is possible to preserve nearly normal overall pump performance in the presence of isolated regional wall dysfunction. It is thus necessary to analyze both in order to characterize ventricular function adequately. Two-dimensional echocardiography is well suited for both analyses because it can accurately resolve endocardial and epicardial targets of both ventricles in multiple planes. The challenge for clinical application of this technique is twofold: first, to refine technically the process of imaging and display so that reliable data can be obtained from a majority of subjects; and second, to create accurate, reproducible formulas to interpret the data and make them meaningful to the clinician. The current state of the art of echocardiography enables formation of left ventricular images that are useful for analytic purposes in about 70 percent of adults and nearly all children. Although further refinement of image quality is both desirable and possible, the present state of development has been sufficient to stimulate a great deal of basic and clinical research in quantitative image analysis. This research forms the foundation for this chapter, which deals with various approaches to quantitation of ventricular pump performance and regional function using two-dimensional echocardiography.

VENTRICULAR PUMP PERFORMANCE

Virtually all indices of left ventricular pump performance have been derived from measurements of volume and pressure. Traditionally this has required cardiac catheterization and left ventriculography. The indices derived from volume measurements have proven to be of greatest clinical value.[1] End-diastolic volume is useful in the evaluation and followup of patients with left ventricular volume overloading

Supported in part by the Medical Research Service of the United States Veterans Administration.

lesions (such as aortic and mitral regurgitation) or myocardial disease (such as primary, ischemic, and secondary). In both of these disease processes, effective stroke volume delivered to the systemic circulation is initially reduced. In the case of left ventricular volume overload, the total stroke volume actually delivered to the circulation is reduced by the regurgitant volume; in myocardial disease the total left ventricular stroke volume is directly diminished by reduced myocardial contractility. As a compensatory mechanism, the left ventricle dilates to maintain an effective stroke volume and hence cardiac output. In general, end-diastolic volume increases in direct proportion to the severity of the underlying lesion and for that reason is a useful clinical tool.

End-systolic volume depends on both the end-diastolic volume and myocardial contractility. Thus it is often ambiguous as an isolated measurement. When both end-diastolic and end-systolic volumes (EDV and ESV) are measured, however, total left ventricular stroke volume (SV) can be estimated:

$$SV_{(cc)} = EDV_{(cc)} - ESV_{(cc)} \tag{1}$$

In the absence of valvular regurgitation, effective cardiac output (CO) can be estimated from stroke volume and heart rate (HR):

$$CO_{cc/min} = HR_{beats/min} \times SV \tag{2}$$

Once both end-diastolic volume and end-systolic volume have been measured, the ejection fraction (EF) can be calculated as the ratio of stroke volume to end-diastolic volume:

$$EF\% = \frac{SV}{EDV} \times 100\% \tag{3}$$

The ejection fraction is a particularly useful index of left ventricular function because it has been shown to be the best single predictor of prognosis in both coronary and valvular heart disease, whether treated medically[2,3] or surgically.[4,5]

Models for Volume Determination

Angiographic estimates of left ventricular volume are usually based on the assumption that the left ventricle approximates the geometry of an ellipsoid—i.e., a three-dimensional figure created by rotating an ellipse on its long axis (Figure 8-1). The volume of such a figure can be calculated if the lengths of its three hemiaxes, a, b, and c, are known:

$$Volume = \frac{4}{3}\pi a \times b \times c \tag{4}$$

In the earliest application of this model, measurements of the hemiaxes were estimated directly from angiographic anteroposterior and lateral projections of the left ventricle. Dodge and coworkers,[6] in comparing angiographic volume with the true volume of barium-filled left ventricles from fresh autopsy hearts, found that accuracy was enhanced if the minor axes were derived arithmetically from idealized ellipses of the same area and length as the two respective angiographic projections. The area of an ellipse is the product of π and its two hemiaxes. Thus, if c is the major hemiaxis, a the minor hemiaxis in the anteroposterior plane, b the minor hemiaxis

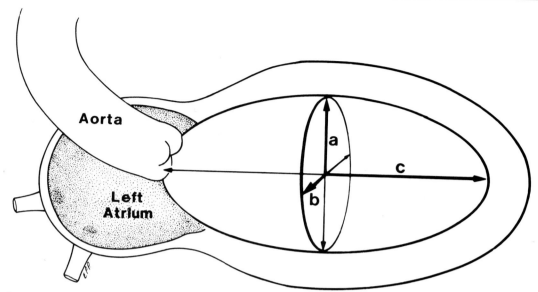

Figure 8-1. The ellipsoid model for left ventricular volume. This model is commonly employed for estimating left ventricular volume from both angiographic and echocardiographic images. The minor hemiaxes, a and b, can be either directly measured from appropriate views or derived from the respective area and largest length of the appropriate views.

in the lateral plane, and A_{AP} and A_{lat} the respective measured angiographic areas, the minor hemiaxes can be expressed as follows:

$$a = \frac{A_{AP}}{\pi c} \qquad (5)$$

$$b = \frac{A_{lat}}{\pi c} \qquad (6)$$

Then, by substitution in equation (4), volume can be calcuated as follows:

$$\text{Volume} = \frac{4}{3}\pi \times \frac{A_{AP}}{\pi c} \times \frac{A_{lat}}{\pi c} \times c \qquad (7)$$

which can be simplified to:

$$\text{Volume} = \frac{4\,A_{AP}A_{lat}}{3\pi c} \qquad (8)$$

This formula is commonly referred to as the *biplane area–length volume model.* In applications where angiography is performed only in a single plane, the formula is simplified by assuming that both minor hemiaxes (a and b) are equal. Thus volume can be derived from the length and area of the single ventricular silhouette:

$$\text{Volume} = \frac{4A^2}{3\pi c} \qquad (9)$$

This is commonly referred to as the *single plane area–length volume model.*

An alternative approach to determining left ventricular volume employs the concept of *Simpson's rule* whereby the volume of a solid may be estimated by first

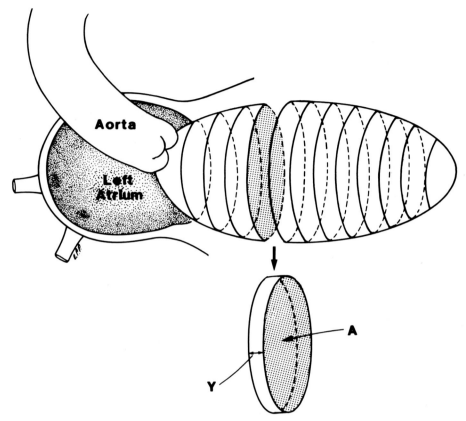

Figure 8-2. Diagram of the Simpson's rule model for left ventricular volume with the left ventricle sliced perpendicular to the long axis. The volume of the total left ventricle is the sum of volumes of individual slices, each with known thickness (y) and area (A).

subdividing along one axis into a series of slices each with a finite thickness and measurable area and then determining the volume of that slice. The volume of each slice is simply the product of its area and thickness; the volume of the complete solid is the sum of volumes of all its slices. The greater the number of slices, the greater is the accuracy of the volume determination. With Simpson's rule, the left ventricle can be envisioned as a series of slices from the base to the apex—analogous to a stack of coins with uniform thickness but variable area (Figure 8-2). Determining volume by this method using Dodge's barium filled hearts[6] proved to be slightly less accurate than the area–length method. Although Simpson's rule is theoretically attractive, it is cumbersome and laborious to apply and has not gained wide acceptance among clinical angiographers.

Two-Dimensional Echocardiographic Measurements of Left Ventricular Volume

Image formation in angiography and ultrasound is fundamentally different. Angiographic images are silhouettes or shadows, whereas ultrasound images are tomographic slices. Nevertheless, there is ample evidence that left ventricular dimensions measured from the two techniques correlate well provided that the ultrasound section is properly oriented. Figure 8-3 shows a plot of 100 corresponding linear measurements from right anterior oblique angiograms and two-dimensional echocardiograms performed in our laboratory.[8] The echocardiographic long axis (using the apical four-chamber view) was measured from the midpoint of the mitral valve to the apex and the short axis (using a parasternal short-axis view at mitral valve level) was measured at the tips of the mitral valve leaflets perpendicular to the long axis. Echocardiographic and angiographic measurements were made at end-diastole and end-systole for a total of four measurements per technique in each patient. The plot shows excellent agreement (r = 0.92, SEE (standard error of the estimate) = 0.97 cm); however, the echocardiographic measurements consistently tended to underestimate the angiographic measurements, which is not surprising in view of the differences in projection in the respective techniques. An x-ray silhouette displays the ventricle at its largest area perpendicular to the x-ray beam. The analogous ultrasound slice very likely may be smaller unless it is perfectly oriented through the central axis of the ventricle. Angiographic images are ordinarily traced at the outermost boundary of contrast which tends to include trabeculae within the cavity profile. Echocardiographic images are traced along the innermost edge of endocardial echoes, which would tend to exclude trabeculae from the cavity. Despite these differences the correlation in measurement between the two techniques is good enough that formulae for angiographic volume should apply equally well to echocardiographic volume determination.

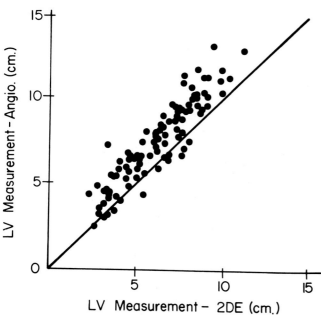

Figure 8-3. Correlation of 100 analogous measurements of left ventricular dimensions made from angiograms (Angio) and echocardiograms (2DE) in 25 patients. The short axis from parasternal view at mitral valve level and long axis from apical four-chamber view were measured at end-diastole and end-systole and compared to analogous measurements from the right anterior oblique angiogram (r = 0.92, SEE = 0.97). (From Moynihan PF, Parisi AF, Folland ED, et al: A system for quantitative evaluation of left ventricular function with two-dimensional ultrasonography. Med Instrum 14:113, 1980. With permission.)

The earliest attempt at estimating left ventricular volumes from echocardiography utilized left ventricular short-axis dimensions from M-mode echocardiograms. This method employed the single plane area–length volume formula, which required several assumptions: (1) that the left ventricular dimension in the standard position at the level of the chordae tendineae coincides with the minor axis of the left ventricle, (2) that both minor axes are equal in length, and (3) that the long axis is twice the length of the minor axis. This approach is commonly referred to as the "cube method" for left ventricular volume determination.[9] If D represents the dimension (at end-diastole or end-systole), then volume can be estimated as follows:

$$\text{Volume} = \frac{4}{3} \pi \times \frac{D}{2} \times \frac{D}{2} \times D \qquad (10)$$

which simplifies to:

$$\text{Volume} = D^3 \qquad (11)$$

Modifications of this formula have been proposed in order to compensate for systematic deviations from the above assumptions present in unusually large and small ventricles.[10,11] Although formulae based on the cube assumption produce fair correlations with angiographic volume (r = 0.64–0.74),[9–11] they suffer from the inherent inaccuracy of making multiple geometric assumptions in an attempt to derive three-dimensional data from a single measurement. Furthermore, these fair correlations are true only in the absence of asynergy.

Two-dimensional echocardiography offers considerable advantage over the M-mode technique because it enables direct measurement of left ventricular contours and dimensions in the planes of all three hemiaxes. It also allows use of other volume formulations, such as Simpson's rule. Studies have shown that correlations between angiographic and echocardiographic volumes are improved if two-dimensional, rather than M-mode methods, are utilized.[12–15] Furthermore, equally good correlations (r = 0.80–0.90) with angiographic volumes have been obtained in groups of patients with and without ventricular asynergy.[16,17] There is considerable technical flexibility in measuring left ventricular volumes by two-dimensional echocardiography. Good correlations have been obtained between angiographic volumes and echocardiographic volumes determined from Simpson's rule[13,15,16,18–21] and single plane and biplane area–length methods.[12–15,17,22]

With Simpson's rule, tomographic slices of the ventricle are taken perpendicular to the long axis as illustrated in Figure 8-2, or parallel to the long axis as illustrated in Figure 8-4. Studies where slices have been taken perpendicular to the left ventricular long axis are limited by insufficient standardized landmarks in short axis to allow full application of Simpson's rule.[13,15,16,18,20] Consequently, since the number of adequate tomograms is usually limited, the application of this method is often described as a "modified" Simpson's rule. In our own laboratory, we have found that tomograms recorded at the mitral leaflet tips and papillary muscle bodies are sufficiently reproducible for this application.[13,15] Studies where slices are taken parallel to the long axis have allowed a more classic application of Simpson's rule. Schiller and coworkers[19] successfully employed this approach in 30 of 42 patients who underwent biplane angiography and had technically adequate two-dimensional echocardiograms in the apical two-chamber and the parasternal short-axis views. The tomograms were obtained at 20 levels along the vertical axis common to both views (Figure 8-4). The total volume was calculated from the sum of these 20

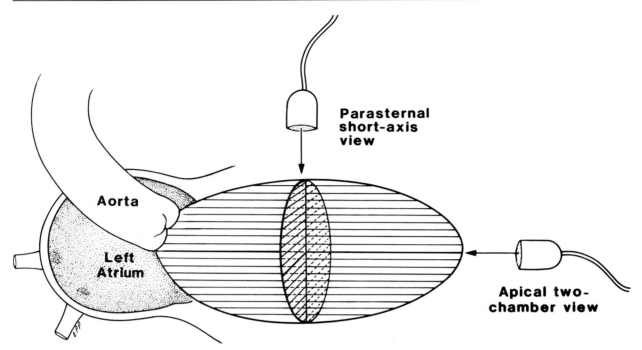

Figure 8-4. The Simpson's rule model for left ventricular volume with slices taken parallel to the long axis. This approach has been successfully used with parasternal short-axis and apical two-chamber echocardiographic views.[19] See text for details.

tomograms. Using this method for both the echocardiographic and angiographic images, they obtained correlations of r = 0.90 for end-systolic volume and r = 0.80 for end-diastolic volume. The echocardiographic volumes tended to underestimate the angiographic volumes.

Volume applications employing the ellipsoid model have been tested using both direct measurement of the minor axis[18] and derived estimates of the minor axis from the previously discussed area–length formula.[12–14,18] Silverman et al[14] found in children that the correlation of the angiographic method with the biplane area–length echocardiographic method was greater than with Simpson's rule. On the other hand Mercier et al,[21] using Simpson's rule and assuming the ventricle to be truncated cone, truncated ellipse, hemisphere cylinder, and ellipsoid plane, found equal accuracy in estimates of left ventricular volume. However, the ellipsoid biplane formula best estimated left ventricular ejection fraction.[21] Simpson's rule was found by Wyatt and coworkers[18] and in our own laboratory[13,15] to correlate better with angiographic determinations.

We have estimated left ventricular volume by two-dimensional echocardiography in a series of 50 patients undergoing single plane angiography. Apical four-chamber and parasternal short-axis views at both mitral valve and papillary muscle levels were employed, as illustrated in Figure 8-5. Volume was estimated using the five formulae illustrated in Figure 8-6. The best correlation with angiography resulted from the modified Simpson's rule formula. The correlation for all volumes combined was r = 0.84, with an SEE of 43 ml (Figure 8-7). In general, correlations with angiographic volume are improved by using the area–length method as compared

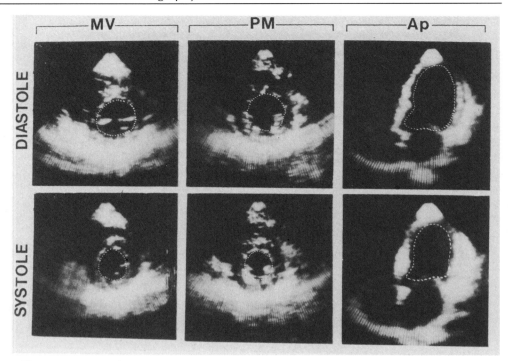

Figure 8-5. Examples of echocardiographic images of a normal heart at end-diastole and end-systole from the parasternal short-axis mitral valve (MV) and papillary muscle (PM) views and the apical four-chamber view (Ap). The endocardial outlines have been traced as described in the text for volume[13,15] and regional wall motion[33–35] analysis. Because of echo dropout, tracing of these outlines required fast- and slow-motion playback of frames immediately preceding and succeeding the respective end-diastolic and end-systolic frames.

to the direct minor axis measurement, and by using biplane as compared to single plane imaging.[13,15,18]

A summary of angiographic–echocardiographic correlations using various two-dimensional methods is presented in Table 8-1. The smallest standard error of the estimate SEE (15 ml/m^2 for end-diastolic volume) has been published by Schiller and coworkers[19] using the Simpson's rule method described earlier. Despite their good correlations the SEE appears rather large, especially since the SEE for single plane versus biplane cineangiography in the same patients has been reported by Kennedy et al[23] to be only 21 ml for end-diastolic volume and 13 ml for end-systolic volume. Appropriate judgment should be exercised, therefore, in applying these echocardiographic estimates of left ventricular volume to individual patients.

Left Ventricular Ejection Fraction

The reliability of the echocardiographic estimate of ejection fraction depends upon the accuracy of the method used for measuring end-diastolic and end systolic volumes. M-mode echocardiography is a particularly weak method because of the adverse influence of left ventricular asynergy on its accuracy. Fair correlations with angiographic ejection fraction have been obtained in patients with symmetrical contraction patterns (r = 0.64–0.74), but poor correlations have been found in

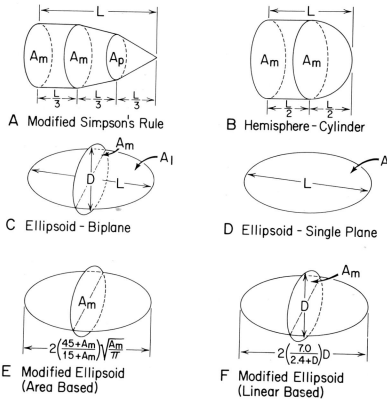

A Modified Simpson's Rule

B Hemisphere-Cylinder

C Ellipsoid - Biplane

D Ellipsoid - Single Plane

E Modified Ellipsoid (Area Based)

F Modified Ellipsoid (Linear Based)

Figure 8-6. Summary of the geometric models employed by Parisi et al[13,15] to generate left ventricular volumes from two-dimensional echocardiographic data. Model A, a modification of the Simpson's rule scheme shown in Figure 8-2 employing only three slices, proved to agree most closely with angiographic volume and ejection fraction. A denotes area measurements, L the long-axis length from the apical view, and D the septal-lateral diameter from the high cross-section of the ventricle. The subscripts m, p, and l refer to the mitral valve, papillary muscle, and long-axis sections, respectively. (From Parisi AF, Moynihan PF, Folland ED, et al: Approaches to determination of left ventricular volumes and ejection fraction by real-time two-dimensional echocardiography. Clin Cardio 2:259, 1979. With permission.)

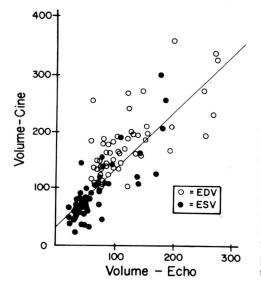

Figure 8-7. Relationship of end-diastolic volumes (EDV) and end-systolic volumes (ESV) as measured by cineangiography (Cine) and two-dimensional echocardiography (Echo) using the modified Simpson's rule approach shown in Figure 8-6A (r = 0.84, SEE = 43 ml). (From Folland ED, Parisi AF, Moynihan PF, et al: Assessment of left ventricular ejection fraction and volumes by real-time, two-dimensional echocardiography. A comparison of cineangiographic and radionuclide techniques. Circulation 60:765, 1979. By permission of the American Heart Association, Inc.)

173

Table 8-1
Comparison Between Echocardiographic and Angiographic Volumes and Ejection Fractions

Investigators	Method	No. of Patients	EDV r	EDV SEE	ESV r	ESV SEE	EF r	EF SEE	Comments
Teicholz et al[25]	B scan	25	—	—	—	—	0.87	—	14 out of 25 had asynergy
Folland et al[13]	Modified Simpson's rule	35	0.76	43 ml	0.86	32 ml	0.78	0.10	20 out of 35 had asynergy
Parisi et al[15]	Modified Simpson's rule	50	0.82	39 ml	0.90	29 ml	0.80	0.09	25 out of 50 had asynergy
Carr et al[12]	Biplane area-length	22	0.93	—	—	—	0.93	—	23 out of 24 volumes clustered; EDV r fell to 0.46 if 1 patient excluded; 6 out of 22 had asynergy
Schiller et al[19]	Modified Simpson's rule	30	0.80	15 ml/m²	0.90	8.5 ml/m²	0.87	0.08	16 out of 30 had asynergy
Chaudry et al[24]	Biplane ellipsoid model, three hemiaxes directly measured	30	0.86	—	0.91	—	0.73	—	20 out of 30 had coronary artery disease
Nixon et al[20]	Modified Simpson's rule	9	0.88	12 ml	0.93	9 ml	0.79	4	Standard errors were small in part because of the low variability of data in this group of normal subjects
Ohuchi et al[17]	Single plane area-length	38	0.84 (for all volumes)				0.88	—	Patients with and without asynergy
		18	0.86 (for all volumes)				0.88	—	Only patients with asynergy

EDV denotes end-diastolic volume; ESV, end-systolic volume; EF, ejection fraction; r, correlation coefficient; SEE, standard error of the estimate.

ischemic heart disease patients with segmental contraction abnormalities.[9–11] Angiographic ejection fractions correlate well in most studies employing two-dimensional echocardiography (r = 0.73–0.93; see Table 8-1).[24,25] In contrast to M-mode, two-dimensional echocardiographic estimates are relatively accurate even in the presence of asynergy. They have correlated well with angiography using either Simpson's rule or the area–length method. In our series of 50 patients, a modified Simpson's rule algorithm (Figure 8-6A) provided good results (r = 0.80, SEE = 9 percent) despite the fact that 25 patients had documented asynergy.[15] In 35 of our patients who also had ejection fraction measurement by radionuclide angiocardiography, the SEE (10 percent) approached that of the radionuclide technique (7 percent) when each method was compared to the cineangiographic ejection fraction.[13]

REGIONAL FUNCTION

Regional abnormalities of left ventricular wall motion are a hallmark of both acute and chronic ischemic heart disease. Wall motion has traditionally been evaluated by contrast angiography. For clinical purposes, qualitative assessment of the various segments outlined in the right anterior oblique and left anterior oblique projections has sufficed. In this approach each segment can be described as normal, hypokinetic, akinetic or paradoxical. This empirical approach is subject to inaccuracy and potential observer bias.

Quantitative techniques for regional wall motion analysis have been demonstrated to be superior to qualitative methods[26] and several approaches to the problem have been evaluated.[27,28] The issues of (1) whether to use a hemiaxis or radial coordinate system and (2) whether or not to use separate coordinates for diastole and systole have not been settled. Nonetheless, it appears that "cavity–area shrinkage" during systole is superior to "linear dimension–change" as a method of quantifying angiographic regional wall motion.[27] Quantifying the degree and extent of regional wall motion abnormalities permits a systematic assessment of the effects of ischemic heart disease on myocardial performance and provides an objective basis for examining left ventricular function serially in the course of illness or after therapeutic interventions.

Qualitative Wall Motion

To analyze regional wall motion, M-mode echocardiography is considerably limited by its unidimensional nature and restriction to the interventricular septal–posterolateral left ventricular plane from the parasternal position. Two-dimensional echocardiography, however, is potentially more ideal for analyzing regional left ventricular motion because it visualizes the left ventricle in tomographic planes at continuously variable levels from three different transducer positions (parasternal, apical, and subcostal). In suitable subjects virtually all regions of the left ventricle are accessible to this high-resolution technique. Although both two-dimensional and M-mode echocardiography are not technically feasible in some patients, the capability of utilizing the apical and subcostal windows for two-dimensional studies makes this approach successful where M-mode echocardiography has failed. Echocardiography is probably the best noninvasive modality today for analysis of regional

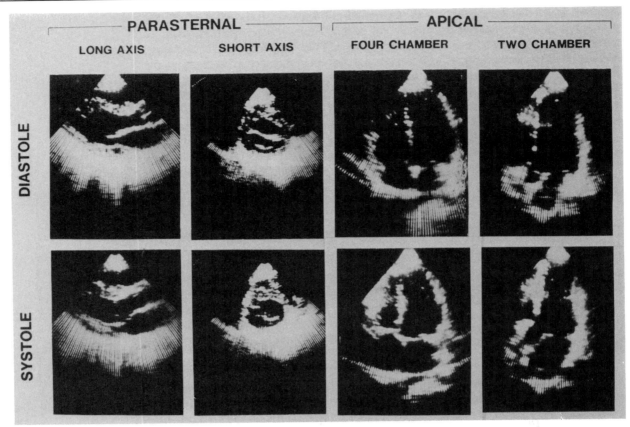

Figure 8-8. Four views of a normal heart at end-diastole and end-systole. These views are commonly employed for qualitative and quantitative assessment of ventricular volume. Note the relative relationship of left ventricular and right ventricular size and that the right ventricle conforms to the dominant shape of the left ventricle.

function because it permits higher resolution (less than or equal to 5 mm) than does radionuclide angiography (1 cm).[29]

Four specific views are best used for wall motion analysis because they are reproducible and relate well to the physician's anatomic concepts of left ventricular anatomy. These are the *parasternal long-* and *short-axis views* and the *apical four-chamber* and *two-chamber views* (Figure 8-8). The parasternal short-axis view can be studied reproducibly at two levels: the mitral valve and papillary muscle (see Figure 8-5). These views obviously lend themselves well to qualitative description of individual segments, similar to cineangiography. Clinical studies of regional wall motion abnormalities have been reported using such qualitative approaches.[25,30–32] Heger et al[31] have reported excellent agreement between the location of echocardiographic left ventricular segments that were qualitatively assessed as abnormal and the presence of the electrocardiographic Q waves in acute myocardial infarction patients. The same investigators[32] also found that qualitative scores of echocardiographic regional asynergy correlated well with the presence of pulmonary congestion and low cardiac output in acute myocardial infarction patients.

Quantitative Wall Motion

Two-dimensional echocardiography lends itself equally well to quantitative assessment of regional wall motion. We have developed a quantitative approach to regional wall motion analysis that is based on a radial axis system at both mitral valve and papillary muscle levels of the parasternal short-axis view and on a long axis in the apical two- or four-chamber view for assessing the apical segment[33] (Figure 8-9). Endocardial outlines are traced on celluloid at end-diastolic and end-systolic frames displayed on a video screen. These are verified by slow- and fast-action playback in a manner similar to cineangiography. Outlines at the lower cross-section levels are traced to include papillary muscles within the confines of the LV silhouette. Figure 8-10 shows three typical tracings for normal, anteroseptal, and inferior wall infarctions as they appear after entry into a computerized digitizing system. After manually identifying the midpoint of the septum (point S, Figure 8-9), the area of the diastolic frame is bisected to point L and the remaining radii automatically constructed from the midpoint by a computer system. Changes in axis lengths and sector areas are automatically measured as the systolic image contracts over the diastolic axis system. We found "percent–area shrinkage" of segments to be a more reproducible and less variable method that "linear axis shortening" for quantitating wall motion.[34]

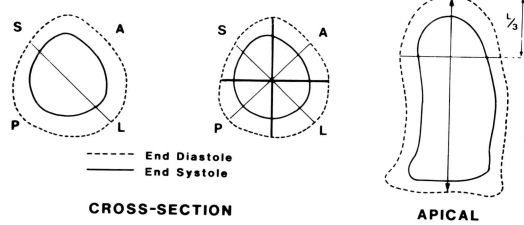

– – – – End Diastole
——— End Systole

CROSS-SECTION   APICAL

Figure 8-9. Quantitative evaluation of regional left ventricular wall motion. This is a scheme used by Moynihan et al[39] for quantitative assessment of regional wall motion. Parasternal short-axis sections are obtained at end-diastole and end-systole at both mitral valve and papillary muscle levels. "Percent-area shrinkage" of eight segments is then measured as the systolic outline superimposes on the radial system set up for the diastolic outline. The operator marks the midpoint of the septum, S, which then determines the septal-lateral (L) axis in such a fashion as to divide the diastolic figure into equal halves. The remaining radii are then generated by computer. A designates anterior and P posterior. Apical motion is viewed from the apical four-chamber view. The apical segment is defined by the perpendicular line to the left ventricular long axis (L) drawn one-third the way (L/3) from the apex. (From Moynihan PF, Parisi AF, Feldman CL: Quantitative detection of regional left ventricular contraction abnormalities by two-dimensional echocardiography. I. Analysis of methods. Circulation 63:754, 1981. By permission of the American Heart Association, Inc.)

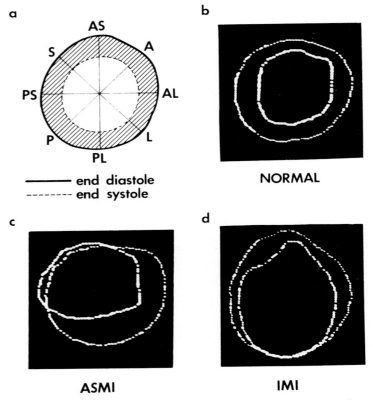

Figure 8-10. Quantitative evaluation of regional ventricular wall motion. Computer displays of three typical endocardial tracings from parasternal images. Panel a displays the radial axis system for orientation. (Abbreviations are the same as in Figure 8-9.) Panel b depicts a normal ventricle with uniform inward excursion on all axes. Panel c depicts an anteroseptal myocardial infarction (ASMI). Note the paradoxical motion of the septum. Panel d depicts an inferior myocardial infarction (IMI). Note the lack of systolic excursion in the posterior (P), posterolateral (PL), and lateral (L) segments.

This finding agrees with the conclusion of Gelberg and coworkers in their angiographic study.[27] Using this approach normal area shrinkage was defined for each of 17 segments, 8 at each short-axis level and 1 at apical level, from 10 healthy volunteers. Thirty-eight patients with documented ischemic heart disease (20 with definite myocardial infarctions, 18 with angiographically normal wall motion) were similarly studied and were grouped by infarction location for comparison to the normals (Figure 8-11).[35] While the patients without infarction failed to differ substantially from normal volunteers, patients with anterior and inferior infarction deviated significantly from the normal range in appropriate regions. Employing a mean ± 2 standard deviation range as normal, this approach has a 95 percent sensitivity for detecting and correctly localizing infarction and an 89 percent specificity for identifying patients with normal wall motion.[35]

Wall Thickening

Ultrasound offers a dimension of analysis of regional function not possible with angiographic or radionuclide techniques because it provides an image of the myocardial wall as well as the ventricular cavity. Echocardiography therefore makes it

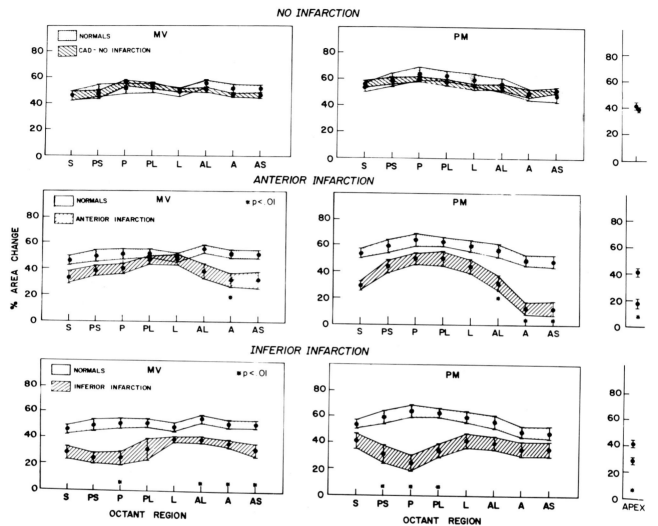

Figure 8-11. Quantitative evaluation of regional left ventricular wall motion. Comparison of normals and coronary artery disease (CAD) patients by percent-area change using the method of Parisi et al.[34,35] The stippled bands represent normal area change for the various segments ± standard error of the mean in 10 healthy volunteers. The crosshatched bands represent CAD patients without infarction (top), with anterior infarction (middle), and with inferior infarction (bottom). Apical contraction is noted at the far right. The small solid squares at the bottom of the panels just above the designation of segment location denote a significant difference from the normal segmental area change. MV denotes mitral valve level; PM, papillary muscle level; S, septal segment; PS, posteroseptal segment; P, posterior segment; PL, posterolateral segment; L, lateral segment; AL, anterolateral segment; A, anterior segment; AS, anteroseptal segment. (Adapted from Parisi AF, Moynihan PF, Folland ED, et al: Quantitative detection of regional left ventricular contraction abnormalities by two-dimensional echocardiography. II. Accuracy in coronary artery disease. Circulation 63:761, 1981. By permission of the American Heart Association, Inc.)

179

possible to follow the changes in thickness of various segments of myocardium during contraction. Systolic wall thickening may be a superior index of regional myocardial function because it is not influenced by motion of the heart within the chest. Lieberman and coworkers[36] have employed two-dimensional echocardiography to study segmental left ventricular function in dogs with experimental myocardial infarction. By analyzing regional myocardial thickening as well as endocardial motion they found that myocardial thickening was more precise than endocardial motion in discriminating between infarcted and noninfarcted zones of myocardium. (See also Chapter 15.)

Myocardial Echo Density

An additional approach to regional ventricular function which is unique to ultrasound is analysis of sonic reflectance of myocardium. It has long been recognized by M-mode echocardiographers that infarcted myocardium is not only akinetic but is also qualitatively different from normal myocardium. Infarcted regions are generally thinner and more echo-dense than normal regions. In two-dimensional studies infarcted regions produce particularly "hard" echoes (Figure 8-12). Dogs with experimental myocardial infarction have shown excellent concordance between regions of increased echo density and corresponding regions of infarction identified by wall motion defects and pathologic scar.[37] (See also Chapter 17.)

RIGHT VENTRICULAR FUNCTION

The shape of the right ventricle is not easily characterized by mathematical models. For this reason, as well as other technical considerations, no single method of quantitative right ventricular cineangiography has gained widespread acceptance or use. The same geometric considerations also complicate echocardiographic analysis of the right ventricle. M-mode measurements of right ventricular dimensions are

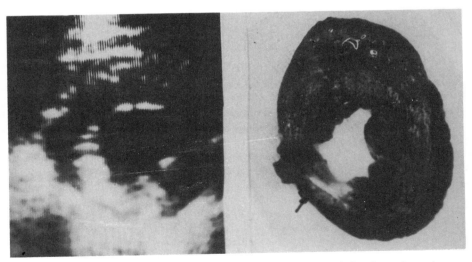

Figure 8-12. Short-axis cross-section of an experimentally infarcted dog heart by echocardiography (left) and the analogous pathology specimen (right). Note the location of the pale, infarcted tissue in the pathology specimen and the presentation of this infarction as an area of bright "hard" echos in the in vivo echo image.

particularly variable because of the crescentic profile that the ventricle assumes as it lies against the well-rounded interventricular septum. The apparent transverse dimension is highly dependent upon transducer position and angulation. Two-dimensional echocardiography offers considerable advantage over the M-mode technique in this regard. In particular, the apical four-chamber view provides a good image of the right ventricle—one that is free from adjacent crystal artifact that complicates the parasternal view. The right ventricle can be assessed qualitatively and quantitatively from the apical view.

Bommer and coworkers[38] measured right ventricles in parasternal long-axis and short-axis views and in the apical four-chamber view. They found good correlation between echocardiographically determined axes' dimensions and actual displacement volumes of eight silicone rubber casts of normal postmortem human right ventricles. In studies in living patients they found good separation between echocardiographic dimensions and areas of 25 normal subjects when compared to 25 patients with right ventricular volume overload. Two-dimensional echocardiography provided better separation of normals from abnormals than did the M-mode technique. The planimetered area (normal $= 18 \pm 1.2$ cm^2) and short-axis measurement at midventricle (normal $= 2.8 \pm 0.2$ cm) provided the best discrimination between the two groups of subjects.

Qualitative assessment of the right ventricle is possible by virtue of comparison with the left ventricle. Normally the transverse dimension in the four-chamber view is smaller than that of the left ventricle. The normal right ventricle in the parasternal short-axis view is crescent-shaped, dominated by the shape of the left ventricle, and smaller in transverse dimension (Figure 8-8). Figure 8-13 displays the heart of a 29-year-old woman with primary pulmonary hypertension. Note that the transverse right ventricular dimensions are comparable to the left ventricular dimensions. Furthermore, the right ventricle has altered the usual round shape of the left ventricle in the parasternal short-axis view. Left-to-right intracardiac shunts dilate the right ventricle and increase right ventricular wall motion due to the disproportionate volume overload. The septum is therefore dominated by right rather than left ventricular contraction and then moves anteriorly, rather than posteriorly, during systole. This accounts for the "paradoxical" motion of the septum seen in such hearts on M-mode display. Figure 8-14 displays the heart of a young man with an atrial septal defect and a large left-to-right shunt. Note the increased right ventricular wall motion compared to that seen in the patient with pulmonary hypertension in Figure 8-13.

Recently Wann and associates[39] presented preliminary data using digital subtraction contrast echocardiography to measure right ventricular ejection fraction. Presaline-contrast two-dimensional images were digitized and subtracted from digitized postcontrast images, which resulted in all structures being masked except the contrast. Right ventricular ejection fraction was determined from the areas of right ventricle occupied by contrast in systole and diastole. There was a good correlation in a small number of patients between right ventricular ejection fractions determined by digital subtraction contrast echocardiography and by first-pass radionuclide angiography.

CLINICAL APPLICATION

As mentioned previously, the clinical application of cardiac ultrasound is limited somewhat in adults by the technical inability to obtain satisfactory images in some subjects. This is particularly true in older subjects and those with chronic obstructive

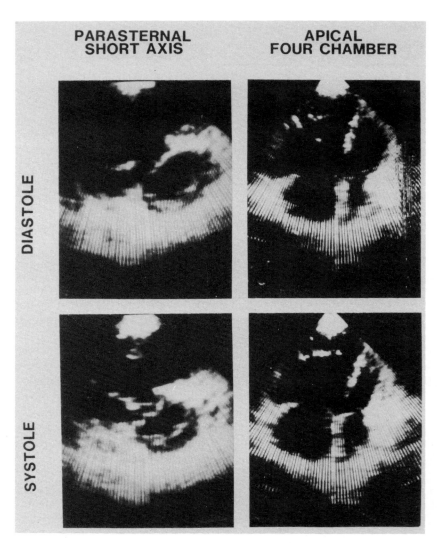

Figure 8-13. Right ventricular function: pure pressure overload from primary pulmonary hypertension. Note the increased size and dominance of the right ventricle relative to the left. In short-axis views the left ventricle assumes an oval configuration due to compression by the large, hypertrophic right ventricle. There is relatively little right ventricular contraction from diastole to systole.

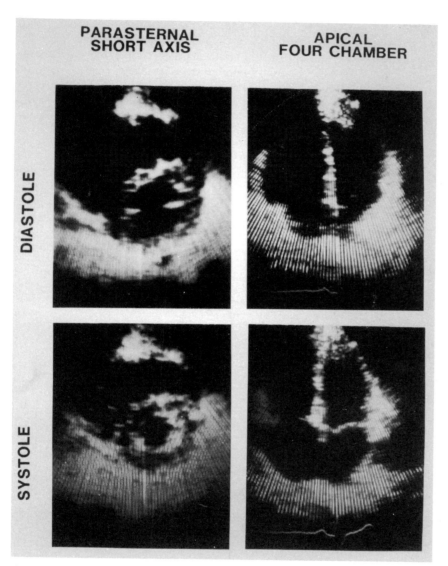

PARASTERNAL SHORT AXIS

APICAL FOUR CHAMBER

DIASTOLE

SYSTOLE

Figure 8-14. Right ventricular function: pure volume overload from a large atrial septal defect. As in pressure overload, the right ventricle is grossly enlarged and causes the left ventricle to assume an oval configuration in the short-axis view. In contrast to Figure 8-13, there is dramatic contraction of this dilated right ventricle in systole consistent with its grossly increased stroke volume.

pulmonary disease. The clinical use of quantitative methods for estimating left ventricular volume, ejection fraction, and wall motion has been further limited by the laborious process of tracing the end-diastolic and end-systolic images and entering them into appropriate processing systems. Several developments now appearing in the latest generation of ultrasound equipment may simplify the process sufficiently that quantitative methods will become everyday clinical practice.[40] Built-in image microprocessors have improved the definition of endocardial borders and allow for easy display of end-diastolic and end-systolic images. Interactive video display systems enable immediate tracing of borders without transferring to external tape or disc recording systems. Built-in microprocessors provide the capability of immediate computation of volume, ejection fraction, and wall motion data. These developments suggest that quantitative assessment of left ventricular pump performance and regional wall motion may become a reality for routine clinical evaluation of most patients in the near future.

REFERENCES

1. Kreulen TM, Bove AA, McDonough MT, et al: The evaluation of left ventricular function in man. A comparison of methods. Circulation 51:677–688, 1975
2. Nelson GR, Cohn PF, Gorlin R: Prognosis in medically treated coronary artery disease. Influence of ejection fraction compared to other parameters. Circulation 52:408–412, 1975
3. Murray JA, Chinn N, Peterson DR: Influence of left ventricular function on early prognosis in atherosclerotic heart disease (Abstract). Am J Cardiol 33:159, 1974
4. Cohn PF, Gorlin R, Cohn LH, et al: Left ventricular ejection fraction as a prognostic guide in surgical treatment of coronary and valvular heart disease. Am J Cardiol 34:136–141, 1974
5. Hammermeister KE, Kennedy JW: Predictors of surgical mortality in patients undergoing direct myocardial revascularization. Circulation 49,50(Suppl II):112, 1974
6. Dodge HT, Sandler M, Ballew AN, et al: Use of biplane angiocardiography for the measurement of left ventricular volume in man. Am Heart J 60:762–776, 1960
7. Chapman CB, Baker O, Reynolds J, et al: Use of biplane cinefluorography for measurement of ventricular volume. Circulation 18:1105–1117, 1958
8. Moynihan PF, Parisi AF, Folland ED, et al: A system for quantitative evaluation of left ventricular function with two-dimensional ultrasonography. Med Instrum 14:111, 1980
9. Pombo JF, Troy BL, Russell RO Jr: Left ventricular volumes and ejection fraction by echocardiography. Circulation 43:480–490, 1971
10. Fortuin NJ, Hood WP Jr. Sherman ME, et al: Determination of left ventricular volumes by ultrasound. Circulation 44:575–584, 1971
11. Teichholz LE, Kreulen T, Herman MV, et al: Problems in echocardiographic volume determinations: Echocardiographic-angiographic correlations in the presence or absence of asynergy. Am J Cardiol 37:7–11, 1976
12. Carr KW, Engler RL, Forsythe JR, et al: Measurement of left ventricular ejection fraction by mechanical cross-sectional echocardiography. Circulation 59:1196–1206, 1979
13. Folland ED, Parisi AF, Moynihan PF, et al: Assessment of left ventricular ejection fraction and volumes by real-time, two-dimensional echocardiography. A comparison of cineangiographic and radionuclide techniques. Circulation 60:760–766, 1979
14. Silverman NH, Ports TA, Snider AR, et al: Determination of left ventricular volume in children: Echocardiographic and angiographic comparisons. Circulation 62:548–557, 1980
15. Parisi AF, Moynihan PF, Folland ED, et al: Approaches to determination of left ventricular volumes and ejection fraction by real-time two-dimensional echocardiography. Clin Cardiol 2:257–263, 1979
16. Gueret P, Meerbaum S, Wyatt HL, et al: Two-dimensional echocardiographic quantitation of left ventricular volumes and ejection fraction. Importance of accounting for dyssynergy in short axis reconstruction mode. Circulation 62:1308–1318, 1980
17. Ohuchi Y, Kuwako K, Umeda T, et al: Real-time, phased-array, cross-sectional echocardiographic evaluation of left ventricular asynergy and quantitation of left ventricular function. A comparison with left ventricular cineangiography. Jpn Heart J 21:1–15, 1980

18. Wyatt HL, Heng MK, Meerbaum S, et al: Cross-sectional echocardiography II. Analysis of mathematical models for quantifying volume of the formalin-fixed left ventricle. Circulation 61:1119–1125, 1980

19. Schiller NB, Acquatella H, Ports TA, et al: Left ventricular volume from paired biplane two-dimensional echocardiography. Circulation 60:547–555, 1979

20. Nixon JV, Saffer SI: Three-dimensional echoventriculography (Abstract). Circulation 57,58:II-57, 1978

21. Mercier JC, DiSessa TG, Jarmarani JM, et al: Two-dimensional echocardiographic assessment of left ventricular volume and ejection fraction in children. Circulation 65:962–969, 1982

22. Gehrke J, Leeman S, Raphael M, et al: Non-invasive left ventricular volume determination by two-dimensional echocardiography. Br Heart J 37:911–916, 1975

23. Kennedy JW, Trenholme SE, Kasser IS: Left ventricular volume and mass from single plane cine-angiocardiogram. A comparison of anteroposterior and right anterior oblique methods. Am Heart J 80:343–352, 1970

24. Chaudry KR, Ogawa S, Pauletto FJ, et al: Biplane measurements of left ventricular volumes using wide-angle, cross-sectional echocardiography (Abstract). Am J Cardiol 41:391, 1978

25. Teichholz LE, Cohen MV, Sonnenblick EH, et al: Study of left ventricular geometry and function by B-scan ultrasonography in patients with and without asynergy. N Engl J Med 291:1220–1226, 1974

26. Chaitman BR, DeMots H, Bristow JD, et al: Objective and subjective analysis of left ventricular angiograms. Circulation 52:420–425, 1975

27. Gelberg HJ, Brundage BH, Glantz S, et al: Quantitative left ventricular wall motion analysis: A comparison of area, chord, and radial methods. Circulation 59:991–1000, 1979

28. Ingels NB, Daughters, GT, Stinson EB, et al: Evaluation of methods for quantifying left ventricular segmental wall motion in man using myocardial markers as a standard. Circulation 61:966–972, 1980

29. Borer JS, Bacharach SL, Green MV, et al: Effect of nitroglycerin on exercise-induced abnormalities of left ventricular regional function and ejection fraction in coronary artery disease. Circulation 57:314–320, 1978

30. Kisslo JA, Robertson D, Gilbert BW, et al: A comparison of real-time, two-dimensional echocardiography and cineangiography in detecting left ventricular asynergy. Circulation 55:134–141, 1977

31. Heger JJ, Weyman AE, Wann LS, et al: Cross-sectional echocardiography in acute myocardial infarction: Detection and localization of regional left ventricular asynergy. Circulation 60:531–538, 1979

32. Heger JJ, Weyman AE, Wann LS, et al: Cross-sectional echocardiographic analysis of the extent of left ventricular asynergy in acute myocardial infarction. Circulation 61:1113–1118, 1980

33. Parisi AF, Moynihan PF, Folland ED, et al: Assessment of regional wall motion in coronary artery disease by two-dimensional echocardiography in Lanceé CT (ed): Proceedings of the Third International Symposium on Echocardiology. The Hague, Martinus Nijhoff, 1979

34. Moynihan PF, Parisi AF, Feldman CL: Quantitative detection of regional left ventricular contraction abnormalities by two-dimensional echocardiography. I. Analysis of methods. Circulation 63:752–760, 1981

35. Parisi AF, Moynihan PF, Folland ED, et al: Quantitative detection of regional left ventricular contraction abnormalities by two-dimensional echocardiography. II. Accuracy in coronary artery disease. Circulation 63:761–767, 1981

36. Lieberman AN, Weiss JL, Jugdutt BI, et al: Two-dimensional echocardiography and infarct size: Relationship of regional wall motion and thickening to the extent of myocardial infarction in the dog. Circulation 63:739–746, 1981

37. Moynihan PF, Khuri S, Karaffa SA, et al: Characteristics of remote myocardial infarction (MI) in a canine model by two-dimensional echocardiography (2DE) (Abstract). Circulation 62(Suppl III): 101, 1980

38. Bommer W, Weinert L, Neumann A, et al: Determination of right atrial and right ventricular size by two-dimensional echocardiography. Circulation 60:91–100, 1979

39. Wann LS, Stickels K, Bamrah VS, et al: Digital subtraction contrast echocardiography—A new technique for measuring right ventricular ejection fraction (Abstract). Circulation 66(Suppl II):II-29, 1982

40. Garcia E, Gueret P, Bennett M, et al: Real time computerization of two-dimensional echocardiography. Am Heart J 101:783–792, 1981

CHAPTER 9

Ischemic Heart Disease

Natesa G. Pandian, David J. Skorton, and Richard E. Kerber

With the technical assistance of Robert Kieso

Recent advances in ultrasound technology have made two-dimensional echocardiography a highly valuable tool for studying alterations in the structure and function of the myocardium in ischemic heart disease. This chapter reviews the experimental and clinical applications of two-dimensional echocardiography of ischemic and infarcted myocardium.

EXPERIMENTAL APPLICATIONS OF ECHOCARDIOGRAPHY

Abnormalities in regional left ventricular wall motion occur very rapidly when a coronary artery is ligated. Since the original description of such alterations by Tennant and Wiggers,[1] the usefulness of wall motion abnormalities as an early indicator of ischemia or infarction has undergone considerable investigation.[1-13] A variety of approaches have been used to demonstrate ischemic regional myocardial dysfunction, including slow-motion movies,[2] mercury-in-silastic length gauges sutured to the epicardium,[3,8-10] radiopaque markers,[4] and ultrasonic sonomicrometers.[5,6] These techniques have shown abnormalities in endocardial motion and wall thickening. All have certain limitations: they are invasive, myocardial function may be altered by the techniques themselves, or repeated and precise measurements are not always possible.

To avoid the limitations of these techniques, echocardiography has been applied to the study of regional left ventricular ischemia. Stefan and Bing[14] used M-mode echocardiography in a canine model of myocardial ischemia and demonstrated decreased posterior left ventricular endocardial excursion and velocity. A series of investigations in our laboratory using M-mode echocardiography have demonstrated the feasibility of identifying segmental dyskinesis in experimentally induced myocardial ischemia. Ligation of either the circumflex coronary artery[15-19] or the left

Supported in part by National Heart, Lung, and, Blood Institute grant 14388, American Heart Association Grant 80-G-36, and the Veterans Administration Merit Review.

Dr. Skorton is a recipient of a Veterans Administration Research Associate Career Development Award.

anterior descending coronary artery[15] produced characteristic systolic expansion and thinning in the posterior wall or septum, respectively. The abnormalities correlated well with the severity of the perfusion defect produced by coronary occlusion. Beneficial and adverse changes in wall motion and thickening of ischemic myocardium caused by pharmacologic agents[17,20] or arterial pressure manipulations[17] have been studied by echocardiography. In 1981 Likoff and associates[21] obtained epicardial M-mode echograms from multiple sites on both ventricles in patients with coronary artery disease during coronary surgery and demonstrated a marked heterogeneity of myocardial wall motion, even in areas without transmural myocardial infarction or ventriculographic abnormalities. Nonetheless, they found that coronary artery occlusion produced prompt systolic wall thinning. Furthermore, when compared to strain gauges, the echograms were found to be more sensitive and equally specific for ischemia.

Two-Dimensional Echocardiographic Technique

Current interest centers on the use of two-dimensional rather than M-mode echocardiography because of its unique advantage of employing multiple views and permitting examination of large areas of myocardium. Two-dimensional studies of experimental myocardial ischemia and infarction have been performed by a number of investigators.[22–28] Myocardial ischemia has been evaluated by studying wall thickening and motion abnormalities with echocardiography during partial and complete coronary artery occlusion in open-chest and closed-chest dogs.[29–33]

Excellent-quality echo images can be obtained in both open- and closed-chest animals with the use of Wyatt and colleagues' technique[34] (Figure 9-1). Using phased-array two-dimensional echocardiography, we routinely record tomographic images in the long-axis view of the left ventricle and in four short-axis planes. Regional wall

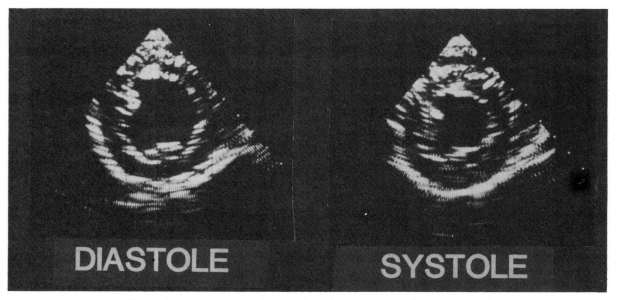

Figure 9-1. Assessment of regional thickening by two-dimensional echocardiography. Short-axis tomographic cross-sections of the left ventricle at papillary muscle level obtained by two-dimensional echocardiography in a dog. All regions show systolic thickening.

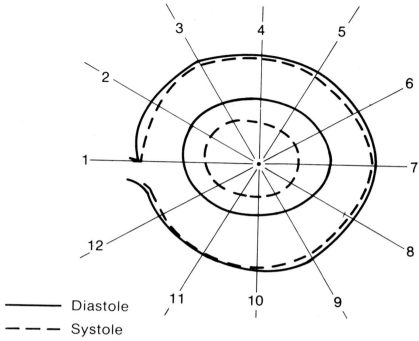

——— Diastole

— — — Systole

Figure 9-2. One approach to two-dimensional echocardiographic analysis utilizes the right ventricular free wall–interventricular septum junction as an initial landmark, from which the left ventricle is divided into 12 equal wedge-shaped regions. The systolic changes in individual radii, individual myocardial segments, and individual cavity areas can be assessed using computerized techniques.

thickening is analyzed from endocardial (excluding papillary muscles) and epicardial outlines on the short-axis tomographic sections: 12 radii are generated by a computer at 30° intervals, dividing the short-axis cavity into 12 equal wedge-shaped regions containing the left ventricular cavity and myocardium (Figure 9-2). The process is performed on end-diastolic and end-systolic images using a computerized contour analysis program. The percentage of change in cavity area and the percentage of myocardial segment thickening during systole are calculated for each segment. Estimates of left ventricular volume and mass can also be obtained from short- and long-axis sections using the formulae validated by Wyatt et al.[34] A similar approach has been described by other investigators[56,57] (see Chapter 8).

Detection and Localization of Regional Wall Motion Abnormalities

Abnormalities of regional wall motion during ischemia can be readily detected by two-dimensional echocardiography. Meerbaum and associates[22] observed that endocardial wall motion abnormalities characteristically appear early after coronary occlusion. Two-dimensional echocardiography correlated well with force-gauge mapping in assessing dysfunctional myocardium. Dyskinesis and increased brightness in the involved myocardium were noted on echocardiograms following experimental myocardial infarction.[24,27,28] Lieberman et al[26] found that changes in systolic wall thickening were more precisely identified echocardiographically than alterations in endocardial motion during ischemia. These studies indicated that two-dimensional echocardiography was useful in detecting wall motion and thickening abnormalities during myocardial ischemia.

To determine whether two-dimensional echocardiography was useful in detecting transient ischemia due to fixed coronary stenosis, we used the technique of Folts et al[35] to create severe circumflex coronary artery stenosis (90 percent reduction in diameter). Two-dimensional echocardiograms were compared to ultrasonic sonomicrometers for detecting systolic thinning produced by stress-induced myocardial ischemia.[29] All the myocardial wall segments thickened in systole in control recordings and remained normal despite the 90 percent reduction in coronary artery diameter. Only when isoproterenol and aortic constriction were added to induce myocardial ischemia, however, did segmental dyskinesis develop (Figure 9-3). Dyskinesis was not present in sonomicrometers when two-dimensional echo abnormalities were absent. In another study nitroglycerine decreased the extent of myocardial dyskinesis following coronary occlusion, whereas phenylephrine worsened left ventricular dysfunction.[24] These studies suggest that two-dimensional echocar-

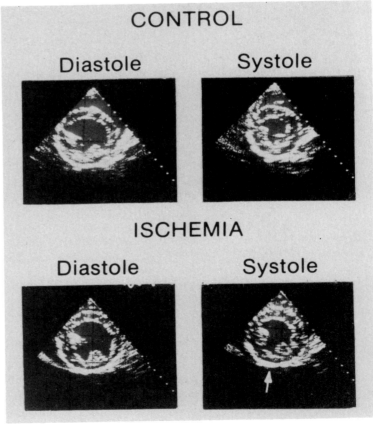

Figure 9-3. Use of two-dimensional echocardiography to demonstrate induced myocardial ischemia in experimental coronary stenosis. In a dog with a 90 percent circumflex coronary stenosis, resting perfusion and systolic thickening were maintained (control). When isoproterenol and acute aortic constriction were superimposed, however, ischemia occurred—as indicated by systolic thinning of the myocardium between the papillary muscles (arrow).

diography is a very sensitive method for detecting transient dyskinesis due to myocardial ischemia and provides a useful tool for therapeutic intervention and clinical investigation.

Wall Dynamics and Myocardial Perfusion

In studies to find whether a quantitative relationship exists between systolic contraction abnormalities (assessed by two-dimensional echocardiography) and reduced perfusion (measured by radiolabeled microsphere), abnormal systolic wall thinning was observed only when increased myocardial oxygen demand (produced by isoproterenol or aortic constriction) or a low aortic pressure (produced by nitroglycerine, nitroprusside, or hemorrhage) were superimposed upon a 90 percent or greater coronary stenosis. Normal systolic thickening at rest as assessed by two-dimensional echocardiography did not exclude the presence of severe coronary artery stenosis. Transient systolic thinning of a segment during stress indicated that severe coronary artery stenosis was present, and myocardinal perfusion of that segment was only 25 percent of normal. These results are similar to those found by Lieberman et al[26] in their model of complete coronary occlusion.

Estimation of Infarct Size and Risk Area

Evaluation of infarct size by two-dimensional echocardiography is under current study. Several investigators have found that endocardial wall motion abnormalities characteristically appear within minutes after coronary occlusion. Meltzer et al[24] compared the extent of dyskinesis early after left anterior descending artery occlusion to infarct size measured by technetium pyrophosphate scans and nitroblue tetrazolium staining. They found a good correlation between endocardial motion abnormalities detected by echocardiography and infarct size. Meerbaum and colleagues[22] also found a good correlation between two-dimensional echocardiography and force-gauge mapping when assessing the extent of myocardial dysfunction. However, they as well as others noted that wall motion abnormalities detected by two-dimensional echocardiography consistently overestimated infarct size.[22,27,30,36] Lieberman et al,[26] using two-dimensional echocardiography, found that endocardial motion was less precise than wall thickening in distinguishing the infarct zone from normal zones.

Systolic wall thinning was only observed in segments in which the infarct extended to greater than 20 percent of transmural thickness. Once the transmural extent of infarct increased from 21 to 100 percent there was no significant augmentation in the degree of systolic thinning. The presence of any degree of systolic thickening indicated less than 20 percent infarction of transmural thickness.

Blumenthal et al[37] employed two-dimensional echocardiography to study the functional properties of ischemic myocardium after pretreatment with prostacycline, ibuprofen, or dipyridamole. Treated dogs had smaller infarcts, but the apparently "salvaged" but histologically normal myocardium remained functionally abnormal for many days.

Direct Imaging of Coronary Arteries

The ability to image the coronary arteries in a beating heart would have important clinical and experimental applications. Toward this end Sahn et al[38] have developed a new method for imaging coronary arteries in open-chested humans during surgery. Using a 9-mHz transducer, they were able to record and localize coronary arterial obstructions in a beating heart during surgery. This method may allow the intraoperative verification and localization of atherosclerotic lesions and aid in accurate placement of saphenous vein bypass grafts.

Study of Myocardial Perfusion

More recently two-dimensional echocardiography has been used to directly assess myocardial perfusion. DeMaria et al[39] injected carbon dioxide and a suspension of microbubbles selectively into a coronary artery and noted the microbubbles opacifying the corresponding left ventricular myocardium. Using echo videodensitometry to analyze myocardial perfusion, Bommer et al.[40] found that reduced perfusion resulting from coronary occlusion could be detected by contrast echocardiography (see Chapter 14). This approach has promise for quantifying abnormalities in regional myocardial perfusion. The safety of these contrast agents has yet to be determined in humans.

CLINICAL APPLICATIONS
OF ECHOCARDIOGRAPHY

Regional Asynergy

M-Mode Echocardiographic Findings

An important application of cardiac ultrasound in man has been the detection of dyskinesis related to coronary artery disease.[41–44] Corya et al[41] showed that 84 percent of patients with acute myocardial infarction studied by M-mode echocardiography had abnormal left ventricular endocardial motion within the electrocardiographic site of infarction. The loss of normal systolic thickening has also been used as an M-mode marker of acute infarction. Corya et al[43] noted that patients with acute infarction lost normal systolic thickening and developed systolic thinning (Figure 9-4). Although systolic thinning was a relatively specific finding it was not very sensitive, being present in only 12 of 40 acute infarction patients.

Other M-mode studies have focused on patients with chronic coronary artery disease. Jacobs et al[44] demonstrated with M-mode echocardiography abnormal endocardial motion in the majority of patients with dysynergy seen on angiographic studies. A number of investigators[44–47] have similarly found that patients with left anterior descending coronary (LAD) artery narrowing have reduced motion of the interventricular septum. Other causes of abnormal septal motion must be excluded, however, before using this criterion to predict the presence of LAD coronary disease.

There are major limitations of M-mode echocardiography in the detection of dyskinesis attributed to coronary artery disease. The M-mode technique samples only a relatively small portion of the left ventricle at any given time. Several areas, such as the apex and lateral wall, are inaccessible to the M-mode ultrasound beam. The complex rotational and transitional motion of the heart is difficult to appreciate by M-mode studies and may influence wall motion analysis. Two-dimensional echocardiography overcomes most of these limitations.

Two-Dimensional Echocardiographic Findings

Two-dimensional echocardiography has been extensively applied to the study of patients with ischemic heart disease. The early studies of Teichholz et al[48] used a gated B-scan technique to display a two-dimensional cardiac image. These workers were able to demonstrate asynergic segments which corresponded well to those

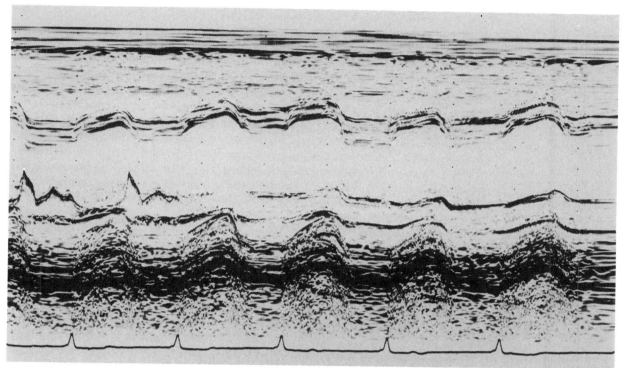

Figure 9-4. An M-mode echocardiogram taken just below the mitral valve from a patient with an anteroseptal myocardial infarction. Systolic thinning and paradoxical systolic motion of the interventricular septum are evident.

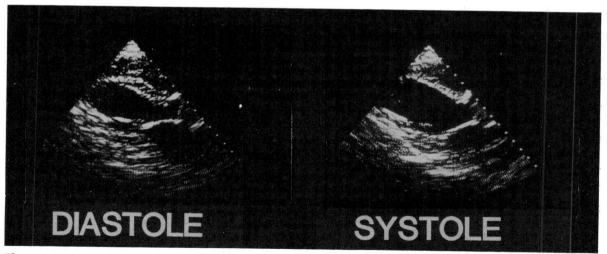

DIASTOLE   SYSTOLE

Figure 9-5. Same patient as in Figure 9-4. Parasternal long-axis view in diastole and systole. Abnormal systolic motion and thinning of the interventricular septum are seen in this patient with an anteroseptal myocardial infarction.

seen in angiographic ventriculograms. This technique was soon supplanted by real-time two-dimensional echocardiography. Kisslo et al[49] compared real-time two-dimensional echocardiography and cineangiography in detecting left ventricular asynergy and found substantial agreement between the two techniques in identifying asynergic segments (Figure 9-5). Heger and coworkers[50] studied wall motion in 44 patients with acute myocardial infarction and devised a wall motion index from each segment to derive an overall assessment of left ventricular asynergy. The wall motion index correlated well with the severity of hemodynamic impairment.

More recently, Weiss et al[36] have compared two-dimensional echocardiographic studies with postmortem studies in patients who died of acute myocardial infarction. They found that all transmurally infarcted segments were either akinetic or dyskinetic on two-dimensional echocardiography (Figure 9-6). Normal wall motion excluded transmural infarction. Akinesis appeared to be a sensitive indicator of transmural infarction but was not specific: 8 percent of the akinetic or dyskinetic segments in the border zone were histologically normal, and 29 percent of these segments exhibited subendocardial infarction. Hypokinesis was even less useful, being seen either in subendocardial infarction or in normal myocardium. Two-dimensional echocardiography appeared to overestimate the amount of myocardial scar, a finding which is in agreement with the results of animal studies in our laboratory.[18,30] The overestimation of the amount of scar by the two-dimensional technique may be due to transient ischemia or to a tethering effect in adjacent noninfarcted areas.

An important concern in the identification of contraction abnormalities by two-dimensional echocardiography is the problem of heterogeneity of normal function. Although complete absence of motion (nonthickening) or expansion (bulging) is clearly abnormal and can indicate ischemia or infarction, reduction of normal thickening and motion (hypokinesis) can occur without ischemia. In other words, because of biological heterogeneity, hypokinesis is difficult to interpret. It is problematic, then, to set a normal lower limit on segmental myocardial thickening. This issue has been explored in depth in human studies by Pandian et al,[57] Moynihan et al,[59] and Parisi et al;[60] the studies confirmed that a marked degree of heterogeneity of

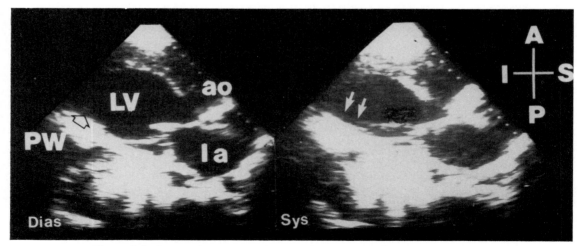

Figure 9-6. Long-axis parasternal view of a patient with a previous inferior myocardial infarction. Note the inferior posterior wall (PW), which is akinetic during systole (double arrows). Note systolic thickening of the septum and absence of inferior posterior wall thickening.

contraction, demonstrable by various methods of echocardiographic analysis, is normally present.

In another important study,[51] two-dimensional echocardiography was utilized prospectively to detect regional expansion and thinning of the infarct zone following acute myocardial infarction. Infarct expansion that occurred within 3 weeks of transmural infarction appears to contribute to left ventricular dilatation. The significant increase in ventricular size due to infarct expansion appears to predict progressive ventricular enlargement due to lengthening of the infarcted and noninfarcted zone.[52,53] This capability may permit the echocardiographer to make the antemortem diagnosis of impending cardiac rupture in some cases, which may be lifesaving.

Recently investigators have also shown that two-dimensional echocardiography can be helpful in the initial evaluation of the acute chest pain syndrome; patients in whom regional wall motion abnormalities were not detected by echocardiography did not develop acute myocardial infarction or complications during their subsequent hospital course.[58]

Detection of Coronary Artery Disease by Stress Echocardiography

The studies previously discussed are based on the presence of preexisting infarcted or fibrotic areas with motion abnormalities detectable in a state of rest by echocardiography. Of course, many patients have coronary arterial stenosis that is clinically significant but does not reduce resting state blood flow. Accordingly, myocardial function at rest is preserved in these individuals, but it may deteriorate when exercise causes myocardial oxygen requirements to rise out of proportion to the ability of the stenotic artery to supply nutrient flow to the affected area. Experimental studies, previously discussed in this chapter, have provided a basis for the clinical use of echocardiography to detect ischemia during stress interventions. Using M-mode echocardiography, Mason et al[53] studied patients with coronary artery disease at rest and during supine bicycle exercise at increasing work loads until angina or ischemic EKG changes appeared. Upon regional left ventricular thickening analysis, it was found that mean systolic thickening in wall segments supplied by stenotic coronary arteries fell instead of rising during exercise. Crawford and colleagues[54] measured left ventricular dimensions and normalized rate of fractional shortening during isometric handgrip and isotonic (upright bicycle) exercise in normal subjects. Both of these studies showed that echocardiography could be successfully accomplished in selected subjects during various forms of exercise.

More recently, Wann and colleagues[55] have applied two-dimensional echocardiography to study endocardial wall motion in patients before and during exercise using a 30° mechanical sector scanner. They performed echocardiograms at rest, during supine bicycle exercise and after sublingual nitroglycerin in 28 patients. Technically adequate studies during exercise were obtained in 20 (71 percent) of these patients. Ten patients had new areas of reversible asynergy: all 10 were demonstrated to have significant stenosis of the corresponding coronary arteries. These workers demonstrated that the technique of exercise echocardiography is technically feasible and may be clinically useful in the detection of occult coronary artery disease. Other workers have utilized wide-angle two-dimensional echocardiography to detect wall motion abnormalities following handgrip exercise. This method has a high specificity in detecting coronary artery disease and is useful in predicting severely stenotic or multiple vessel coronary artery lesions.[56]

Assessment of Global Left Ventricular Size and Performance

The theory and practical applications of two-dimensional echocardiography in the assessment of global left ventricular size and function have been discussed in detail in Chapter 8. Gueret et al[63] have studied this problem in detail in dogs and have shown that when regional asymmetry of contraction is present, two-dimensional echocardiographic quantification of left ventricular volumes may be obtained with a simplified model, using the formula:

$$\text{Volume} = 5/6 \text{ area} \times \text{length}$$

However, the cross-section used for the area determination *must* reflect the geometric distortion of the ventricle. That is, if the dyssynergy occurs at the papillary muscle level, this section must be used in the volume formula. If a mitral valve section were used above the area of ischemia, the calculated volumes would not accurately reflect true left ventricular volumes. Additional clinical investigation is required to further establish and apply the knowledge gained from these experimental studies.

Complications of Ischemic Heart Disease and Acute Myocardial Infarction

Acute myocardial infarction is frequently accompanied by complications which may be detectable by two-dimensional echocardiography. Complications involve either extensive contraction abnormalities which become chronic and progress to ventricular dilatation or aneurysm, rupture of the interventricular septum producing an acute ventricular septal defect, flail mitral leaflet secondary to papillary muscle rupture, or extensive papillary muscle dysfunction.

Drobec and coworkers[64] reported their two-dimensional echocardiographic findings in 30 patients with complicated acute myocardial infarction: 2 patients had a ventricular septal rupture and 1 had a flail mitral valve. Heger and associates[65] found that of 23 patients with acute myocardial infarction studied by two-dimensional echocardiography, 6 had either acute mitral regurgitation or a ventricular septal rupture.

Papillary Muscle Dysfunction and Rupture

Mintz et al[66] have studied 9 patients with papillary muscle rupture or dysfunction. In papillary muscle rupture there is severe prolapse, usually of the anterior mitral leaflet, giving the appearance of a flailing systolic motion. In some cases a mass may be seen attached to the anterior leaflet (Figure 9-7) or posterior leaflet. Papillary muscle dysfunction is typically found to occur in the setting of an inferior myocardial infarction: motion of the mitral valve anterior leaflet is normal, but posterior leaflet motion is restricted and the leaflet is retracted and held in a rigid semi-closed position. Left ventricular contraction abnormalities (dyskinesis or akinesis) in the posterior-basal area are generally associated with this abnormal posterior leaflet motion. In all of these cases significant mitral regurgitation was documented angiographically.[66]

Ventricular Septal Rupture

Mintz and associates[66] studied 5 patients with acute ventricular septal rupture and found that the site of septal rupture is usually the center of a septal aneurysm, with

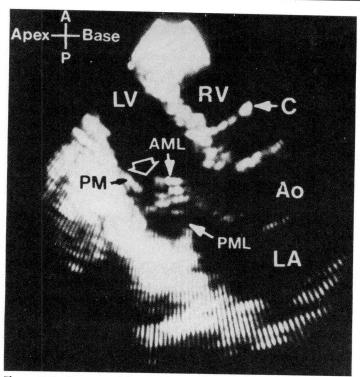

Figure 9-7. Parasternal long-axis view in diastole of a patient with papillary muscle rupture. A mass representing the head of the ruptured papillary muscle (PM) is attached to the anterior mitral leaflet (AML). The open arrow depicts the point of rupture. Ao denotes aortic root; LA, left atrium; C, catheter; LV, left ventricle; PML, posterior mitral leaflet; RV, right ventricle. (From Mintz GS, Victor MF, Kotler MN, et al: Two-dimensional echocardiographic identification of surgically correctable complications of acute myocardial infarction. Circulation 64:91, 1981. By permission of the American Heart Association, Inc.)

the surrounding septal tissue appearing denser and thinner than normal myocardium. During systole this septal aneurysm bulges into the right ventricle with widening of the defect (Figure 9-8A). No abnormalities of mitral leaflets or papillary muscles are generally seen in these patients. Scanlon et al[67] and Farcot et al[68] have also reported on the two-dimensional echocardiographic findings in ventricular septal rupture. As opposed to a congenital ventricular septal defect, acutely acquired ventricular septal rupture due to myocardial infarction may be multiple and/or serpiginous (Figure 9-8B), making it somewhat difficult to visualize by two-dimensional echocardiography. Contrast echocardiography for the detection of the left-to-right shunts may be helpful, but streaming effects may reduce its utility in ventricular septal rupture as compared to its usefulness in atrial septal defects.

Ventricular Aneurysms

The evaluation of chronic ventricular aneurysms by two-dimensional echocardiography was described by Weyman and associates in 1974.[69] Typically these are located at the apex of the ventricle (Figure 9-9); less commonly they are found in the true posterior wall (Figure 9-10) or the septum. They may be well defined or the margins may be less well demarcated. The fully developed aneurysm shows systolic

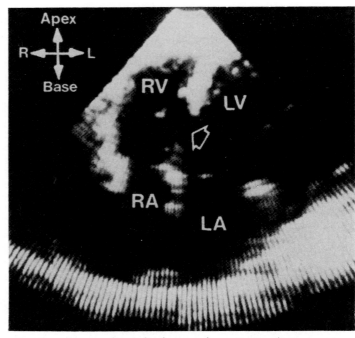

Figure 9-8A. Apical four-chamber view, end-systolic frame, of a patient with acute antero-septal myocardial infarction and ventricular septal rupture (arrow). (From Mintz GS, Victor MF, Kotler MN, et al: Two-dimensional echocardiographic identification of surgically cor-rectable complications of acute myocardial infarction. Circulation 64:91, 1981. By permission of the American Heart Association, Inc.)

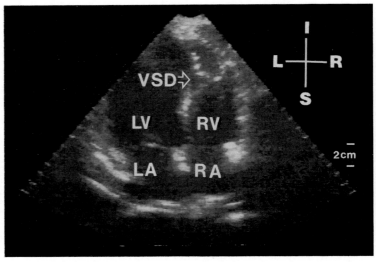

Figure 9-8B. Apical four-chamber view (reversed) in systole. Note rupture of the midseptum (VSD) into the right ventricle. The patient had a massive anterior septal infarction.

198

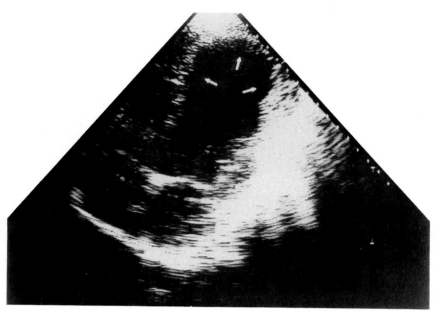

Figure 9-9. Apical four-chamber view. A large apical aneurysm (arrows) is evident in the left ventricle.

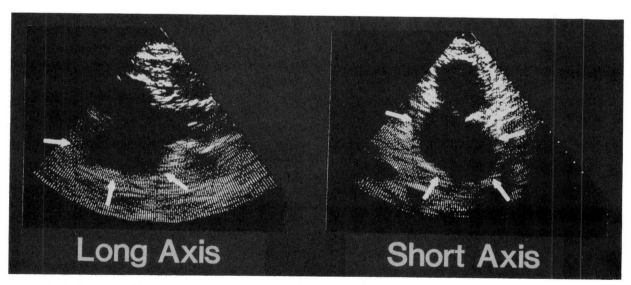

Figure 9-10. Parasternal long-axis and short-axis views. A left ventricular aneurysm (arrows) is located in the true posterior wall. Note the wide neck and fundus of the aneurysm.

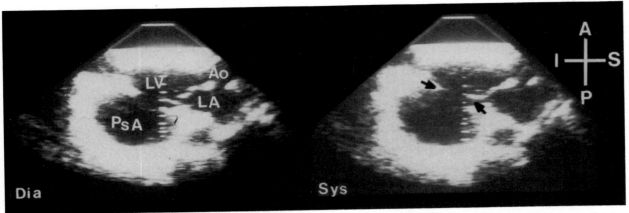

Figure 9-11. Parasternal long-axis view of a patient with a posterior-basal myocardial infarction resulting in a pseudoaneurysm (PsA). Note the wide body and narrow neck (black arrows) of the pseudoaneurysm. Note also the thrombus filling the inferior portion of the fundus. (Courtesy of Dr. Philip Liebson.)

expansion or bulging as the rest of the myocardium contracts inwardly. Akinesis rather than dyskinesis, however, may also be present.

Pseudoaneurysms—caused by rupture of the ventricular wall and sealing of the perforation by pericardium, a rim of thrombus, and fibrous tissue—have also been reported using two-dimensional echocardiography. The key to differentiating the two entities involves visualization of the typically narrow neck of the pseudoaneurysm (Figure 9-11) as opposed to the normally wide margin surrounding a true aneurysm (see Figure 9-10).[70] In addition, the pseudoaneurysms more commonly are filled with thrombus.

Left Ventricular Thrombus

Left ventricular thrombus is common in myocardial infarction, particularly within a left ventricular aneurysm. The two-dimensional echocardiographic appearance of ventricular thrombus is generally a distinct mass of echoes clearly seen in both systole and diastole that appears to be discrete, projecting into the ventricular cavity and usually contiguous with the endocardium or occasionally attached to an atrioventricular valve (Figure 9-12).[71] Well-defined contraction abnormalities are usually present in the underlying left ventricular myocardium (Figures 9-13 and 9-14). Echocardiographic "noise" sometimes causes confusion because it is usually less well defined than a thrombus, does not move with the underlying ventricular wall, and often is present only in systole or diastole in a single echocardiographic review.

Coronary Artery Visualization

The ability to visualize the proximal coronary arteries by two-dimensional echocardiography has been an exciting development in the assessment of ischemic heart disease. Weyman et al[72] and others have shown that the two-dimensional technique can be used to visualize the orifices of the left and often also the right coronary artery.[73] Ultrasonic contrast techniques, using intravascular catheters that were selectively inserted into the coronary ostia, have validated the echocardiographic

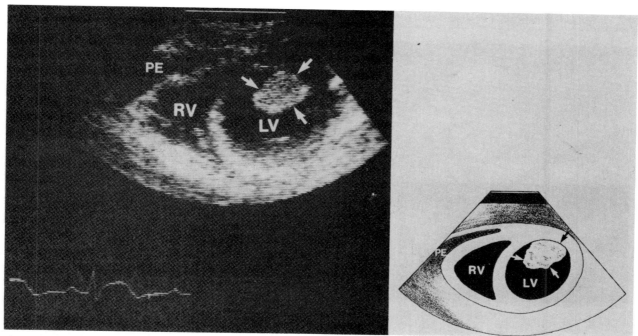

Figure 9-12. Apical short-axis view of left ventricular apical thrombus (arrows) 7 days after actue anterior myocardial infarction at left; artist's drawing at right. Such thrombi are usually seen within a left ventricular aneurysm or are associated with contraction abnormalities of the underlying left ventricular myocardium. PE denotes pericardial effusion. (From Asinger RW, Mikell FL, Sharma B, et al: Observations on detecting left ventricular thrombus with two-dimensional echocardiography. Am J Cardiol 47:145, 1981. With permission.)

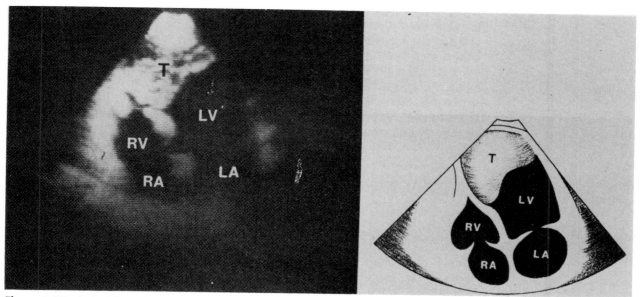

Figure 9-13. Apical four-chamber view of left ventricular apical thrombus (T) 10 days after acute myocardial infarction at left; artist's drawing at right. The thrombus is observed to fill the fundus of a large apical aneurysm. (From Asinger RW, Mikell FL, Sharma B, et al: Observations on detecting left ventricular thrombus with two-dimensional echocardiography. Am J Cardiol 47:145, 1981. With permission.)

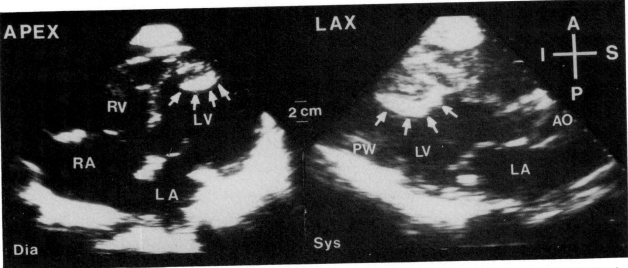

Figure 9-14. Apical four-chamber view (APEX) and parasternal long-axis view (LAX) of a patient with a large apical thrombus 10 days after an extensive anterior septal myocardial infarction. Note the discrete echo mass (arrows) contiguous with the anterior wall endocardium.

observations. This technique has been used to detect proximal coronary artery stenosis, especially left main coronary artery lesions.[73,74] It is clear that left main coronary stenosis has been detected in some patients by two-dimensional echocardiography, but the true sensitivity and specificity of the technique used in this manner has not been well established.

Recent work has suggested that identifying high-intensity echoes from arterial plaques may materially aid the accuracy of this potentially useful application. In one small study left main coronary artery disease was detected with the echocardiographic criteria of either asymmetric high-intensity wall density or disruption of the arterial lumen in 12 (75 percent) of 16 patients.[75] Recently coronary artery fistulas have also been detected by identifying the dilated coronary artery by two-dimensional echocardiography.[76]

REFERENCES

1. Tennant R, Wiggers CJ: The effect of coronary occlusion on myocardial contraction. Am J Physiol 112:351, 1935
2. Prinzmetal M, Schwartz LL, Corday E, et al: Studies on the coronary circulation. VI. Loss of myocardial contractility after coronary artery occlusion. Ann Intern Med 31:429, 1949
3. Wyatt HL, Forrester JS, da Luz PL, et al: Functional abnormalities in non-occluded regions of myocardium after experimental coronary occlusion. Am J Cardiol 37:366, 1976
4. Heikkila J, Tabakin BS, Hugenholtz PG: Quantification of myocardial function in normal and infarcted regions of the left ventricle. Cardiovasc Res 6:516, 1972
5. Theroux P, Franklin D, Ross J Jr, et al: Regional myocardial function and electrophysiological alterations after brief coronary artery occlusion in conscious dogs. J Clin Invest 56:978, 1975
6. Heyndrickx G, Millar RW, McRitchie RJ, et al: Regional myocardial function and electrophysiological alterations after brief coronary artery occlusion in conscious dogs. J Clin Invest 56:978, 1975

7. Sayen JJ, Sheldon WF, Peirce G, et al: Polarographic oxygen, the epicardial electrogram and muscle contraction in experimental acute regional ischemia. Circ Res 6:779, 1958

8. Tabooks CJ, Randall WC: Local ventricular bulging after acute coronary occlusion. Am J Physiol 201:451, 1961

9. Schelbert HR, Corbell J, Burns JW, et al: Observations on factors affecting local forces in the left ventricular wall during acute myocardial ischemia. Circ Res 39:306, 1971

10. Yosidar S: Experimental studies of coronary insufficiency 1. Changes in myocardial contractility in the ischemic area of the ventricle following acute coronary occlusion. Jpn Circ J 33:1253, 1969

11. Puri PS, Bing RJ: Effect of drugs on myocardial contractility in the intact dog and in experimental infarction. Am J Cardiol 21:886, 1968

12. Hood WB Jr, Covell J, Abelmann H, et al: Persistence of contractile behavior in acutely ischemic myocardium. Cardiovasc Res 3:249, 1969

13. Tyberg JV, Forrester JS, Wyatt HL, et al: An analysis of segmental ischemic dysfunction utilizing the pressure length loop. Circulation 49:748, 1974

14. Stefan G, Bing RJ: Echocardiographic findings in experimental myocardial infarction of the posterior left ventricular wall. Am J Cardiol 30:629, 1972

15. Kerber RE, Abboud FM: Echocardiographic detection of regional myocardial infarction. An experimental study. Circulation 47:997, 1973

16. Kerber RE, Marcus ML, Wilson R, et al: Effects of acute coronary occlusion on the motion and perfusion of the normal and ischemic interventricular septum: An experimental echocardiographic study. Circulation 54:928, 1976

17. Kerber RE, Abboud FM: Effect of alterations of arterial pressure and heart rate on segmental dyskinesis during acute myocardial ischemia and following coronary reperfusion. Circ Res 36:145, 1975

18. Kerber RE, Marcus ML, Ehrhardt J, et al: Correlation between echocardiographically demonstrated segmental dyskinesis and regional myocardial perfusion. Circulation 52:1097, 1975

19. Kerber RE, Marcus M, Abboud FM: Effect of inotropic agents on the localized dyskinesis of acutely ischemic myocardium: An experimental ultrasound study. Circulation 49:1038, 1974

20. Komer RR, Edalji A, Hood WB: Effects of nitroglycerine on echocardiographic measurements of left ventricular wall thickness and regional myocardial performance during acute coronary ischemia. Circulation 59:926, 1979

21. Likoff M, Reichek N, Macoriak J et al: High frequency epicardial echo mapping of segmental myocardial performance at multiple sites on right and left ventricles (Abstract), Am J Cardiol 47:403, 1981

22. Meerbaum S, Wyatt HL, Heng MK, et al: Quantification of ischemic dysfunctioning myocardium in dogs (Abstract). Circulation 56 (Suppl III):III-89, 1977

23. Heng MK, Lang TW, Toshimitsu T, et al: Quantification of myocardial ischemic damage by two-dimensional echocardiography (Abstract). Circulation 56(Suppl III):III-125, 1977

24. Meltzer RS, Woythaler JN, Buda AJ, et al: Two-dimensional echocardiographic quantification of infarct size alteration by pharmacologic agents. Am J Cardiol 44:257, 1979

25. Meltzer R, Jang G, Woythaler JN, et al: Correlation of 2-dimensional echocardiographic measurement of infarct size with anterior descending coronary distributional area in canine hearts. Circulation 60(Suppl II):II-152, 1979

26. Lieberman AN, Weiss JL, Jugdutt BI, et al: Two-dimensional echocardiography and infarct size: Relationship of regional wall motion and thickening to the extent of myocardial infarction in the dog. Circulation 63:739, 1981

27. Weyman AE, Franklin TD, Egenes KM, et al: Correlation between extent of abnormal regional wall motion and myocardial infarct size in chronically infarcted dogs. Circulation 56(Suppl III):III-72, 1977

28. Kisslo J, Ideker R, Harrison L, et al: Serial wall changes after acute myocardial infarction by two-dimensional echo. Circulation 60:(Suppl II):II-151, 1979

29. Pandian N, Kerber R: Ultrasonic sonomicrometers vs. 2-D echocardiography in the detection of transient myocardial dyskinesis. Circulation 62(Suppl III):III-328, 1980

30. Pandian N, Koyanagi S, Eastham C, et al: Relationships between two-dimensional echocardiographic wall thickening abnormalities, infarct size and coronary risk area in dogs. Circulation 62(Suppl III):III-186, 1980

31. Pandian N, Kerber R: Two-dimensional echocardiographic assessment of wall thinning and its relation to perfusion during graded coronary stenosis. Am J Cardiol 47:1384, 1981

32. Pandian N, Kieso R, Kerber R: Relationship between myocardial blood flow by layer and abnormalities of wall thickening on two-dimensional echocardiograms. Experimental studies (Abstract). Clin Res 30:597A, 1981

33. Pandian N, Koyanagi S, Skorton D, et al: Effect of left ventricular hypertrophy on two-dimensional echocardiographic evaluation of infarct size and risk area in dogs (Abstract). Circulation 64(Suppl IV):IV-204, 1981
34. Wyatt HL, Heng MK, Meerbaum S, Cross-sectional echocardiography. I. Analysis of mathematic models for quantifying mass of the left ventricle of dogs. Circulation 60:1104, 1979
35. Folts JD, Gallagher J, Rowe GG: Hemodynamic effects of controlled degrees of coronary artery stenosis in short-term and long-term studies in dogs. J Thorac Cardiovasc Surg 73:722, 1977
36. Weiss JL, Bulkley BH, Hutchins GM, et al: Two-dimensional echocardiographic recognition of myocardial injury in man: Comparison with post-mortem studies. Circulation 63:401, 1981
37. Blumenthal DS, Becker LS, Bulkley BH, et al: Impaired function of "salvaged" myocardium. Clin Res 29:178A, 1981
38. Sahn DJ, Barratt-Boyes B, Graham K, et al: Cross-sectional ultrasonic imaging of the coronary arteries in open chest humans; the evaluation of coronary atherosclerotic lesions at surgery. Am J Cardiol 47:403, 1981
39. DeMaria AN, Bommer WJ, Riggs K, et al: Echocardiographic visualization of myocardial perfusion by left heart and intracoronary injection of echo contrast agents. Circulation 62(Suppl III):III-143, 1981
40. Bommer WJ, Rason J, Tickner G, et al: Quantitative regional myocardial perfusion scanning with contrast echocardiography. Am J Cardiol 47:403, 1981
41. Corya BC, Rasmussen S, Knoebel SB, et al: Echocardiography in acute myocardial infarction. Am J Cardiol 36:1, 1975
42. Corya BC, Feigenbaum H, Rasmussen S, et al: Anterior left ventricular wall echos in coronary artery disease. Linear scanning with a single element transducer. Am J Cardiol 34:652, 1974
43. Corya BC, Rasmussen S, Feigenbaum H, et al: Systolic thickening and thinning of the septum and posterior wall in patients with coronary artery disease, congestive cardiomyopathy, and atrial septal defect. Circulation 55:109, 1977
44. Jacobs JJ, Feigenbaum H, Corya BC, et al: Detection of left ventricular asynergy by echocardiography. Circulation 48:263, 1973
45. Dortimer AC, DeJoseph RL, Shiroff RA, et al: Distribution of coronary artery disease: Prediction by echocardiography. Circulation 54:724, 1976
46. Joffe CD, Brik H, Teichholz LE, et al: Echocardiographic diagnosis of left anterior descending coronary artery disease. Am J Cardiol 40:11, 1977
47. Gordon MJ, Kerber RE: Interventricular septal motion in patients with proximal and distal left anterior descending coronary artery lesions. Circulation 55:338, 1977
48. Teichholz LE, Cohn MD, Sonnenblick E: Study of left ventricular geometry and function by B scan ultrasonography in patients with and without asynergy. N Engl J Med 291:1220, 1974
49. Kisslo JA, Robertson D, Gilbert BW, et al: The comparison of real-time two-dimensional echocardiography and cineangiography in detecting left ventricular asynergy. Circulation 54:134, 1977
50. Heger JJ, Weyman AE, Wann LS, et al: Cross-sectional echocardiographic analysis of the extent of left ventricular asynergy in acute myocardial infarction. Circulation 61:1113, 1980
51. Eaton LW, Weiss JL, Bulkley BH, et al: Regional cardiac dilatation after acute myocardial infarction. Recognition by two-dimensional echocardiography. N Engl J Med 300:57, 1979
52. Erlebacher JA, Weiss JL, Eaton LW, et al: Late effects of infarct dilatation on heart size: A two-dimensional study. Am J Cardiol 49, 1120–1126, 1982
53. Mason SJ, Weiss JL, Weisfeldt ML, et al: Exercise echocardiography: Detection of wall motion abnormalities during ischemia. Circulation 59:50, 1979
54. Crawford MH, White DH, Amon KW: Echocardiographic evaluation of left ventricular size and performance during hand grip and supine and upright bicycle exercise. Circulation 59:1188, 1979
55. Wann LS, Farris JV, Childress RH, et al: Exercise cross-sectional echocardiography in ischemic heart disease. Circulation 60:1300, 1979
56. Mitamura H, Ogawa S, Hori S, et al: Two dimensional echocardiographic analysis of wall motion abnormalities during handgrip exercise in patients with coronary artery disease. Am J Cardiol 48:711–719, 1981
57. Pandian N, Skorton D, Collins S, et al: Heterogeneity of segmental left ventricular wall thickening and exercusion in two-dimensional echocardiograms in normal humans. Am J Cardiol 47:452, 1981
58. Horowitz RS, Morganroth J, Parrotto C, et al: Immediate diagnosis of acute myocardial infarction by two-dimensional echocardiography. Circulation 65:323–329, 1982
59. Moynihan PF, Parisi AF, Feldman CL: Quantitative detection of regional left ventricular contraction abnormalities by two-dimensional echocardiography. I. Analysis of methods. Circulation 63:752, 1981

60. Parisi AF, Moynihan PF, Folland ED, et al: Quantitative detection of regional left ventricular contraction abnormalities by two-dimensional echocardiography. II. Accuracy in coronary artery disease. Circulation 63:761, 1981

61. Folland ED, Parisi AF, Moynihan PF, et al: Assessment of left ventricular ejection fraction and volume by real-time two-dimensional echocardiography. A comparison of cineangiographic and radionuclide technique. Circulation 60:716, 1979

62. Schiller NB, Acquatella H, Ports TA, et al: Left ventricular-volume from paired biplane two-dimensional echocardiography. Circulation 60:547:1979

63. Gueret P, Meerbaum S, Wyatt HL, et al: Two-dimensional echocardiographic quantitation of left ventricular volume and ejection fraction. Importance of accounting for dysenergy in short axis reconstruction models. Circulation 62:1308, 1980

64. Drobec M, Morgan CD, Gilbert BW, et al: Complicated acute myocardial infarction. The importance of two-dimensional echocardiography (Abstract). Am J Cardiol 43:387, 1979

65. Heger J, Weyman AE, Noble R, et al: An analysis of site, extent and hemodynamic consequences of acute myocardial infarction by cross-sectional echocardiography (Abstract). Circulation 56(Suppl III):III-152, 1977

66. Mintz GS, Victor MF, Kotler MN, et al: Two-dimensional echocardiographic identification of surgically correctable complications of acute myocardial infarction. Circulation 64:91, 1981

67. Scanlan JG, Seward JB, Tajik AJ: Visualization of ventricular septal rupture utilizing wide angle two-dimensional echocardiography. Mayo Clin Proc 54:381, 1979

68. Farcut JC, Borsante L, Rigaud M, et al: Two-dimensional echocardiographic visualization of ventricular septal rupture after acute anterior myocardial infarction. Am J Cardiol 45:370, 1980

69. Weyman AE, Peskoe SM, Williams ES, et al: Detection of left ventricular aneurysms by cross-sectional echocardiography. Circulation 54:936, 1976

70. Catherwood E, Mintz GS, Kotler MN, et al: Two-dimensional echocardiographic recognition of left ventricular pseudoaneurysm. Circulation 62:294, 1980

71. Asinger RW, Mikell FL, Sharma B, et al: Observations on detecting left ventricular thrombus with two-dimensional echocardiography. Am J Cardiol 47:145, 1981

72. Weyman AE, Feigenbaum H, Dillon JC, et al: Noninvasive visualization of the left main coronary artery by cross-sectional echocardiography. Circulation 54:169, 1976

73. Rogers EW, Feigenbaum H, Weyman AE, et al: Evaluation of left coronary artery anatomy in vitro using cross-sectional echocardiography. Circulation 62:782, 1980

74. Rogers EW, Feigenbaum H, Weyman AE, et al: Possible detection of atherosclerotic coronary calcification by two-dimensional echocardiography. Circulation 62:1046, 1980

75. Rink LD, Feigenbaum H, Godley RW, et al: Echocardiographic detection of left main coronary artery obstruction. Circulation 65:719–724, 1982

76. Yoshikawa J, Katao H, Yanagihara K, et al: Noninvasive visualization of the dilated main coronary arteries in coronary artery fistulas by cross-sectional echocardiography. Circulation 65:600–603, 1982

CHAPTER 10

Primary and Secondary Cardiomyopathies

James B. Seward and Abdul J. Tajik

Over the past several years echocardiography has become increasingly more important in recognizing the various cardiomyopathies and assessing them anatomically and functionally.[1] M-mode echocardiography reliably differentiates the basic subgroups of cardiomyopathies (dilated, hypertrophic, and restrictive) and can indicate degrees of global and regional myocardial function. Secondary cardiomyopathies such as amyloidosis,[2] Friedreich's ataxia,[3,4] glycogen-storage disease, and Fabry's disease[5] have received less attention; but in the proper clinical setting they can also be recognized and characterized noninvasively. In particular, two-dimensional echocardiography[6] provides a better diagnostic tool for recognizing the spectrum of myocardial pathology and for separating the primary and secondary cardiomyopathies from diseases with similar clinical presentations.

The following discussion illustrates the echocardiographic features of the primary and the common secondary cardiomyopathies. It is our experience that two-dimensional echocardiography, with its ability to portray anatomic and functional patterns of the various cardiomyopathies, is superior to angiography and other present-day imaging modalities.

PRIMARY CARDIOMYOPATHIES

Three groups of primary cardiomyopathies are recognized as to their anatomic presentation; in order of frequency they are the dilated (Figure 10-1A), the hypertrophic (Figure 10-1B), and the primary restrictive types (Figure 10-1C). Each of these cardiomyopathies has characteristic clinical and echocardiographic features. Where applicable, more commonly encountered secondary cardiomyopathies are also discussed.

Dilated Cardiomyopathy

Characteristics of dilated cardiomyopathy are increased left ventricular chamber dimensions and reduced left ventricular systolic performance (Figures 10-2 and 10-3). Because the disease involves the entire heart, two-dimensional echocardiography can better assess global ventricular function. However, some patients with dilated cardiomyopathy have regional wall motion abnormalities indistinguishable from

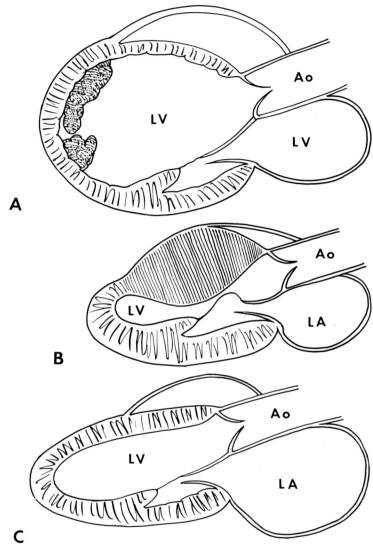

Figure 10-1. Two-dimensional echocardiographic features of primary cardiomyopathies. A: Idiopathic dilated cardiomyopathy—dilation of all chambers, global hypokinesis, reduced opening and closing excursion of valve leaflets, and frequent association of cavitary thrombus. B: Hypertrophic cardiomyopathy—asymmetric myocardial hypertrophy, normal-dimensioned left ventricle, systolic anterior motion of mitral valve, enlarged left atrium, highly refractile appearance of involved myocardium, and normal systolic contraction of uninvolved myocardium. C: Restrictive cardiomyopathy—normal ventricular cavity dimensions, enlarged (often massive) atrial dimensions, normal to moderately depressed ventricular systolic function. LV denotes left ventricle; Ao, aorta; LA, left atrium.

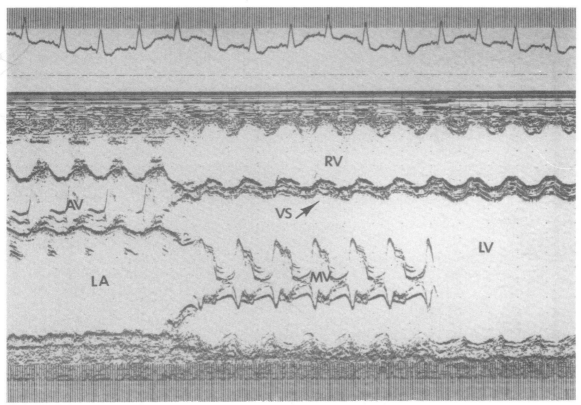

Figure 10-2. M-mode echocardiogram of dilated cardiomyopathy. All chambers are dilated. Myocardial walls show reduced excursion and reduced systolic contraction (thickening). Mitral Value (MV) often assumes a position in mid-left ventricle cavity. Premature systolic closure of aortic valve (AV) and delayed opening of mitral valve are consistent with reduced output and myocardial dysfunction. VS denotes ventricular septum.

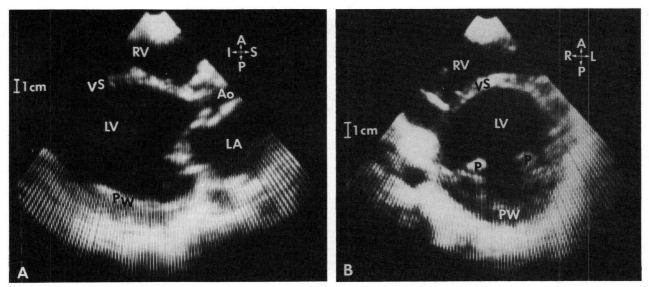

Figure 10-3. Two-dimensional echocardiographic features of dilated cardiomyopathy: parasternal long-axis (A) and short-axis (B) views. Markedly increased cavitary dimensions. Septal and posterior walls (PW) appear thin in comparison to increased cavities. Myocardium often appears hyper-refractile. RV denotes right ventricle; P, papillary muscle.

ischemic heart disease. Thus, an absolute distinction between end-stage ischemic cardiomyopathy and idiopathic dilated cardiomyopathy cannot always be made by echocardiography. At this stage of disease, however, absolute distinction is not clinically necessary.

More importantly, echocardiography can detect early global manifestations of a dilated cardiomyopathy and distinguish it from "segmental" ischemic heart disease or myocardial dysfunction secondary to valvular heart disease. This distinction depends on a detailed two-dimensional echocardiographic examination of segmental wall motion as well as cardiac valves and chambers. Two-dimensional echocardiography can exclude other secondary disease states whose presentation may resemble that of an enlarged, dilated heart, such as valvular heart disease, cardiac tumor, infective endocarditis, and intracardiac shunts.

Not only the left ventricle but also the right ventricle and the atria are increased in dimension (see Figure 10-1A). The myocardium is often highly refractile, a feature thought to represent myocardial scarring and fibrosis. Although thinning of the myocardium is part of the myopathy, more typically the myocardium is nearly normal in thickness; it appears thin, however, in comparison to the inordinately dilated cardiac chamber.

Another feature of dilated cardiomyopathy is the reduced global systolic performance. The two-dimensionally directed M-mode examination best reveals the relevant changes in global and regional function (i.e., ejection fraction, fractional shortening.[7] Myocardial wall excursion is reduced, and valve motion may reflect a low cardiac output state and reduced myocardial performance (i.e., premature systolic closure of the semilunar valves, delayed end-diastolic closure and reduced opening velocity of the atrioventricular valves). When functional incompetence of the atrioventricular valves is also present, myocardial wall may have normal or reduced excursion but abnormal systolic wall thickening.[8] Among patients with dilated cardiomyopathy, approximately 30 percent have an echo-detected ventricular thrombus,[9,10] which is usually confined to the apex of the ventricle (Figure 10-4).

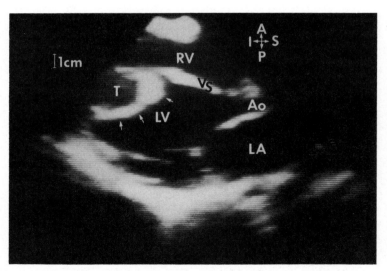

Figure 10-4. Dilated cardiomyopathy with large apical septal thrombus (T, arrows) having central echolucency. Left ventricle and left atrium are enlarged. (From Reeder GS, Tajik AJ, Seward JB: Left ventricular mural thrombus: Two-dimensional echocardiographic diagnosis. Mayo Clin Proc 56:82–86, 1981. With permission.)

In summary, two-dimensional echocardiography and simultaneous M-mode examination, by excluding other diseases, measuring global ventricular function, and delineating its complications, have supplanted cardiac catheterization in the diagnosis and characterization of dilated cardiomyopathy.

Hypertrophic Cardiomyopathy

There are two forms of hypertrophic cardiomyopathy: the obstructive and the nonobstructive type.[1] The obstructive form accounts for approximately 9 of 10 cases. Echocardiographic features of the obstructive form consist of systolic anterior motion of the mitral valve, cavitary obliteration, and midsystolic closure of the aortic valve. In occasional cases, obstructive features become evident only with vasoactive maneuvers such as the valsalva.[11] Both the obstructive and nonobstructive forms, however, are characterized by asymmetric septal hypertrophy (septal thickness 1.3 or more times posterior wall thickness), reduced ventricular diastolic compliance, small-to normal-sized left ventricular cavity, and normal or increased systolic function.[12,13] The two entities, although different in their clinical manifestation, appear to have similar prognoses.

In obstructive hypertrophic cardiomyopathy, the hypertrophy characteristically affects the ventricular septum, resulting in septal thickness exceeding posterior wall thickness by a factor of 1.3 or greater (asymmetric septal hypertrophy; see Figure 10-5).[12] M-mode echocardiography may erroneously overestimate septal thickness if the ultrasound beam is obliquely angulated through the septum.[14] The hypertrophic myocardium contracts poorly and appears highly refractile on two-dimensional echocardiography (Figures 10-5A, B). This refractile change is thought to be related to the myopathic process—possibly fibrosis, myocardial cell disarray or increased connective tissue content.

The ventricular cavity is invariably small; the uninvolved myocardium contracts either hyperdynamically or normally. The papillary muscles are usually of normal dimension. Although congestive heart failure may develop, a dilated left ventricle or reduced systolic ventricular performance is rare.

The level of ventricular obstruction can be best appreciated by two-dimensional echocardiography. Frequently the papillary muscles abut on the ventricular septum and obliterate the midcavity (Figure 10-6). An explanation for the systolic anterior motion of the mitral valve is the Venturi effect produced by the increased left ventricular outflow turbulence resulting in a transient lowering of pressure in the left ventricular outflow tract, which pulls the mitral structures superiorly during systole.[16,17] That portion of the mitral valve apparatus that shows systolic anterior motion varies from the body of the mitral leaflets to the heads of the papillary muscles and their chordae tendineae[18] (Figure 10-7). Rodger described systolic anterior motion as a complex of echoes from the chordae tendineae, the papillary muscle, and the anterior mitral leaflet, the latter structure being the furthest from and not impinging upon the septum.[19]

Two-dimensional echocardiography is superior to M-mode for appreciation of the varied distribution of the hypertrophic process[20] (Figure 10-8). Older patients typically have a more localized basal septal hypertrophy; younger ones characteristically have a more extensive myopathic process with fusiform hypertrophy of the ventricular septum.[21] During youth the incidence of echo-detected right ventricular outflow obstruction is also higher.[22,23] Infrequently encountered forms include apical septal involvement and isolated free wall hypertrophy.[24] An observation that has not been adequately emphasized is that the majority of patients with hypertrophic cardiomyopathy also have left ventricular lateral free wall involvement.

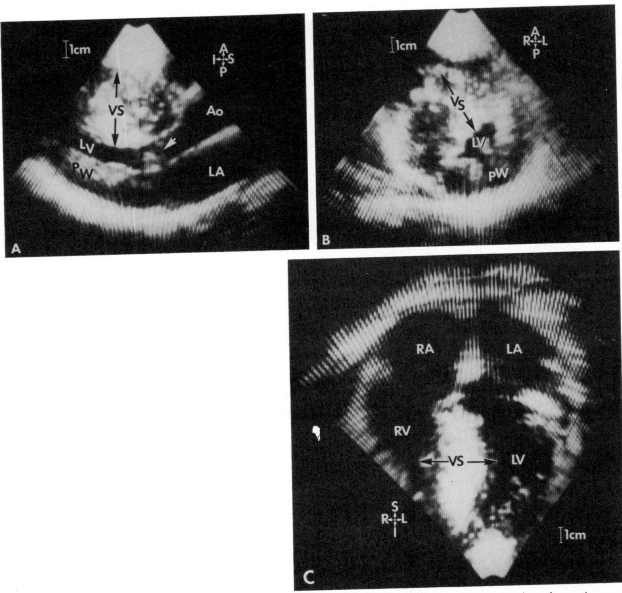

Figure 10-5. Two-dimensional echocardiographic features of hypertrophic obstructive cardiomyopathy. A: Parasternal long-axis view showing large fusiform hypertrophic segment of ventricular septum (VS, black arrows). The posterior wall (PW) is of nearly normal thickness. This systolic frame also demonstrates systolic anterior motion of mitral valve (white arrow). B: Parasternal short-axis view illustrating distribution of septal hypertrophy (VS, arrows). Note that papillary muscles appear normal in dimension. Septal or myocardial hypertrophy extends from lower septum to anterior free wall of left ventricle. Only the posterior wall appears to be totally spared. C: Apical four-chamber view showing hypertrophied ventricular septum. Septal thickness appears to begin at the base of the heart and extend in a fusiform manner, ending just short of the apex.

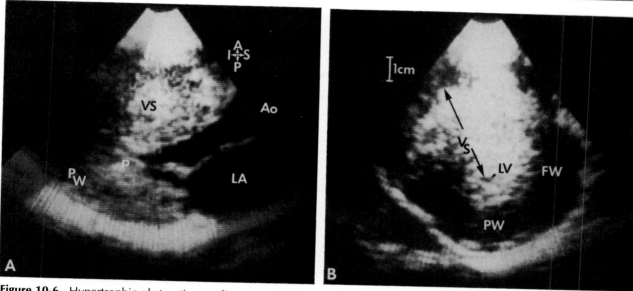

Figure 10-6. Hypertrophic obstructive cardiomyopathy. A: Parasternal long-axis view showing systolic cavitary obliteration at the level of the papillary muscle (p). Note the marked increase in ventricular septal (VS) thickness. B: Parasternal short-axis view of left ventricle shows nearly complete cavitary obliteration (LV, small arrow). This systolic frame shows asymmetric septal hypertrophy, and the free wall (FW) and posterior wall (PW) also appear significantly thickened.

Preoperative knowledge of the distribution of myocardial hypertrophy is important when surgical myectomy or myotomy is indicated. With preoperative echocardiographic mapping of the hypertrophic process, the surgeon can better anticipate the level as well as the extent of the resection required. Such planning will reduce the chance of an ineffectual surgical procedure and obviate iatrogrenic complications such as ventricular septal defect. Postoperative two-dimensional echocardiography can be very useful in evaluating the anatomic and functional result of myotomy procedure.[25]

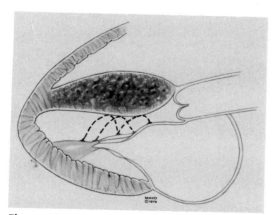

Figure 10-7. Variable appearance of systolic anterior motion of mitral valve. Mitral valve apparatus shows various motion abnormalities from the body of the mitral leaflets to the head of the papillary muscle and their support apparatus.

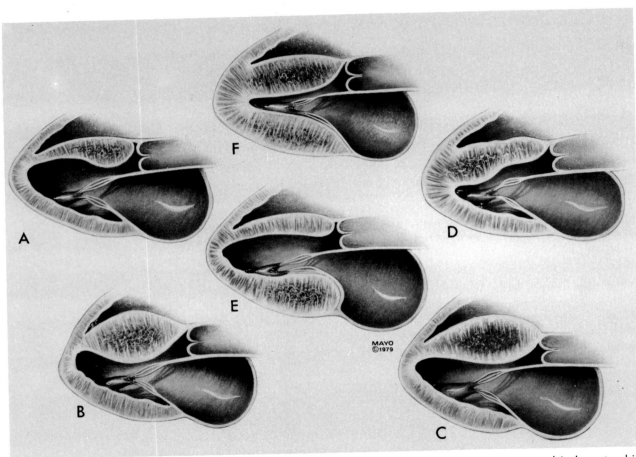

Figure 10-8. Variable distribution of myocardial hypertrophy encountered in hypertrophic cardiomyopathy. A, B, and C show common kinds of septal hypertrophy. Less frequently encountered variants are apical hypertrophy (D) and isolated free wall or posterior basal hypertrophy (E). F is more generalized hypertrophy as encountered with the nonobstructive form of hypertrophic cardiomyopathy.

Restrictive Cardiomyopathy

Primary Type

Primary restrictive cardiomyopathy is a poorly understood entity (Figure 10-9). Most accounts describe Loeffler's endocarditis—which is characterized by eosinophilia, an associated febrile state often resembling active endocarditis, ventricular thrombus, normal ventricular dimensions, and biventricular dysfunction[26,27] (Figure 10-9A). A second entity, endomyocardial fibrosis, is more commonly encountered in tropical zones of the world and is characterized by normal cardiac dimensions, reduced ventricular compliance, predominance of right ventricular involvement, and left ventricular inflow obstruction secondary to thrombus.[1,28] In our practice these two forms of restrictive cardiomyopathy are very rare, and their presentation is not often classic. Under such circumstances the two-dimensional echocardiogram often is very helpful. Because of massive accumulation of cavitary thrombus, there usually is a history of systemic embolization (Figure 10-10).

By far the more common primary restrictive cardiomyopathy encountered in the United States is a nondilated myopathy with clinical features of reduced ventricular compliance; often systolic ventricular function is preserved.[1,29,30] There usually is no inordinate increase in the incidence of cavitary thrombus or systemic embolization. The echocardiogram typically reveals normal ventricular dimensions, dilated atria, normal or moderately depressed global systolic function, and normal myocardial thickness often associated with a highly refractile pattern suggesting scarring or fibrosis (see Figure 10-9B).

Primary restrictive cardiomyopathy (nondilated, nonhypertrophic ventricles) is the most challenging entity of this group. A correct diagnosis can be made confidently on the basis of clinical and echocardiographic examination in the majority of cases; but in practice a diagnosis of restrictive cardiomyopathy based on two-dimensional echocardiography usually is followed by invasive studies such as cardiac catheterization (including endomyocardial biopsy)—and in selected cases by thoracotomy—as one must exclude the possibility of constrictive pericarditis in this situation.

Secondary Type: Amyloid Heart Disease

Of secondary restrictive cardiomyopathies, amyloid heart disease is the most common subgroup encountered. Others forms which have been studied echocardiographically include hemochromatosis and glycogen storage disease.[31-34] Usually amyloid cardiomyopathy appears in older patients who have heart failure characterized by prominent right-heart findings of ascites and peripheral edema.[2] Echocardiographically, the myocardium appears thickened and hyper-refractile with variable reduction in ventricular performance (Figures 10-9C and 10-11).

Other features of amyloid heart disease include pericardial effusion, uniform increase of myocardial wall thickness (particularly notable in the right ventricular myocardium), thickened highly refractile valve leaflets, and a thickened atrial septum.[35] Usually there is uniform increase in myocardial wall thickness; occasionally, however, there is asymmetric hypertrophy of the septum or free wall of the left ventricle. Right or left ventricular involvement may predominate. A granular echocardiographic appearance of the myocardium is said to be characteristic but is not pathognomonic of this disease. It may also be encountered with other hypertrophic states, including hypertrophic cardiomyopathy, infiltrative myopathies such as gly-

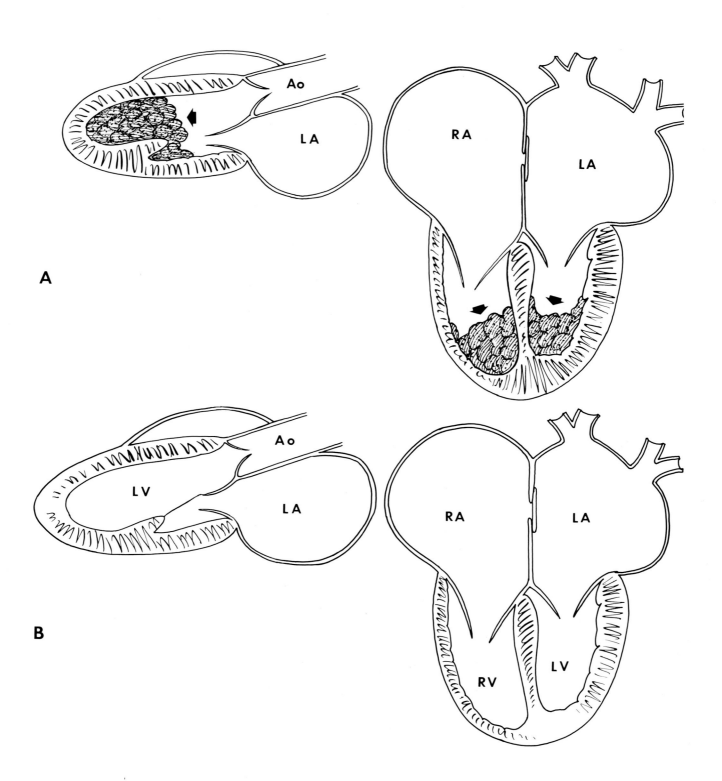

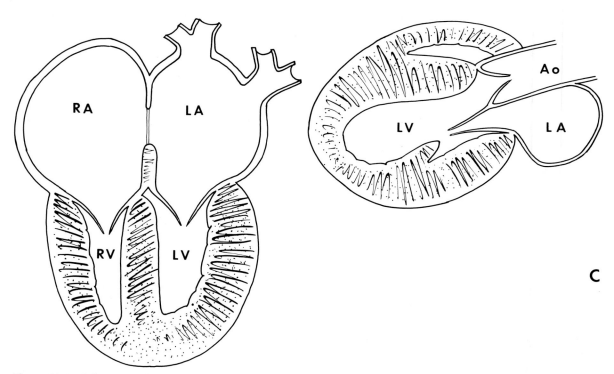

Figure 10-9. Subgroups of restrictive cardiomyopathy. A: Obliterative myopathy characteristic of Loeffler's endocarditis and endomyocardial fibrosis typified by normal ventricular dimensions, large accumulations of cavitary thrombus (arrows), moderate reduction in systolic ventricular performance, and dilated atria. B: Idiopathic restrictive cardiomyopathy (nondilated cardiomyopathy)—normal ventricular dimensions, normal to moderately reduced systolic ventricular performance, usually no evidence of cavitary thrombus, frequent association with marked atrial dilatation. C: Amyloid heart disease—increased myocardial wall thickness involving both ventricles and both atria and their septa. Generalized granular appearance and hyper-refractile echo are characteristic.

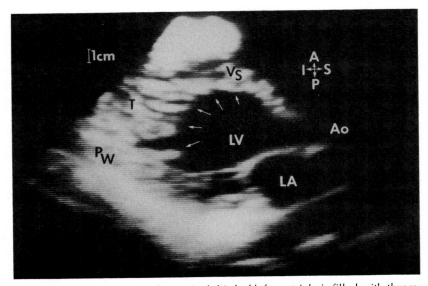

Figure 10-10. Obliterative cardiomyopathy. Apical third of left ventricle is filled with thrombus (arrows, T). Left atrium is markedly dilated. (Right ventricular cavity had similar massive accumulation of thrombus material.) (From Reeder GS, Tajik AJ, Seward JB: Left ventricular mural thrombus: Two-dimensional echocardiographic diagnosis. Mayo Clin Proc 56:82–86, 1981. With permission.)

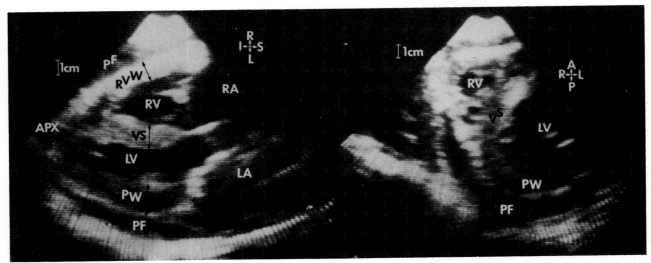

Figure 10-11. Amyloid heart disease: four-chamber and short-axis views. All myocardial walls are thickened; there are a general increase in refractile pattern and a moderate-sized pericardial effusion (PF). Of particular note is the increased thickness of right ventricular wall (RVW). (From Siqueira-Filho AG, Cunha CLP, Tajik AJ, et al: M-mode and two-dimensional echocardiographic features in cardiac amyloidosis. Circulation 63:188–196, 1981. By permission of American Heart Association, Inc.)

cogen-storage disease, hypertension or post-renal-transplant states, Fabry's disease, and hemochromatosis.

Especially important for a correct echocardiographic interpretation is clinical assessment. Amyloid heart disease is more common among elderly patients who present with biventricular heart failure. The electrocardiographic voltage is usually low in this disease, whereas it is increased in hypertrophic cardiomyopathy. With due attention to the clinical presentation as well as the typical electrocardiographic features, the characteristic two-dimensional echocardiogram can be virtually diagnostic of amyloid heart disease.

REFERENCES

1. Seward JB, Tajik AJ: Primary cardiomyopathies: Classification, pathophysiology, clinical recognition and management. Cardiovasc Clin 10:199–230, 1980
2. Siqueira-Filho A, Cunha CLP, Tajik AJ, et al: M-mode and two-dimensional echocardiographic features in cardiac amyloidosis. Circulation 63:188–196, 1981
3. Pasternac A, Krol R, Petitclerc R, et al: Hypertrophic cardiomyopathy in Friedreich's ataxia: Symmetric or asymmetric? Can J Neurol Sci 7:379–382, 1980
4. St John Sutton MG, Olukotun AY, Tajik AJ, et al: Left ventricular function in Friedreich's ataxia: An echocardiographic study. Br Heart J 44:309–316, 1980
5. Bass JL, Shrivastava S, Grabowski GA, et al: The M-mode echocardiogram in Fabry's disease. Am Heart J 10:807–812, 1980
6. Tajik AJ, Seward JB, Hagler DJ, et al: Two-dimensional real-time ultrasonic imaging of the heart and great vessels: Technique, image orientation, structure identification, and validation. Mayo Clin Proc 53:271–303, 1978
7. Quinones MA, Waggoner AD, Reduto LA, et al: A new, simplified and accurate method for determining ejection fraction with two-dimensional echocardiography. Circulation 64:744–753, 1981
8. Levisman JA: Echocardiographic diagnosis of mitral regurgitation in congestive cardiomyopathy. Am Heart J 93:33–39, 1977
9. Reeder GS, Tajik AJ, Seward JB: Left ventricular mural thrombus: two-dimensional echocardiographic diagnosis. Mayo Clin Proc 56:82–86, 1981
10. Asinger RW, Mikell FL, Sharma B, et al: Observations on detecting left ventricular thrombus with two-dimensional echocardiography: Emphasis on avoidance of false positive diagnoses. Am J Cardiol 47:145–156, 1981
11. Gilbert BW, Pollick C, Adelman AG, et al: Hypertrophic cardiomyopathy: subclassification by M-mode echocardiography. Am J Cardiol 45:861–872, 1980
12. Kansal S, Roitman D, Sheffield LT: Interventricular septal thickness and left ventricular hypertrophy: An echocardiographic study. Circulation 60:1058–1065, 1979
13. St John Sutton MG, Tajik AJ, Gibson DG, et al: Echocardiographic assessment of left ventricular filling and septal and posterior wall dynamics in idiopathic hypertrophic subaortic stenosis. Circulation 57:512–520, 1978
14. Fowles RE, Martin RP, Popp RL: Erroneous diagnosis of asymmetric septal hypertrophy due to angled interventricular septum (Abstract). Am J Cardiol 43:348, 1979
15. Silverman KJ, Hutchins GM, Weiss JL, et al: Catenoid shape of the interventricular septum in idiopathic hypertrophic subaortic stenosis: Two dimensional echocardiographic confirmation. Am J Cardiol 49:27–32, 1982
16. Sabbah HN, Alam M, Anbe DT, et al: Mid-systolic closure of the aortic valve in hypertrophic obstructive cardiomyopathy: A pressure-related phenomenon induced by turbulent blood flow. Cathet Cardiovasc Diagn 6:397–404, 1980
17. Henry WL, Clark CE, Griffith JM, et al: Mechanism of left ventricular outflow obstruction in patients with obstructive asymmetrical septal hypertrophy (idiopathic hypertrophic subaortic stenosis). Am J Cardiol 35:337, 1975
18. Tajik AJ, Seward JB, Hagler DJ: Detailed analysis of hypertrophic obstructive cardiomyopathy by wide-angle two-dimensional sector echocardiography (Abstract). Am J Cardiol 43:348, 1979
19. Rodger JC: Motion of mitral apparatus in hypertrophic cardiomyopathy with obstruction. Br Heart J 38:732, 1976
20. Maron BJ, Gottdiener JS, Bonow RO, et al: Hypertrophic cardiomyopathy with unusual locations

of left ventricular hypertrophy undetectable by M-mode echocardiography: Identification by wide-angle two-dimensional echocardiography. Circulation 63:409–418, 1981

21. Krasnow N, Stein RA: Hypertrophic cardiomyopathy in the aged. Am Heart J 96:326–336, 1978
22. Fiddler GI, Tajik AJ, Weidman WH, et al: Idiopathic hypertrophic subaortic stenosis in the young. Am J Cardiol 42:793–799, 1978
23. Cardiel EA, Alonso M, Delcan JL, et al: Echocardiographic sign of right-sided hypertrophic obstructive cardiomyopathy. Br Heart J 40:1321–1324, 1978
24. Yamaguchi H, Ishimura T, Nishiyama S, et al: Hypertrophic nonobstructive cardiomyopathy with giant negative T waves (apical hypertrophy): Ventriculographic and echocardiographic features in 30 patients. Am J Cardiol 44:401–412, 1979
25. Schapira JN, Stemple DR, Martin RP, et al: Single and two-dimensional echocardiographic visualization of the effects of septal myectomy in idiopathic hypertrophic subaortic stenosis. Circulation 58:850, 1978
26. Bell JA, Jenkins BS, Webb-Peploe MM: Clinical, haemodynamic, and angiographic findings in Loffler's eosinophilic endocarditis. Br Heart J 38:541–548, 1976
27. Rodger JC, Irvine KG, Lerski RA: Echocardiography in Loffler's endocarditis. Br Heart J 46:110–112, 1981
28. Somers K, Brenton DP, Sood NK: Clinical features of endomyocardial fibrosis of the right ventricle. Br Heart J 30:309–321, 1968
29. Benotti JR, Grossman W, Cohn PF: Clinical profile of restrictive cardiomyopathy. Circulation 61:1206–1212, 1980
30. Erath HG Jr, Graham TP Jr, Smith CW, et al: Restrictive cardiomyopathy in an infant with massive biatrial enlargement and normal ventricular size and pump function. Cathet Cardiovasc Diagn 4:289–296, 1978
31. Borer JS, Henry WJ, Epstein SE: Echocardiographic observations in patients with systemic infiltrative disease involving the heart. Am J Cardiol 39:184, 1977
32. Smith JW, Clements PJ, Levisman J, et al: Echocardiographic features of progressive systemic sclerosis (PSS): Correlation with hemodynamic and postmortem studies. Am J Med 66:28–37, 1979
33. Gottdiener JS, Moutsopoulos HM, Decker JL: Echocardiographic identification of cardiac abnormality in scleroderma and related disorders. Am J Med 66:391–399, 1979
34. Henry WL, Nienhuis AW, Wiener M, et al: Echocardiographic abnormalities in patients with transfusion-dependent anemia and secondary myocardial iron deposition. Am J Med 64:547–551, 1978
35. Maron BJ, Tajik AJ, Ruttenberg HD, et al: Hypertrophic cardiomyopathy in infants: Clinical features and natural history. Circulation 65:7–17, 1982

CHAPTER 11

Pericardial Disease

Ivan A. D'Cruz

It is generally accepted by clinicians that echocardiography is the method of choice for evaluation of the pericardium. Additionally, echocardiography has the advantage that it can be conveniently performed with short notice at the patient's bedside. M-mode echocardiography has proved quite useful in the routine assessment of patients with suspected pericardial disease. The work of Feigenbaum and associates in 1965 established ultrasound as a feasible and reliable means of detecting pericardial effusions.[1] Subsequent advances in the technique have been useful in the development of the following echocardiographic applications.

A semiquantitative classification of pericardial effusions into small, moderate, and large has been developed using the width of the M-mode echo-free space (representing fluid) posterior and anterior to the heart.[2] Exaggerated motion of the heart is a common feature in patients with large pericardial effusions.[3] This pendular or "swinging" movement presents an unmistakable appearance on the M-mode echocardiogram. In massive effusion this alternation in cardiac position on alternate beats explains the changes in the height of the electrocardiographic complexes (electrical alternans) and the intensity of heart sounds (auscultatory alternans). When cardiac tamponade develops in a patient with a large pericardial effusion, it is usually accompanied by exaggerated respiratory phasic changes in ventricular dimension (right ventricular enlargement during inspiration at the expense of left ventricular compression).[4] Right ventricular compression, abnormal right ventricular wall motion, and other less constant echocardiographic signs have also been described.

Various M-mode echocardiographic patterns have been described in patients with pericardial thickening or sclerosis.[5-7] If a pericardial effusion is also present, the epicardium (visceral pericardium) and parietal pericardium are easily identified as dense, thick layers. If no effusion is present, the visceral and parietal layers fuse and may appear as one of the following:

- It may appear as a single layer, relatively echo-free, that is of constant width and moves parallel to the left ventricular posterior wall. This pattern is distinguished from that of a small pericardial effusion in which there is a fluctuating width (wider in systole than in diastole) to the echo-free space.

- It may appear as a wide layer of dense, stratified linear echoes, representing an advanced degree of sclerosis or even calcification.
- Occasionally the space between the thickened epicardium and parietal pericardium is filled with multiple linear echoes or parallel lines. This third pattern results from dense fibrotic change or organizing pyogenic exudates within the pericardial space.

These M-mode patterns have their counterparts in two-dimensional echocardiography. Yet there is no definite association between any particular pattern and the presence of hemodynamically significant pericardial constriction.

Although several M-mode echocardiographic abnormalities have been described in constrictive pericarditis, this ultrasound diagnosis is much less reliable than that of pericardial effusion. The reason is that all the abnormal findings reported in patients with pericardial constriction are either nonspecific, inconstant or both.[5,8–11] Pericardial thickening is an essential feature. Most patients with thickened pericardium, however, do not exhibit the clinical syndrome of constrictive pericarditis even when the pericardial sclerosis is dense and impressive on the echocardiogram. Abnormal systolic motion of the ventricular septum, of either the paradoxical anterior (type A) or the flat akinetic (type B) variety, is often present. However, numerous other causes of this nonspecific finding must be excluded. After initial rapid ventricular filling, the left ventricular posterior wall remains "flat" during subsequent slow diastolic filling; in normals it drifts posteriorly to the extent of 2 to 4 mm. Premature pulmonic valve opening is only occasionally encountered. An increased mitral E-F slope is a nonspecific and inconstant finding.

The main shortcoming of M-mode echocardiography in evaluating pericardial effusions is that only a limited area of the left ventricular posterior wall and subjacent parietal pericardium can be scanned. The anterior pericardial space (anterior to the right ventricle) visualized by the M-mode technique is even smaller; the pericardial space around the apex and lateral wall of the left ventricle is not generally accessible by the M-mode technique. For this reason two-dimensional echocardiography is superior. On the other hand, the finer resolution and gray-scale display obtainable in high-quality M-mode tracings cannot be matched by current two-dimensional technology. Consequently, the detection of pericardial thickening, intrapericardial fibrin, pericardial exudate, and so forth, which depends on fine details of echocardiographic "texture," is at present still better evaluated by M-mode than two-dimensional echocardiography.

APPLICATION OF TWO-DIMENSIONAL ECHOCARDIOGRAPHY

As two-dimensional echocardiography became available during the late 1970s, its role in the diagnostic assessment of pericardial effusions was explored by several investigators.[6–10,12–16]

Pericardial Effusion

The two-dimensional echocardiographic appearances of pericardial effusion vary with the amount of pericardial fluid present.

With small pericardial effusions (Figure 11-1), the fluid is seen as a narrow slitlike

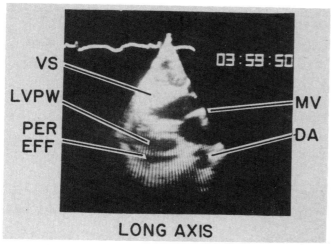

Figure 11-1. Two-dimensional echocardiogram in the long-axis view of a patient with a small pericardial effusion (PER EFF), which appears as a narrow echo-free space posterior to the left ventricular posterior wall (LVPW). Note the small round echo-free space, representing the descending aorta (DA), posterior to the atrioventricular junction, in the same plane as the small pericardial effusion. VS denotes interventricular septum; MV, mitral valve.

space between the left ventricular posterior wall and parietal pericardium in both long-axis and short-axis views. This narrow posterior pericardial space, only a few millimeters wide, is best seen in systole and diminishes or even disappears in diastole (Figures 11-2 and 11-3). This cyclic fluctuation from beat to beat facilitates recognition when viewed in real time or slow motion. Often, close inspection reveals a narrow rim of echo-free space anteriorly, outlining the right ventricular anterior wall. This narrow pericardial space in systole and narrow rim of anterior echo-free space is characteristic of small pericardial effusions.

With moderate pericardial effusions (Figures 11-4 and 11-5) the space behind the left ventricular posterior wall, as well as the echo-free space anteriorly, broadens. In the short-axis view a halo of echo-free space may encircle the entire heart. A similar echo-free space between ventricular myocardium and parietal pericardium will also be evident in other views, such as the apical or subcostal four-chamber view (Figure 11-5) and apical long-axis view (Figure 11-4). In the apical four-chamber view pericardial effusions can easily be missed if a narrow sector-angle of 30° to 60° is used. Here the two-dimensional probe must be rocked from side-to-side to explore the area adjacent to the right and left ventricles. The apical and subcostal views are particularly useful in elderly or emphysematous patients in whom the left lung tends to be interposed between the heart and the chest wall anteriorly, thwarting conventional parasternal scanning.

In large pericardial effusions (Figure 11-6) the echo-free space anterior and posterior to the ventricles is further widened and the ventricles exhibit exaggerated motion within the fluid-filled pericardial sac. Such undue cardiac mobility is unmistakable evidence of a massive accumulation of pericardial fluid and is the two-dimensional echocardiographic equivalent of the "swinging heart" seen on M-mode echocardiography. Oscillatory motion of the heart in large pericardial effusions was studied in detail by Matsuo et al,[15] who detected a rotatory component in addition

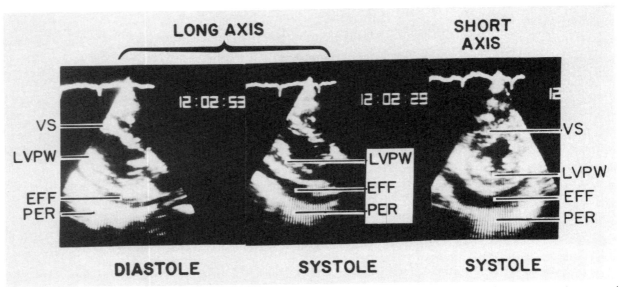

Figure 11-2. Two-dimensional echocardiogram of a patient with a small- to medium-sized pericardial effusion. The long-axis frames are from the same cardiac cycle. The posterior echo-free space is wider in systole (center frame) than in diastole (left). The posterior space is also well seen in short axis (systole). PER indicates pericardium; EFF, pericardial effusion.

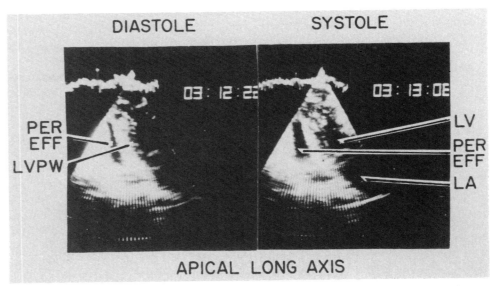

Figure 11-3. Two-dimensional echocardiogram in the apical long-axis view demonstrating a small pericardial effusion as an echo-free space behind the left ventricular posterior wall which is wider in systole than it is in diastole. LV denotes left ventricle; LA, left atrium.

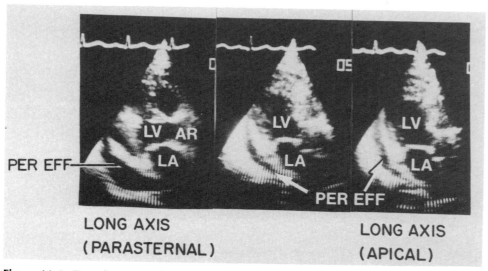

Figure 11-4. Two-dimensional echocardiogram of a patient showing a pericardial effusion as an echo-free space posterior to the heart. The left panel (parasternal long-axis view) is in systole; the right panel (apical long-axis view) is in early diastole; the center panel is recorded at a time intermediate between the two. AR denotes aortic root.

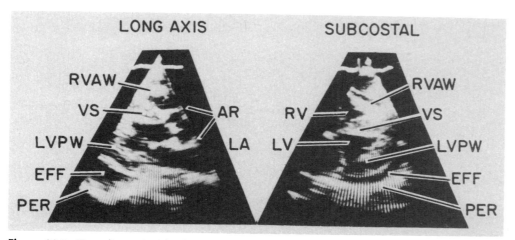

Figure 11-5. Two-dimensional echocardiogram in a patient with a moderate pericardial effusion posteriorly and a very small pericardial effusion anterior to the right ventricular anterior wall (RVAW).

225

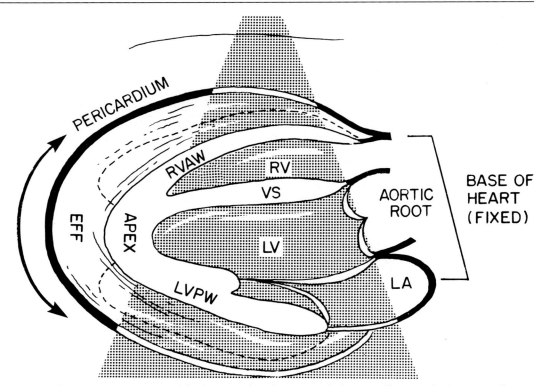

Figure 11-6. Diagram of the heart within the pericardial sac to illustrate the heart oscillating within a large pericardial effusion. The shaded area represents the area visualized in a standard wide-angle two-dimensional echocardiogram. The heart is fixed at its base; however, the ventricles swing freely anteriorly and posteriorly (arrows). The maximum amplitude of oscillation is at the apex.

to the anteroposterior oscillatory motion. Careful examination of the two-dimensional echocardiogram in the long-axis view, in slow motion or frame-by-frame sequence, can also demonstrate alternation of left ventricular alignment from beat to beat (Figure 11-7).

In the earlier years of echocardiography, the statement was often made that pericardial fluid did not extend posterior to the left atrium. In large pericardial effusions, however, it is not unusual to notice the echo-free pericardial space extending into the oblique sinus, a pericardial recess posterior to the left atrium (Figure 11-8). This can be imaged in the parasternal long-axis and short-axis and the apical long-axis and four-chamber views. Two-dimensional echocardiography confirmed the M-mode observation by Lemire et al[16] and Greene et al[17] that an echo-free space may extend behind the left atrium.

Large pericardial effusions are most often due to malignant neoplastic involvement of the pericardium by primary tumors originating in the lung, the breast, or lymphatic tissues. Less commonly, chronic renal failure, recent cardiac surgery, systemic lupus erythematosus, or viral or tuberculous pericarditis is responsible. The largest pericardial effusion in my experience, however, was in a young woman with cholesterol pericarditis (Figure 11-9).

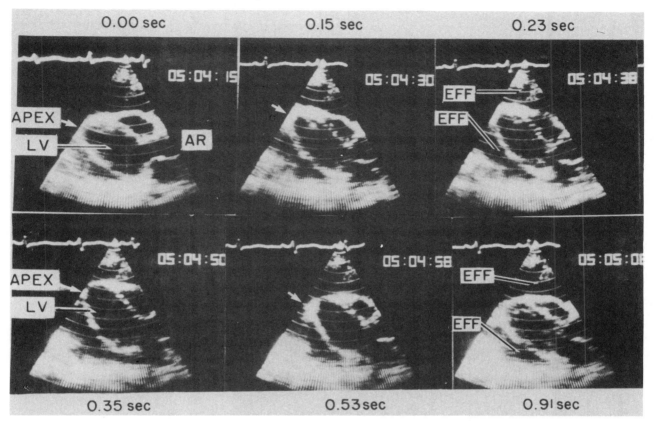

Figure 11-7. Six successive frames in the long axis from a patient with a large pericardial effusion. The ECG shows QRS alternans. Each upper frame corresponds approximately to the frame below at the same stage of the cardiac cycle; the cardiac cycle of the upper frames immediately precedes the cycle of the lower frames. Note that the ventricular position and apex (arrows) are different in two succeeding cardiac cycles. This explains the alternation in QRS amplitude. Cardiac swinging within each cardiac cycle is evident.

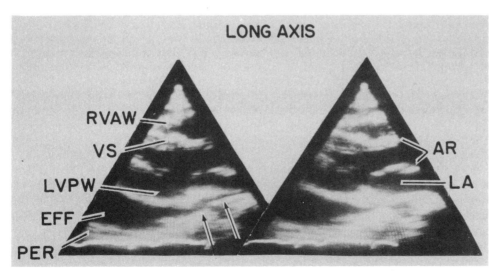

Figure 11-8. Two-dimensional echocardiogram of a patient with a large pericardial effusion. The two frames are serial ones from the same cardiac cycle. Extension of pericardial fluid behind the left atrium (arrows) is present in the left panel; at a different phase of systole the space is no longer present (right panel).

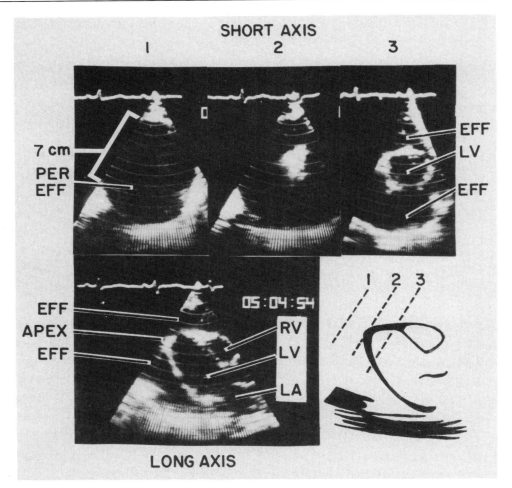

Figure 11-9. Two-dimensional echocardiogram of the same patient as in Figure 11-8. The three upper short-axis frames correspond to the three planes of imaging in the diagram below. The patient has an extremely large pericardial effusion. In frame 1 only the vast expanse of fluid is seen; in frame 2 the tip of the apex appears in the center of the effusion; in frame 3 the left ventricle near its apex is seen in cross-section. The bottom frame demonstrates large anterior and posterior pericardial echo-free spaces in a parasternal long-axis view. The two-dimensional echocardiogram thus depicts the massive amount of pericardial fluid and its uniform distribution around the ventricles (1.5 liters was aspirated).

Pericardial effusions accompanying congestive heart failure are seldom, if ever, large. The finding of a large pericardial effusion in a patient who described few or no symptoms and is free of tachycardia, tachypnea, and orthopnea suggests that the fluid has accumulated gradually and that pericardial tamponade is not imminent. I have encountered such instances complicating myxedema, rheumatoid arthritis, and Dressler's (post-myocardial-infarction) syndrome.

Figure 11-10 shows serial frames in one cardiac cycle from a videotape recording of a patient with a large pericardial effusion. Note specifically the alteration in cardiac position at different points in the cardiac cycle.

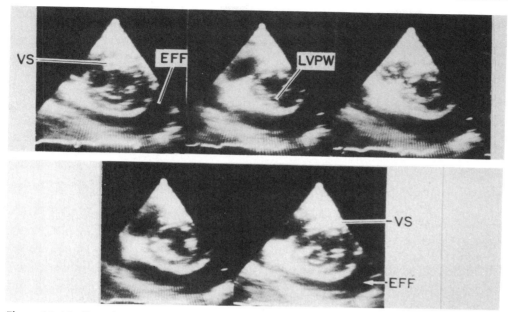

Figure 11-10. Two-dimensional echocardiogram in the parasternal short-axis view in a patient with a large pericardial effusion (top panel: systole; bottom panel: diastole). The large frame-to-frame variation in the pericardial space is due to cardiac "swinging." The frames are serial ones from the same cardiac cycle.

Distribution of Pericardial Fluid

Two-dimensional echocardiography is able to depict the anatomic distribution of fluid within the pericardial sac better than M-mode. In chronic pericarditis the visceral and parietal pericardium may become partly adherent, causing loculation of the pericardial fluid.[13] This information is vital if pericardiocentesis is being planned for diagnostic or therapeutic purposes. It is important to verify that a sufficiently large volume of pericardial fluid is available for aspiration so that the needle is not directed to an area likely to be myocardium. One would like to see a wide echo-free space anterior to the right ventricle if the subxiphoid site is to be used, and around the cardiac apex if the lateral midclavicular or anterior axillary approach is planned. It is prudent to perform echocardiography just prior to pericardiocentesis to ensure that the pericardial fluid has not been reabsorbed or become loculated since the previous examination.

Another practical consideration is not to confuse loculation of pericardial fluid with localization due to gravity. With the patient supine it is common to see pericardial fluid localize posteriorly. If the patient is then reexamined in the sitting position, the fluid appears in the anterior pericardial space; this indicates that it was not loculated.[18]

Quantitation of Pericardial Effusion

Quantitation of the amount of pericardial fluid has been attempted based on the following two assumptions: that the pericardial sac is a prolate ellipsoid, similar in shape to the left ventricle; and that the width of pericardial space visualized posterior to the left ventricle is representative of the width of fluid around the entire heart.

The first assumption is questionable; the second is seldom true. Two-dimensional echocardiographic examination of patients with pericardial effusions often reveals a variable width of fluid around the heart.

In theory, estimating pericardial fluid by two-dimensional echocardiography should be more accurate, although no systematic study has been done. In this method the volume of the pericardial sac is measured, using one of the various formulae used for measuring left ventricular volume, i.e., Simpson's rule or the area–length method. The entire volume of the heart that the ventricles displace, the external ventricular volume, is then measured in a similar manner. The difference between the pericardial sac volume (V_{ps}) and the external ventricular volume (V_v) is the estimated volume of pericardial fluid (V_{pe}):

$$V_{pe} = V_{ps} - V_v$$

Intrapericardial Echoes in Patients with Pericardial Effusions

Bands or strands of fibrin are occasionally visualized floating in the fluid of a large pericardial effusion.[19,20] They appear adherent to the ventricular epicardium (Figure 11-11) and can exhibit an erratic undulating motion in response to cardiac motion and pericardial fluid turbulence. In other instances the intrapericardial adhesions

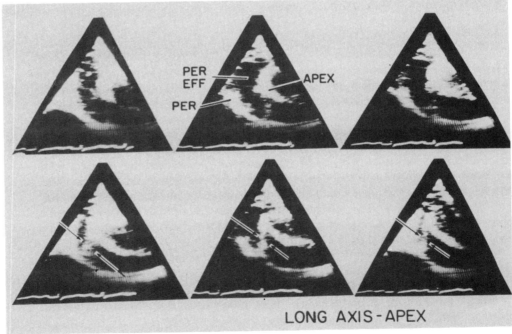

Figure 11-11. The six parasternal (long-axis) frames are of a patient with a large pericardial effusion. A great amount of fluid surrounds the cardiac apex. The arrows indicate a bandlike echo bridging the pericardial space from apex to parietal pericardium; this is a fibrinous adhesion. Note that a "side-lobe artifact" that looks somewhat similar can be seen with phased-array equipment.

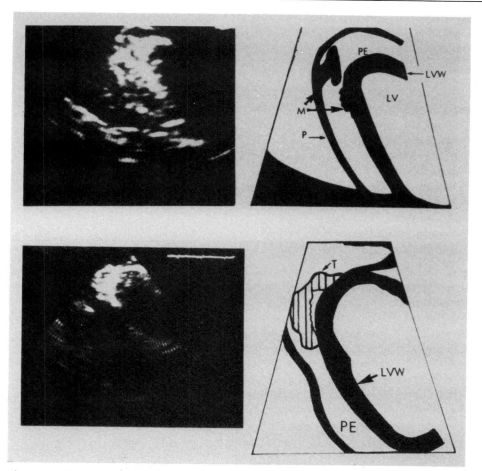

Figure 11-12. Parasternal long-axis views in two patients with surgically proved pericardial metastases. In the top panel a pericardial effusion (PE) is present. Note the abnormal echoes (M) that project into the pericardial space from the pericardium (P) and epicardium. These echoes demonstrate a to-and-fro oscillatory motion during the cardiac cycle, and they probably represent pericardial metastases. In the bottom panel a large, irregular mass (T) protrudes into the pericardial effusion. The mass probably represents pericardial metastasis. LVW denotes left ventricular wall. (From Chandraratna PAN, Aronow WS: Detection of pericardial metastases with cross-sectional echocardiography. Circulation 63:197–199, 1981. By permission of the American Heart Association, Inc.)

appear so echo-dense and taut that they prevent the heart from "swinging." Artifacts due to reverberations from strong epicardial echoes or the side-lobe artifact of phased-array systems could easily be mistaken for intrapericardial adhesions.

Chandraratna et al[21] have described intrapericardial nodules or masses from malignant metastases. They noted that this type of abnormal echocardiographic morphology was typical of metastases (Figure 11-12). At times, however, they are indistinguishable from other linear or bandlike echoes due to fibrinous adhesions or intrapericardial clot.

Echocardiographic Simulators of
Pericardial Effusion

Two-dimensional echocardiography is superior to the M-mode technique in distinguishing between pericardial effusions and other echo-free spaces anterior or posterior to the heart. Other causes of echo-free spaces posterior to the heart are:

- Pleural effusion
- Descending aorta (normal or dilated)[22]
- Dilated coronary sinus[23]
- Pseudoaneurysm of the left ventricle[24,25]
- Subvalvular (submitral) left ventricular aneurysm[26]
- Extension (prolapse) of an enlarged left atrium behind the left ventricle[27]
- Arteriovenous aneurysm involving proximal circumflex coronary artery and coronary sinus[28]
- Pancreatic pseudocyst[29]
- Posterior neoplastic mass spreading from esophagus, lymphoma, lung, etc.

Many of these entities have been reported only once or twice in the echocardiographic literature. Others, however, are common in routine practice and deserve special comment:

A left pleural effusion can present as a large echo-free space posterior to the heart (Figure 11-13). It can be distinguished from pericardial effusion on the M-mode echocardiogram by noting that (1) the retrocardiac echo-free space from a pleural effusion usually extends behind the left atrium, (2) the pleural effusion is not associated with an anterior echo-free space, and (3) the pleural effusion is not accompanied by "swinging" or excessive cardiac motion. Occasionally there are exceptions to these three rules. Two-dimensional echocardiography can help to differentiate a pleural from a pericardial effusion by the characteristic shape of the retrocardiac

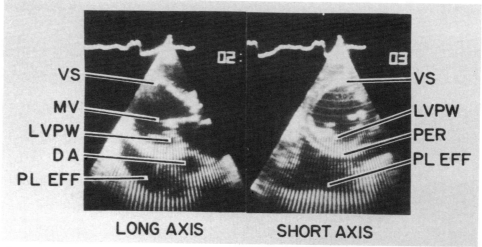

Figure 11-13. Two-dimensional echocardiogram of a patient with a left pleural effusion (PL EFF). An echo-free space is seen posterior to the heart in the parasternal long- and short-axis views. This can be differentiated from a pericardial effusion by its different shape in both views and by the fact that it occupies a plane posterior to the descending aorta.

space in long-axis and short-axis views. The differentiation becomes easier when pericardial and pleural effusions coexist; in this instance the parietal pericardial-pleural interface appears as a well-defined linear echo between an anterior retro-cardiac space (pericardial effusion) and the posterior space (pleural effusion) (Figure 11-14).

Recently the diagnostic usefulness of the descending thoracic aorta as an anatomical landmark has been recognized.[22] The descending aorta can usually be identified in parasternal long-axis view as a round or oval echo-free space posterior to the left atrioventricular junction. Moving the examining plane more obliquely in a superior-inferior orientation allows examination of the descending aorta in the long axis. Pericardial effusions present as an echo-free space anterior to the plane of the descending aorta, whereas pleural effusions present as an echo-free space posterior to the descending aorta. The echo-free space representing the descending aorta can at times be mistaken for a small localized pericardial effusion on the M-mode echocardiogram, but it is easily identified on the two-dimensional echocardiogram by its location, size, and shape.

A dilated coronary sinus, usually associated with a congenital persistent left superior vena cava, can also produce an echo-free space posterior to the atrioventricular junction; it is located somewhat more anterior than the descending aorta and is clearly extracardiac in location.[23]

Pseudoaneurysm of the left ventricle is an uncommon but important complication of acute myocardial infarction; this results from a slow hemorrhage from the damaged left ventricular wall into the pericardial space, forming a localized "false" aneurysm that communicates with the left ventricular chamber through a narrow "neck"[24] (see p. 200). Pseudoaneurysm presents on the M-mode echocardiogram as a large retrocardiac space, either echo-free or partly echo-dense from clots arising within. It is important to recognize this complication early because of the high mortality

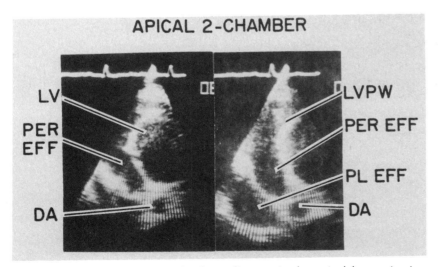

Figure 11-14. Two-dimensional echocardiogram in the apical long-axis view of a patient with a pericardial as well as a left pleural effusion. The pericardial effusion lies in a plane anterior to that of the descending aorta, while the pleural effusion occupies a plane posterior to it.

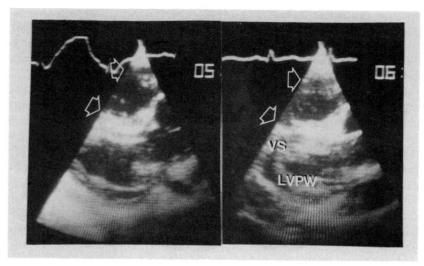

Figure 11-15. Two-dimensional echocardiogram of a 10-year-old child with an anterior mediastinal cystic mass (arrows) simulating an anterior pericardial effusion. Frames are the parasternal long-axis view during diastole (left) and systole (right). Note that the right ventricular chamber at this level has been compressed almost to the point of apparent "obliteration."

associated with myocardial rupture. It may be suspected on two-dimensional echocardiography by (1) a history and echocardiographic evidence of recent inferior wall infarction; (2) demonstrating a communication between the retrocardiac space and the left ventricular cavity, i.e., a break in continuity of the left ventricular posterior wall; or (3) a narrow neck and wide fundus of the pseudoaneurysm filled with clot.

Anterior echo-free spaces, simulating an anterior pericardial effusion, can be caused by:

- Pericardial fat, common in very obese persons
- Loculated pericardial fluid or blood accumulated after cardiac surgery
- Anterior mediastinal cysts (Figure 11-15) or tumors of varied etiology, including thymomas, hamartomas, and Hodgkin's lymphomas, and spread of malignant neoplasms from lung, stomach, testes, or breast (see Figure 12-28)

In size these anterior spaces can vary from 1 to 2 cm in width to huge cysts displacing the heart from its usual location. The presence of an anterior mediastinal cyst or mass can be suspected if a large anterior echo-free space is not accompanied by a posterior space. Moreover, the contour of the anterior space, as depicted by two-dimensional echocardiography, is that of a round cyst or circumscribed mass, whereas an anterior pericardial effusion tends to take on a curvilinear contour around the cardiac structures.

Cardiac Tamponade

Initially it was believed that echocardiography had little use in the diagnosis of cardiac tamponade. It was then shown with M-mode echocardiography that phasic respiratory changes in ventricular dimensions occur in patients with tamponade.

During inspiration the right ventricle enlarges while the left ventricle becomes smaller; during expiration the opposite changes take place.[4] These conspicuous respiratory alterations in ventricular dimension are also noted on two-dimensional echocardiography in either parasternal long-axis, short-axis, or apical four-chamber views. Since these patients usually have large pericardial effusions and "swinging" hearts, it takes an experienced echocardiographer to properly image the ventricular chambers and ventricular septum during phases of respiration.

Schiller et al[30] described right ventricular compression as an additional sign of cardiac tamponade. This finding may, at least in some patients, be indistinguishable from right ventricular collapse or the decrease in right ventricular size during expiration. Phasic respiratory changes in ventricular dimension are now not considered specific for cardiac tamponade, since similar changes have been described in patients with chronic obstructive lung disease, pulmonary embolism, and tracheal obstruction. Right atrial collapse has also proved to be a useful, but not totally specific, sign of tamponade. Nevertheless the occurrence of these echocardiographic changes on serial tracings in patients with large pericardial effusions constitutes a valuable sign to alert the clinician to suspect cardiac tamponade and influence his decision to treat the effusion more aggressively by pericardiocentesis or surgical relief. An interesting manifestation of tamponade, in a patient with septal hypertrophy, was the provocation of abnormal systolic anterior mitral motion (SAM), which disappeared after the tamponade resolved.[31]

Pericardial Thickening and Constriction

Two-dimensional echocardiography is beginning to be useful in the diagnosis of pericardial thickening and constriction. M-mode echocardiography is still probably more helpful than the two-dimensional technique because the various signs considered suggestive of constriction are better detected on M-mode tracings. Abnormal septal systolic and early diastolic motion, loss of left ventricular expansion in mid- to late-diastole, and small to normal ventricular size are still better detected by M-mode echocardiography. A recent study of patients with constrictive tuberculous pericarditis showed some improved utility for the two-dimensional technique.[32] The features typically seen were the following:

- The heart was normal in size or small, the ventricles were decreased in size, and the atria were normal or enlarged.
- The hepatic veins and inferior vena cava were dilated.
- The pericardium was seen as a very dense single or double thickened layer surrounding the heart.
- The thickened pericardium was almost totally immobile.
- The interventricular septum and interatrial septum deviated to the left side of the heart on inspiration.
- A sudden ventricular filling halt was visible (pericardial knock).

Further confirmation of these findings and greater experience should prove two-dimensional superior to M-mode echocardiography.

Pericardial thickening and sclerosis are better seen on the M-mode strip-chart recording, which has better gray-scale shading and finer resolution capability than two-dimensional echocardiography. In children, by using a high-frequency two-dimensional transducer which has finer resolution capability it may be possible to identify thickened epicardium and pericardium (Figure 11-16). Sclerotic pericardium

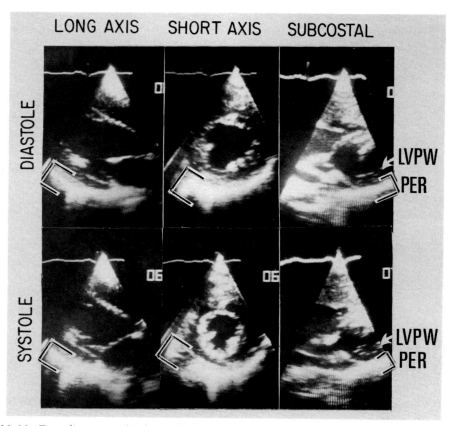

Figure 11-16. Two-dimensional echocardiogram in multiple views of a patient with sclerotic thickened pericardium resulting from acute pericarditis with a pericardial effusion a few weeks earlier. In both systole and diastole a thickened pericardium manifests as a very dense echo, much denser than that of the left ventricular posterior wall. Left ventricular contraction appears normal.

produces unduly dense echoes; progressive increase of the reject (damping) control results in persistence of these dense pericardial echoes long after the left ventricular myocardial echoes have been completely suppressed. Two-dimensional echocardiography is helpful in assessing patients with partial constriction of the ventricles (i.e., after a partial pericardiectomy) by revealing the extent of constriction around the left ventricle.

Echocardiography may have an important role in differentiating constrictive pericarditis from restrictive cardiomyopathy. The resemblance between these two entities, with regard to their clinical, radiological, electrocardiographic, and even hemodynamic presentation, is notorious. Fortunately, their echocardiographic appearances are different (see Chapter 10). Patients with restrictive cardiomyopathy (such as amyloid) have thickened ventricular walls and septum, which often show diminished motion without pericardial thickening; in constrictive pericarditis the pericardium is obviously thickened, whereas the ventricular wall and septum generally are not; overall ventricular wall motion is normal or even exaggerated.

CONCLUSION

It is sometimes said that all instances in which pericardial effusions are diagnosed by two-dimensional echocardiography could also be detected by M-mode echocardiography. While there is some truth in this statement, it must be added that the two-dimensional technique provides additional information about the nature of the effusion that may prove quite useful to the clinician. Hence, two-dimensional echocardiography is routinely used in most laboratories today to complement M-mode echocardiography. Moreover, one does occasionally encounter patients in whom a moderate or even large pericardial effusion is clearly seen on two-dimensional, but for technical reasons is difficult to record on M-mode echocardiography.

In addition to the routine application of the two-dimensional technique in pericardial disease, it is likely that the procedure will be increasingly utilized in intensive care, emergency room, and postoperative recovery settings to exclude or confirm pericardial effusion and to concomitantly assess left ventricular function. Two-dimensional echocardiography employed at the patient's bedside can make a valuable contribution to post-traumatic or postsurgical acute patient care.

REFERENCES

1. Feigenbaum H, Waldhausen JA, Hyde LP: Ultrasound diagnosis of pericardial effusion. JAMA 191:107–110, 1965
2. Horowitz MS, Rosen R, Harrison DC: Echocardiographic diagnosis of pericardial disease. Am Heart J 97:420–427, 1979
3. Feigenbaum H, Zaky A, Grabhorn L: Cardiac motion in patients with pericardial effusion: a study using ultrasound cardiography. Circulation 34:611–619, 1966
4. D'Cruz IA, Cohen HC, Prabhu R, et al: Diagnosis of cardiac tamponade by echocardiography: changes in mitral valve motion and ventricular dimensions, with special reference to paradoxical pulse. Circulation 52:460–465, 1975
5. Schnittger I, Bowden RE, Abrams J, et al: Echocardiography: Pericardial thickening and constrictive pericarditis. Am J Cardiol 42:388–395, 1978
6. Allen JW, Harrison EC, Camp JC, et al: The role of serial echocardiography in the evaluation and differential diagnosis of pericardial disease. Am Heart J 93:560–567, 1977
7. Pool PE, Seagren SC, Abbasi AS, et al: Echocardiographic manifestations of constrictive pericarditis. Abnormal septal motion. Chest 68:684–688, 1975
8. Candell-Riera J, Garcia del Castillo H, Permanyer-Miralda G, et al: Echocardiographic features of the interventricular septum in chronic constrictive pericarditis. Circulation 57:1154–1158, 1978
9. Voelkel AG, Pietro DA, Folland ED, et al: Echocardiographic features of constrictive pericarditis. Circulation 58:871–875, 1978
10. D'Cruz IA, Levinsky R, Anagnostopoulos C, et al: Echocardiographic diagnosis of partial pericardial constriction of the left ventricle. Radiology 127:755–756, 1978
11. Martin RP, Rakowski H, French J, et al: Localization of pericardial effusion with wide angle phased array echocardiography. Am J Cardiol 42:904–912, 1978
12. Chandraratna PA, Aronow WS: Limitations of surgical methods of pericardial drainage. Echocardiographic observations. JAMA 242:1062–1063, 1979
13. Feigenbaum H: Echocardiography (ed 3). Philadelphia, Lea & Febiger, 1981, pp 485–494
14. Ports TA, Schiller NB: Pericardial effusion, in Kisslo JA (ed): Two-Dimensional Echocardiography. New York, Churchill-Livingston, 1980, pp 145–156
15. Matsuo H, Matsumoto M, Hamanaka Y, et al: Rotational excursion of heart in massive pericardial effusion studied by phased-array echocardiography. Br Heart J 41:513–521, 1979
16. Lemire F, Tajik AJ, Giuliani ER, et al: Further echocardiographic observations in pericardial effusion. Mayo Clin Proc 51:13–18, 1976

17. Greene DA, Kleid JJ, Naidu S: Unusual echocardiographic manifestation of pericardial effusion. Am J Cardiol 39:112–115, 1977
18. Friedman MJ, Sahn DJ, Haber K: Two-dimensional echocardiography and B-mode ultrasonography for the diagnosis of loculated pericardial effusion. Circulation 60:1644–1649, 1979
19. Martin RP, Bowden R, Filly K, et al: Intrapericardial abnormalities in patients with pericardial effusion. Findings by two-dimensional echocardiography. Circulation 61:568–572, 1980
20. Chiaramida SA, Goldman MA, Zerma MJ, et al: Echocardiographic identification of intrapericardial fibrous strands in acute pericarditis with pericardial effusion. Chest 77:85–88, 1980
21. Chandraratna PAN, Aronow WS: Detection of pericardial metastases by cross-sectional echocardiography. Circulation 63:197–199, 1981
22. Haaz WS, Mintz GS, Kotler MN, et al: Two-dimensional echocardiographic recognition of the descending thoracic aorta: Value in differentiating pericardial from pleural effusions. Am J Cardiol 46:739–743, 1980
23. Snider AR, Ports TA, Silverman NH: Venous anomalies of the coronary sinus: Detection by M-mode, two-dimensional and contrast echocardiography. Circulation 60:721–727, 1979
24. Catherwood E, Mintz GS, Kotler MN, et al: Two-dimensional echocardiographic recognition of left ventricular pseudoaneurysm. Circulation 62:294–303, 1980
25. Katz RJ, Simpson A, DiBianco R, et al: Noninvasive diagnosis of left ventricular pesudoaneurysm: Role of two dimensional echocardiography and radionuclide gated pool imaging. Am J Cardiol 44:372–377, 1979
26. Hickey AJ, Braye S: Annular subvalvular left ventricular aneurysm mimicking a pericardial effusion on echocardiogram. Aust NZ J Med 9:571–574, 1979
27. Reeves WC, Ciotola T, Babb JD, et al: Prolapsed left atrium behind the left ventricular posterior wall: two-dimensional echocardiographic and angiographic features. Am J Cardiol 47:708–712, 1981
28. Come PC, Riley MF, Fortuin NJ: Echocardiographic mimicry of pericardial effusion. Am J Cardiol 47:365–370, 1981
29. Shah A, Schwartz H: Echocardiographic features of cardiac compression by mediastinal pancreatic pseudocyst. Chest 77:440–443, 1980
30. Schiller NB, Botvinick EH: Right ventricular compression as a sign of cardiac tamponade: An analysis of echocardiographic ventricular dimensions and their clinical implications. Circulation 56:774–779, 1977
31. Schulman P, Come PC, Isaac R, et al: Left ventricular outflow obstruction induced by tamponade in hypertrophic cardiomyopathy. Chest 80:110–113, 1981
32. Lewis BS: Real time two dimensional echocardiography in constrictive pericarditis. Am J Cardiol 48:1789–1793, 1982

CHAPTER 12

Vegetations, Tumors, Masses, and Thrombi

James V. Talano

Vegetations are masses of fibrin and cellular debris that adhere to valvular or other intracardiac structures. Although most frequently infected and related to bacterial or fungal endocarditis, nonbacterial thrombotic endocarditis may occur in association with chronic illness, cancer, or collagen vascular disease. The detection of vegetations on heart valves in the presence of unexplained bacteremia or stroke may explain the pathophysiology of the illness as well as guide therapeutic management. The surgical implications of finding vegetations by cardiac ultrasound in the setting of bacterial endocarditis are just now being examined. It appears certain that this finding increases the likelihood of complications in the patient with endocarditis, yet the presence of a vegetation is not in itself an indication for surgery.

THE M-MODE ECHOCARDIOGRAM IN INFECTIVE ENDOCARDITIS

M-mode echocardiography is a potentially useful adjunct to clinical diagnosis in patients with infective endocarditis.[1,2] Valvular vegetations appear, as in Figure 12-1, as masses of "shaggy" echoes creating an irregular thickening of the valves. The vegetations, which attach to one or more leaflets, often have unrestricted or chaotic motion. Vegetations as small as 2 mm have been correctly identified and located by the M-mode technique (Figure 12-1).[2]

The presence of vegetations on M-mode echocardiograms has become a marker of complicated infective endocarditis. Roy et al[3] found definite vegetations in 22 of 32 patients with clinical infective endocarditis in whom 20 (90 percent) had congestive heart failure, 12 (54 percent) developed emboli and 12 (54 percent) required valve replacement during that hospitalization. Their finding of a *probable* vegetation carried with it a lesser morbidity.[3]

In early M-mode echocardiographic studies, only one-third of patients with clinical infective endocarditis had vegetations detected by M-mode echocardiography. Of the patients with vegetations documented by echocardiography, however, a greater percentage required surgery. In a study by Wann et al,[4] 18 of 22 patients with infective endocarditis and vegetations on M-mode echocardiography urgently re-

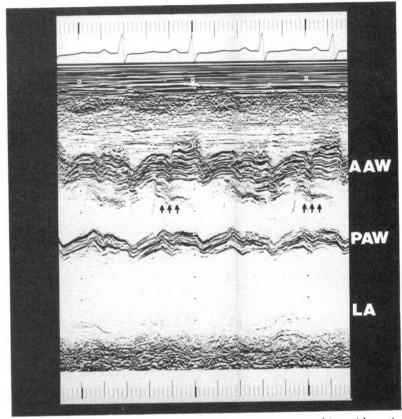

Figure 12-1. M-mode echocardiogram of an aortic valve vegetation on a bicuspid aortic valve. Note the "smudged" diastolic echoes on the eccentric line of closure (arrows). Diastolic fluttering of the aortic valve implies an aortic flail cusp; this was confirmed at surgery. AAW denotes anterior aortic wall; PAW, posterior aortic wall; LA, left atrium.

quired valve replacement.[8] The M-mode echocardiogram is thus important not only in defining the presence or absence of vegetations but also in determining the consequences of the infectious process, such as flail aortic leaflet, flail mitral leaflet or aortic ring abscess.

TWO-DIMENSIONAL ECHOCARDIOGRAPHY IN INFECTIVE ENDOCARDITIS

With two-dimensional echocardiography, spatial characteristics of the target image are obtained by rapidly steering an ultrasound beam through a given field. The images obtained are tomographic views of the heart. The spatial characteristics are such that target recognition is greatly enhanced, resulting in rapid accurate identification of valves and vegetations. The ability of two-dimensional echocardiography to characterize size and morphology of vegetations, recesses or commissures of valves, structures of the right side of the heart, and so forth is superior to that of the M-mode technique (Figure 12-2).[5] This superior ability in imaging is most helpful

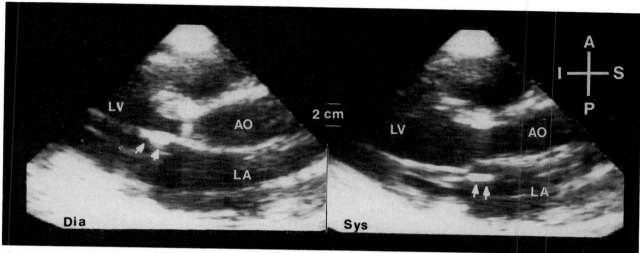

Figure 12-2. Two-dimensional echocardiogram of a mitral valve vegetation in long axis (arrows). Note the anterior leaflet vegetation within the left atrium during systole. The two-dimensional study allows for more precise localization of the vegetations. LV denotes left ventricle; LA, left atrium; AO, aorta.

in identifying the destructive sequelae of vegetations. This is especially true in the presence of flail leaflets, valve ring abscesses, sinus of Valsalva aneurysms, and paravalvular sinus formation. Furthermore, lesions of the right side of the heart which are poorly identified by M-mode are easily detected with two-dimensional echocardiography.[5,6] Thus, although M-mode and two-dimensional echocardiography have proved complementary, the latter technique is more helpful in identifying the complications of infective endocarditis.[7]

Comparison of M-Mode and Two-Dimensional Echocardiography in Infective Endocarditis

Several studies have compared the ability of M-mode and two-dimensional echocardiography to identify vegetations. Wann et al investigated 23 patients with infective endocarditis and found 18 patients with vegetations by M-mode and two-dimensional echocardiography.[11] One patient with prosthetic valve endocarditis had vegetations found only by two-dimensional echocardiography. Although two-dimensional echocardiography did not appear to be more sensitive than M-mode in detecting vegetations, it did provide superior spatial orientation and characterization of the sizes and shapes of vegetations. Mintz et al[7] studied 21 patients with the clinical diagnosis of infective endocarditis, detecting vegetations by M-mode in 10 and by two-dimensional echocardiography in 9. Two-dimensional echocardiography, however, was far superior in detecting complications of infective endocarditis, i.e., flail aortic cusp, ring abscess, and sinus of Valsalva aneurysm. Martin et al[9] found two-dimensional echocardiography to be more sensitive than M-mode (81 percent versus 47 percent) in the detection of vegetations; this was partly owing to a large number of prosthetic valve and tricuspid valve endocarditides in their study—conditions in which the superiority of two-dimensional echocardiography has been shown.[5,8]

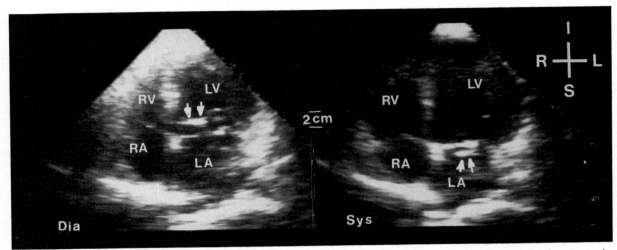

Figure 12-3. Apical four-chamber view in infective endocarditis of the mitral valve. Note the vegetations within the left ventricle (arrows) during diastole. During systole the vegetation is noted within the left atrium (arrows). RA denotes right atrium; RV, right ventricle.

Technical Aspects of Two-Dimensional Examination for Vegetations

An important question relates to who should perform the study in the patient with suspected endocarditis. The initial examination can be performed by the technologist and reviewed by the echocardiographer. If any masses or abnormal findings are noted, however, the two-dimensional procedure should be completed by the echocardiographer. Interaction between the experienced physician and the ultrasound technologist during the two-dimensional procedure is important in order to direct the examination and maximize the likelihood of providing an answer to the clinical question. M-mode and two-dimensional echocardiography is best performed by the echocardiographer who has reviewed the clinical record and assessed the patient clinically, a practice well established for cardiac catheterization.

Proper gain setting is of extreme importance in scanning heart valves for vegetations. Setting the gain too low may cause the echocardiographer to overlook or underestimate the size of a vegetation. Inappropriately high gain settings will increase the size of the target and cause its border to become indistinct and coalesce with adjacent valve tissue.[5] The use of multiple views in addition to the standard parasternal long- and short-axis ones can enhance recognition of a vegetation or the complications associated with vegetations. Not infrequently, use of the apical four-chamber or subxiphoid four-chamber views will allow a lesion or a complication to be more readily recognized (Figure 12-3).

Complications of the Infective Endocarditis Patient with Vegetation

The major consequences of infective endocarditis are (1) congestive heart failure, (2) pulmonary or systemic embolization, (3) valve destruction or dehiscence where the need for surgical intervention is urgent, and (4) death.

Does the size or shape of the vegetation as depicted by two-dimensional echocardiography play a role in predicting the consequence of infective endocarditis?

Two studies[8,10] have analyzed their echocardiographic data for size and shape of lesions, i.e., whether pedunculated or sessile (see Figure 12-2). Neither study has found a clear-cut relationship between size or shape of vegetation and congestive heart failure, embolization, or the need for valve surgery.[11,14] Two-thirds of vegetations remain unchanged in size during medical therapy. Complete disappearance of vegetations rarely occurs with medical therapy but frequently occurs after embolization.[10] Thus, morphology and size of vegetations are well delineated by two-dimensional echocardiography, yet their precise clinical implications are yet to be established.

Congestive Heart Failure

The two-dimensional or M-mode echocardiographic demonstration of a vegetation provides a biologic marker that appears associated with congestive heart failure. In their study of prognostic implications of the echocardiogram in 32 patients with aortic valve endocarditis, Mintz et al[11] found vegetations in 17 patients (53 percent), of whom 12 (71 percent) developed congestive heart failure. Vegetations detected by echocardiography were almost always associated with flail aortic leaflet, a ring abscess, or severe valve destruction.[11] Premature mitral valve closure (an M-mode sign of severe acute aortic regurgitation) was found in only 2 of their 23 patients (9 percent) who urgently required aortic valve replacement. Consequently, although it was specific for severe aortic regurgitation, premature mitral valve closure was an insensitive marker for urgent valve replacement. Similarly Pratt et al,[12] in defining the relationship of vegetations to clinical course in infective endocarditis, found 13 patients with vegetations, all of whom developed congestive heart failure during medical therapy. Twelve (93 percent) required valve surgery before medical therapy could be completed. A larger, more comprehensive series defining the relationship between the presence of vegetations and cardiac failure did not find such a high incidence of congestive heart failure. Stewart et al[10] found only a 32 percent incidence of congestive heart failure in patients with echocardiographic vegetative lesions. These authors suggested that referral patterns and differences in definition of infective endocarditis may account for this discrepancy. In most series reported, however, the presence of new vegetations with clinical congestive heart failure invariably resulted in surgery.[5,6,8,10]

Embolization

The site of valvular vegetation does not appear to influence the occurrence of embolization. Aortic and mitral valve vegetations appear to be equally common as the source of systemic embolization. The rate of embolization is variable in the presence of vegetation and ranges from 30 percent[10] to 80 percent in two recent series.[8] What is certain, however, is that the presence of vegetation carries with it a considerably higher risk of embolization. The absence of vegetation in infective endocarditis markedly reduces the chances of emboli. Successful bacteriologic cure does not preclude an embolic event even several years after successful antimicrobial therapy. Weinstein[13] has reported systemic embolization long after completion of successful antibiotic therapy.

In endocarditis of the right side of the heart pulmonary embolization is common and may require early surgical valvulectomy and replacement for recurrent septic pulmonary emboli. Persistent infection, cardiomegaly, and right-sided heart failure identify a subgroup of patients with tricuspid endocarditis at increased risk.[6]

Consequences of Valve Destruction

An autopsy study of healed endocarditis by Roberts and Buckbinder[14] showed that 65 percent of patients with fatal aortic valve endocarditis and 37 percent of patients with fatal mitral valve endocarditis had significant valve destruction. Davis et al[15] found valvular destruction by M-mode echocardiography in 46 percent of patients with aortic valve and 56 percent of patients with mitral valve vegetations. Consequently, in acute infective endocarditis, almost two-thirds of patients with vegetation present on echocardiography have valvular destruction.[15]

Our Experience[16]

Eighty-two patients with the clinical suspicion of endocarditis were examined by M-mode and two-dimensional echocardiography. Of the 82 patients, 32 satisfied clinical and laboratory criteria for infective endocarditis. Echocardiograms from 28 of 32 patients (88 percent) with infective endocarditis met the criteria established for vegetations on M-mode or two-dimensional echocardiography. Vegetations were diagnosed by both M-mode and two-dimensional techniques in 22 patients (70 percent), by only M-mode in 3 (9 percent) patients, and by only two-dimensional echocardiography in 3 (9 percent) patients. Echocardiograms from 4 patients with infective endocarditis did not meet either the M-mode or the two-dimensional echocardiographic criteria for vegetations.

Fifty patients did not meet the clinical and laboratory criteria for infective endocarditis. Of these, 48 (96 percent) patients had no evidence of cardiac vegetations by either M-mode or two-dimensional criteria. The presence of vegetations correlated well with the diagnosis of infective endocarditis ($p < 0.001$). Given the echocardiographic demonstration of vegetations by M-mode or two-dimensional echocardiography or both, the probability of having infective endocarditis was 94 percent. If vegetations were absent on M-mode or two-dimensional echocardiography or both, the probability of not having infective endocarditis was 92 percent. The sensitivity of echocardiography in detecting vegetations was 88 percent. The specificity of echocardiography in patients presenting with suspected infective endocarditis was 96 percent.

Of the 17 patients that had a complication of their infective endocarditis (embolus, refractory heart failure, urgent requirement for valve surgery, and/or death), 12 (71 percent) had vegetations greater than 5 mm in diameter. Seven of the 8 that suffered embolic events, 6 of the 8 that required surgery, and 7 of the 11 that died had vegetations greater than 5 mm. The absence of complications was statistically related to a vegetation size of 5 mm or less ($p < 0.05$). The probability that a patient with a vegetation of 5 mm or less would suffer a complication of his infective endocarditis was 33 percent. Of the 5 patients who suffered a complication with a vegetation size of 5 mm or less, 2 had prosthetic heart valves and 3 had *Staphylococcus aureus* infections. All but 1 of the 4 patients with aortic vegetations greater than 5 mm died.

Cumulative Experience

Table 12-1 summarizes the cumulative experience of 13 reported studies with a total of 460 patients with infective endocarditis. There were five studies that used M-mode echocardiography alone and eight studies that included M-mode and two-dimensional studies.

Two hundred eighty-one patients (61 percent) had vegetation-positive endocarditis and 179 (39 percent) had vegetation-negative endocarditis. Vegetation-positive and vegetation-negative patients were compared for the presence or absence of complications of endocarditis (congestive heart failure, emboli, urgent need for surgery, and death). Congestive heart failure occurred in 127 of 223 (57 percent) vegetation-positive lesions and in only 39 of 160 (24 percent) vegetation-negative lesions (p < 0.01). Embolization occurred in 74 of 223 (33 percent) patients with vegetation-positive and in only 7 of 160 (4 percent) vegetation-negative patients (p < 0.01). Valve surgery was required in 136 of 257 (53 percent) vegetation-positive patients and in only 17 of 168 (7 percent) vegetation-negative patients (p < 0.01). Death during hospitalization for acute infective endocarditis occurred in 31 (14 percent)

Table 12-1

Cumulative Experience of Complication Rates in Vegetation-Positive and Vegetation-Negative Patients

Author	Total Patients Studied	Patients with Vegetations by M-Mode	Patients with Vegetations by 2D	Complication			
				CHF	Emboli	Surgery	Death
DeMaria, 1976[18]	3	+3 −0	ND	Veg +3 Veg −0	Veg +0 Veg −0	Veg +3 Veg −0	Veg +0 Veg −0
Roy, 1976[3]	32	+22 −10	ND	+20 −9	+14 −0	+12 −4	+4 −0
Wann, 1976[4]	65	+22 −43	ND	+22 −12	+4 −0	+18 −0	+2 −0
Mintz, 1979[7]	32	+17 −15	NE separately	+12 −7	+9 −2	+8 −6	+2 −3
Pratt, 1978[12]	32	+13 −19	ND	+13 −2	+0 −0	+12 −2	+0 −0
Wann, 1979[8]	23	+18 −5	+19 −4	+11 −0	+7 −0	+12 −0	+1 −0
Stewart, 1980[10]	87	+47 −40	+47 −40	+15 −1	+14 −2	+12 −2	+5 −2
Davis, 1980[15]	30	+17 −13	ND	+14 −6	+8 −2	+17 −2	+6 −3
Martin, 1980[9]	42	+17 −25	+34 −8	NE	NE	+21 −0	NE
Berger, 1980[5]	12	+6 −6	+10 −2	+0 −0	+0 −0	+0 −0	+0 −0
Takeda, 1980[17]	35	+18 −17	+24 −11	+12 −2	+10 −1	+11 −1	+1 −1
Bardy, 1981[18]	32	+27 −5	+29 −3	+5 −0	+8 −0	+10 −0	+10 −1
Melvin, 1981[19]	35	+17 −18	+28 −7	NE	NE	NE	NE
Total	460	Veg +244 (53%) Veg −216 (47%)	+191 (72%) −75 (28%)	+127 (57%) −39 (24%)	+74 (33%) −7 (4%)	+136 (53%) −17 (7%)	+31 (14%) −10 (4%)

Abbreviations: ND, not done; NE, not evaluated; +, with vegetation; −, without vegetation.

vegetation-positive patients versus 10 (4 percent) vegetation-negative patients (p < 0.05).

Thus the cumulative experience is that vegetation-positive endocarditis carries with it a more protracted course complicated by the more frequent occurrence of congestive heart failure and embolization. A majority of vegetation-positive patients are likely to require early valve replacement. The in-hospital mortality of these patients is three times that of endocarditis patients free of vegetations.

SPECIFIC SITES OF VEGETATIONS

Aortic Valve

The M-mode diagnosis of aortic valve vegetations is made by recognizing multiple "shaggy" or "smudged" echoes on the aortic cusps with little, if any, restriction of motion. When attached to aortic cusps, the vegetation may appear as abnormal smudged echoes adherent to the cusps in systole. In diastole the echoes may be seen as thickening or smudging on the line of closure of the valve (Figure 12-4). A mobile vegetation can be seen in the left ventricular outflow tract during diastole

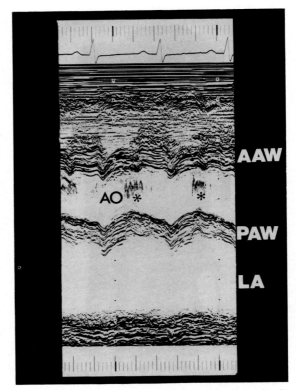

Figure 12-4. M-mode echocardiogram of an aortic valve vegetation (asterisks) noted as "smudged" echoes on the line of closure of the aortic valve (AO denotes aortic valve opening). Note the shaggy, erratic nature of the aortic valve vegetation. At surgery a perforated posterior coronary cusp and vegetation were found.

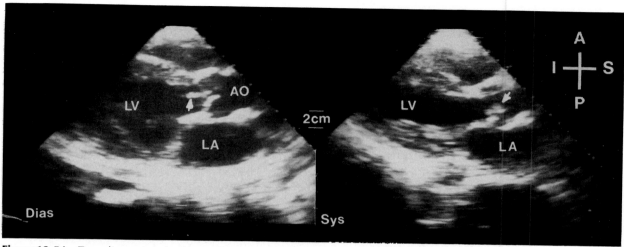

Figure 12-5A. Two-dimensional echocardiograms in parasternal long-axis view in aortic valve endocarditis. Note the cordlike vegetation (arrow) in the left ventricular outflow tract in diastole. During systole the mass of vegetations on the posterior aortic cusp is noted (arrow).

as shaggy erratic echoes just below the aortic valve. They frequently can be seen just anterior, but separate from, the anterior mitral leaflet. This finding in the left ventricular outflow tract is more helpful than observing the echoes on the aortic cusps.

Two-dimensional echocardiography is more helpful than M-mode in evaluating aortic valve vegetations (Figure 12-5). Berger et al[20] recognized three morphological types of vegetations: globular polypoid (most common); irregular elongated (com-

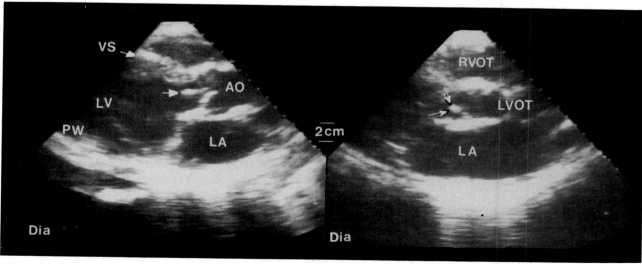

Figure 12-5B. Parasternal long-axis and short-axis views of a vegetation (arrows) in the outflow tract in diastole. VS denotes interventrical septum; PW, left ventricular posterior wall; RVOT, right ventricular outflow tract; LVOT, left ventricular outflow tract.

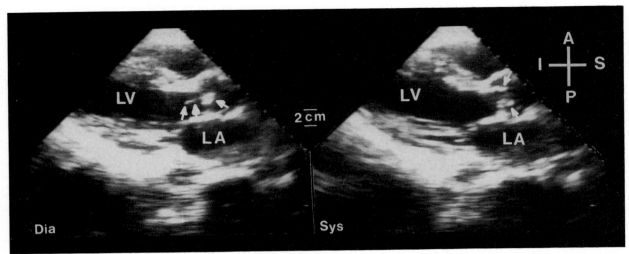

Figure 12-6. Two-dimensional echocardiogram in long-axis view in a patient with aortic valve endocarditis with a flail aortic cusp. Note the portion of the flail cusp (arrows) just anterior to the anterior mitral leaflet in diastole. The vegetation is seen as a polypoid mass (superior arrow) attached to the aortic cusp.

mon); and cordlike (rare). Two-dimensional echocardiography correctly identified vegetations in 12 of 14 patients. In the 2 patients not identified by two-dimensional echocardiography, the lesions were 3 mm or less. In these patients the only echocardiographic finding was mild nonspecific thickening of the aortic cusps. In the study by Mintz et al[11] the finding of aortic valve vegetation, flail aortic cusp, or aortic root abscess by two-dimensional echocardiography was associated with a more severe prognosis (Figure 12-6).

Mitral Valve

Mitral valve vegetations are similarly seen as shaggy or smudged echoes on the leaflets in diastole. The leaflets frequently have shaggy erratic detached echoes in the left atrium during systole or within the mitral valve inflow tract in diastole (Figure 12-7). Even though these echoes are seen within the left atrium behind the anterior mitral leaflet in systole, it is possible that they merely represent a flail leaflet without vegetation (Figure 12-8). Occasionally there is idiopathic rupture of chordae tendineae without vegetation. The flail mitral leaflet may exhibit subtle differences in appearance in each of these states. Vegetations tend to be larger targets with multiple eccentric echoes (Figure 12-9). A single flail leaflet appears thinner, "nonsmudgy," with high-frequency vibrations.

The importance of serial echocardiography has been outlined in two studies. Lundstrom and Bjorkhem[21] showed progressive left atrial and left ventricular enlargement in an infant with mitral regurgitation secondary to mitral valve endocarditis. Bamrah et al[22] demonstrated development of a vegetation on a previously normal mitral valve. A worsening prognosis was found with the development of valvular vegetations. Once the vegetation was recognized by echocardiography, multiple systemic emboli occurred in a patient with *Haemophilus parainfluenzae* mitral valve endocarditis.[22]

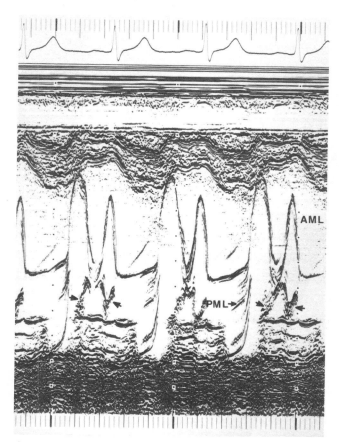

Figure 12-7. M-mode echocardiogram of mitral valve vegetation with a flail posterior mitral leaflet (PML). Note the "mass" of vegetation within the mitral valve inflow tract in diastole (between horizontal arrows). AML denotes anterior mitral leaflet.

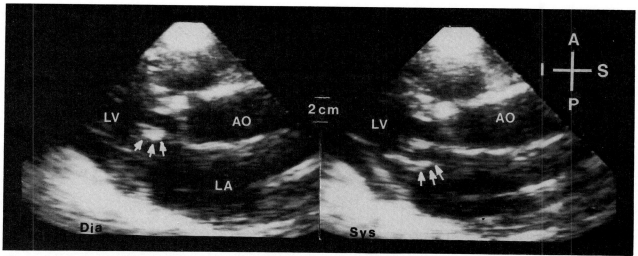

Figure 12-8. Parasternal long-axis view of mitral valve vegetation on the anterior mitral leaflet. Note the polypoid echoes in diastole within the mitral valve inflow tract (vertical arrows). In systole the vegetations are found within the left atrium behind the aorta (arrows). There is marked left atrial enlargement.

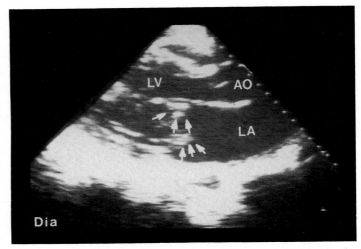

Figure 12-9A. Parasternal long-axis view in diastole of vegetation on the anterior mitral leaflet (top arrows) and posterior leaflet (bottom arrows). Note the flail posterior leaflet within the left atrium during systole.

Tricuspid Valve

Tricuspid valve vegetations can also be recognized by M-mode and two-dimensional echocardiography.[23–25] Their appearance is similar to mitral valve vegetations. Unless the tricuspid valve is specifically examined by M-mode, however, the tricuspid valve vegetations may be missed (Figure 12-10).[23] Kisslo et al[23] compared M-mode and two-dimensional echocardiography in a patient with tricuspid valve endocarditis. The initial examination revealed large vegetations which on followup showed disruption of the chordae tendineae with a flail leaflet. Berger et al[5] found two-dimensional echocardiography superior to M-mode not only in detecting veg-

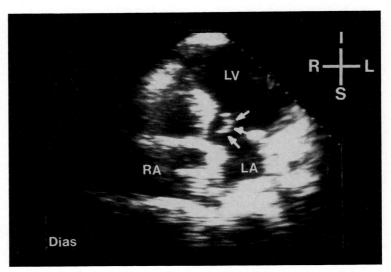

Figure 12-9B. Apical four-chamber view of an anterior mitral leaflet vegetation within the left ventricular inflow tract in diastole (arrows). The large mass of echoes to the right of the arrows is a calcified mitral annulus. Note also left ventricular enlargement.

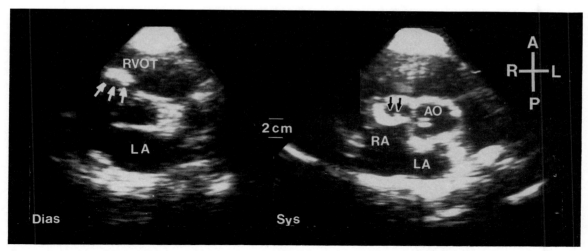

Figure 12-10A. Tricuspid valve vegetation in parasternal short-axis view. Note the vegetations in the right ventricular outflow tract in diastole (white arrows). During systole the vegetations are seen prolapsing toward the right atrium (black arrows). The interatrial septum is not imaged well in this view.

etations but in elucidating the complications of valvular destruction. Tricuspid valve endocarditis has also been detected by two-dimensional echocardiography after pacemaker implantation (Figure 12-11). Many times the pacemaker itself may be confused with a large tricuspid mass by M-mode but is clearly differentiated by two-dimensional echocardiography.[26]

Pulmonary Valve

The pulmonary valve is infrequently the site of vegetative endocarditis.[27–29] Congenital lesions such as pulmonary stenosis and pulmonary regurgitation are frequent prerequisites for development of endocarditis. *Neisseria gonorrhoeae* infrequently

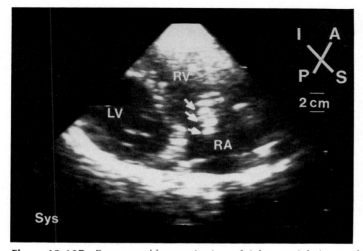

Figure 12-10B. Parasternal long-axis view of right ventricle in systole. Note the large tricuspid valve vegetation in the right atrium (arrows).

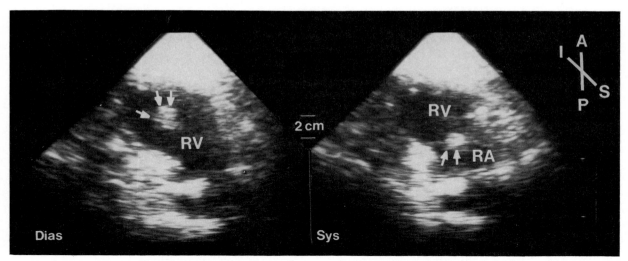

Figure 12-11. Parasternal long-axis view of right ventricular inflow tract of a right ventricular mass due to a large (3 cm) vegetation. Note that the vegetation is seen within the right atrium in systole.

will cause endocarditis (Figure 12-12). However, since it has a particular affinity for the pulmonic valve,[30] the presence of an isolated pulmonic valve vegetation should raise the possibility that *Neisseria gonorrhoeae* may be the cause.[29]

Prosthetic Valve

Prosthetic valve endocarditis is increasingly more common as more valves are being utilized and patients are long-term survivors. Porcine heterografts appear to have a high attack rate (Figure 12-13). In one series, an attack rate over a 32-month

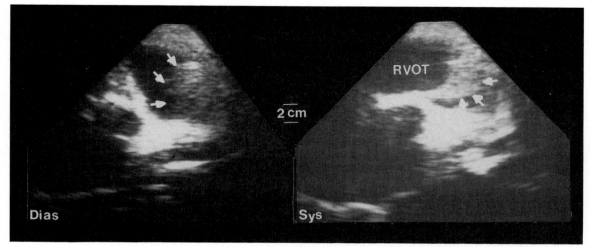

Figure 12-12. Parasternal short-axis view just superior to the aortic valve of a polymicrobial pulmonic valve endocarditis. Note the large vegetation within the right ventricular outflow tract in diastole (arrows, down). During systole the vegetation is seen within the pulmonary artery (arrows, up).

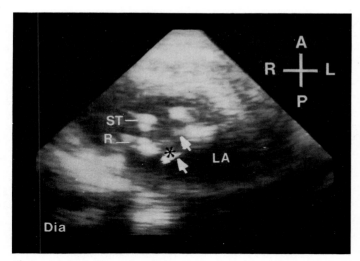

Figure 12-13A. Parasternal short-axis view of porcine mitral valve endocarditis. The vegetation (asterisk) is seen as a light mass of echoes within the valve orifice in diastole (arrow, top) and within the left atrium (arrow, bottom). ST denotes valve stents; R, valve ring.

period with *Staphylococcus epidermidis* suggests that nosocomial infection may be the cause of such an increased rate.[31] Echocardiographic details of prosthetic valve endocarditis are discussed in Chapter 7.

CARDIAC MASSES

Cardiac masses include, in addition to vegetations (see preceding discussion), artificial devices—i.e., pacemaker wires, catheters, and intracardiac patches—tumors, and thrombi. Two-dimensional echocardiography has proved quite useful in the detection of intra- and extracardiac masses. Compared to nuclear imaging and cine-

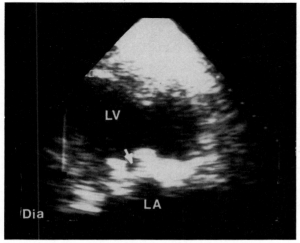

Figure 12-13B. Porcine mitral valve vegetation in apical long-axis view. The vegetations are noted within the valve orifice during diastole (arrow).

angiography, it can better identify the precise location of the mass, its relationship to adjoining structures, and its tissue characteristics—all of which should prove useful in the diagnosis. At this time, its sensitivity and reliability make two-dimensional echocardiography the procedure of choice. Whether nuclear magnetic resonance will improve sensitivity in diagnosis and tissue characterization remains to be determined.

Catheters

Catheters in the right side of the heart are a common source of "mass" echoes.[32–34] These catheter echoes are frequently confused with echoes from the anterior leaflet of the tricuspid valve (Figure 12-14). Echoes from a Swan-Ganz catheter in the right side of the heart are at times confused with a right atrial mass, vegetations, or a pacemaker wire (Figure 12-15).[33–35] Yarnal and Smiley[35] have theorized that the abnormal echoes are from the catheter and the distorted movements of the anterior tricuspid leaflets.

Transvenous right heart pacing catheters can be visualized using M-mode and two-dimensional echocardiography in the majority of patients with catheters at the right ventricular apex or in the coronary sinus.[36] Using both techniques, Reeves et al[36] reported that pacing catheters may appear as linear echoes in the right ventricle during mitral valve recording adjacent or superior to the tricuspid valve. Uncommonly, they may appear anterior to the aortic root and pulmonic valve as a redundant loop of catheter in the right ventricular outflow tract. Occasionally the pacing catheter can mimic a right atrial myxoma (Figure 12-16).[35,36]

Coronary sinus catheters are detected as linear images or echoes recorded in the area of the interatrial septum behind the tricuspid valve. These echoes have a typical late-diastolic anterior–posterior sharp motion (Figure 12-17A). On two-dimensional study they appear near the base of the atrial septum in the apical two-chamber view.[36] Since these catheters are strong reflectors of ultrasound they produce artificial

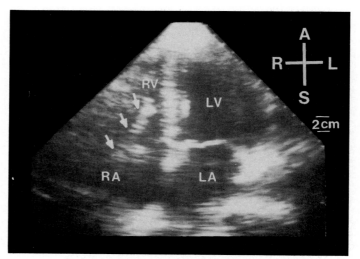

Figure 12-14. Apical four-chamber view of a right ventricular pacing catheter across the tricuspid valve (arrows). Note the catheter appears as a linear echo which is sometimes confused with a vegetation. They are usually not as mobile as vegetations, however.

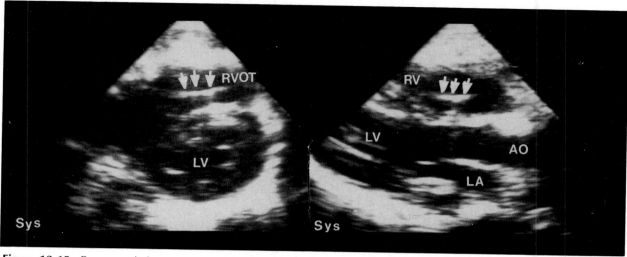

Figure 12-15. Parasternal short-axis view, mitral valve level (left panel) and long-axis view (right panel) of a Swan-Ganz catheter within the right ventricle and right ventricular outflow tract. Note the linear density of the catheter in the right ventricular outflow tract. The catheter appears in the right ventricle adjacent to the tricuspid valve as a linear or round structure.

reverberatory echoes from repeating reflections of the beam. These reverberations are identified as a shadowy effect posterior to the catheter.[37]

Two-dimensional echocardiography can be also useful in the diagnosis of pacemaker perforation of the right ventricular free wall. Using the subcostal or apical four-chamber view the pacing catheter can be visualized through the right ventricular apex with the tip of the catheter outside the cardiac border.[37] Gondi and Nanda[37] also reported perforated interventricular septum and apical ventricular septum (Figure 12-17B).

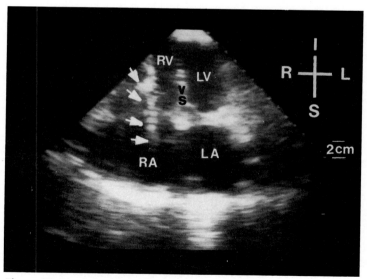

Figure 12-16. Apical four-chamber view of a pacing catheter within the right ventricle, across the tricuspid valve and right atrium (arrows).

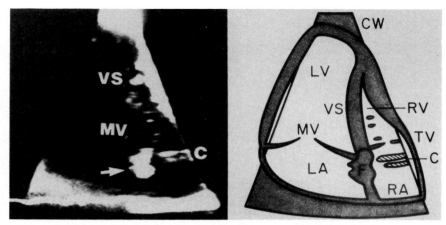

Figure 12-17A. Apical four-chamber view of a patient with a pacing catheter in the coronary sinus (C). CW denotes chest wall; F, central fibrous junction; MV, mitral valve; TV, tricuspid valve. (From Reeves WC, Nanda NC, Barold SS: Echocardiographic evaluation of intracardiac pacing catheters: M-mode and two-dimensional studies. Circulation 58:1055, 1978. By permission of the American Heart Association, Inc.)

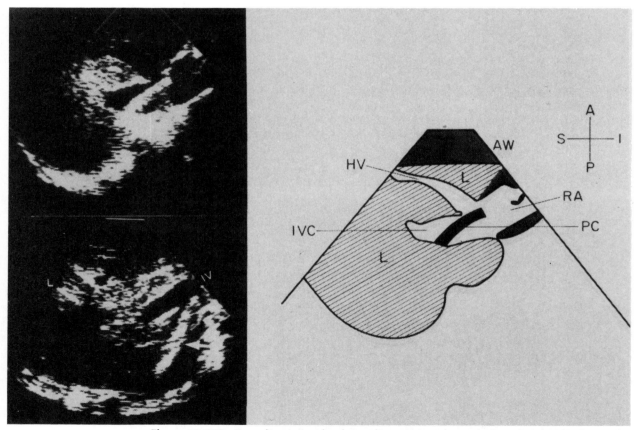

Figure 12-17B. Two-dimensional echocardiogram in subcostal view showing (top) a perforated pacing catheter into the inferior vena cava. Further examination (bottom) of the liner region reveals the catheter tip (arrow) in a hepatic vein. AW denotes anterior wall. Other abbreviations as in Figure 12-17A. (From Gondi B, Nanda NC: Real-time, two-dimensional echocardiographic features of pacemaker perforation. Circulation 64:103, 1981. By permission of the American Heart Association, Inc.)

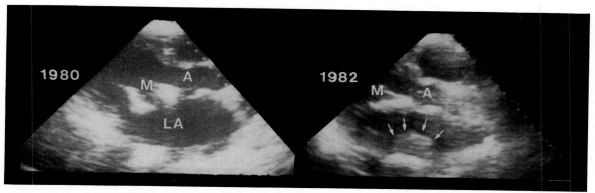

Figure 12-18. Parasternal long-axis views of porcine mitral valve and left atrium in 1980 and 1982. Note the large left atrial mass or thrombus noted within the left atrium in 1982. A, aortic valve; M, porcine mitral valve.

Thrombi

Left Atrial Thrombi

Left atrial thrombi are seen most frequently in patients with mitral valve disease. The common sites of these thrombi are at or near the left atrial appendage and at the posterior left atrial wall. When seen by two-dimensional echocardiography they appear as a homogeneous round or oval mass with specular echoes from within the thrombus (Figure 12-18).[38–41] The M-mode diagnosis is often quite difficult owing to the similarity between the clot and normal left atrial posterior wall. By providing the spatial relationships and multiple views of chambers, two-dimensional echocardiography allows differentiation of an abnormal echo arising from normal cardiac structures such as the interatrial septum or pulmonary vein.

Mikell et al[42] reported the superiority of two-dimensional over M-mode echocardiography in patients with left atrial thrombi and prosthetic mitral valves. The criteria which they found helpful in diagnosing left atrial thrombi were (1) an echo-producing mass confined clearly to the left atrial cavity, and (2) presence of the mass in multiple echocardiographic views (Figure 12-18).

Given the improvements noted with two-dimensional echocardiography, it may supplant the need for cineangiography in diagnosing left atrial thrombi. Recently, a ball thrombus was diagnosed by two-dimensional echocardiography when the M-mode echocardiogram did not visualize the thrombus. The change in Q-M$_1$ interval (Q wave of ECG to mitral closure sound) and systolic ejection time of the aortic valve when the tumor "prolapsed" into the left ventricle outflow tract also helped in the diagnosis.[43]

Left Ventricular Thrombi

Two-dimensional echocardiography has proven more helpful than M-mode in the diagnosis of left ventricular thrombus. Most ventricular clots are located at the left ventricular apex—an area not generally examined well by M-mode echocardiography (Figure 12-19). The detection of clots by two-dimensional echocardiography may be difficult because of similar acoustic impedance of fresh thrombus and surrounding blood (Figure 12-20).[44–46] Mikell et al[42,47] studied acute left ventricular thrombi in an in vivo canine model of acute infarction. Left ventricular thrombi

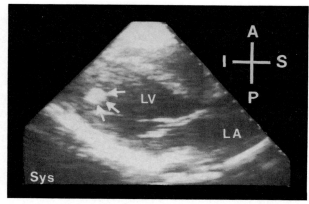

Figure 12-19A. A parasternal long-axis view of the left ventricle in a patient with a ventricular thrombus following an inferior apical infarction. The transducer is angulated laterally to image the thrombus (arrows). Note the difference in acoustic impedence of the thrombus and surrounding cavitary blood.

could be imaged by two-dimensional echocardiography within hours. The thrombi were easily differentiated from surrounding blood and adjacent myocardium. Thrombi as small as 6 mm were highly reflective and were detected by two-dimensional echocardiography.

The echocardiographic appearance of the mural portion of the thrombus is either flat and parallel to the endocardial surface or spherical and protruding into the ventricular cavity. In their study[47] the size of the thrombus rather than the acoustic properties were the limiting factors.

In patients with acute myocardial infarction, left ventricular thrombus is seen in about half of patients who demonstrate dyskinetic and akinetic apical segments.[45] From several studies it is now apparent that apical left ventricular thrombi are the most common source in patients who manifest systemic embolization following acute myocardial infarction.[48–50] Two-dimensional echocardiography can correctly predict

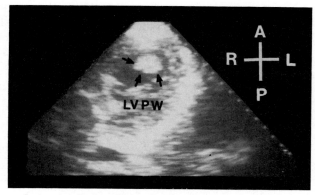

Figure 12-19B. Short-axis parasternal view at the papillary muscle of the same patient. An oblique cut is made through the left ventricular posterior wall (LVPW). Note the thrombus at the apex (arrows).

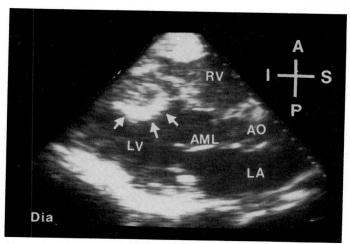

Figure 12-20A. A parasternal long-axis view of the left ventricle of a patient with a large recent anterior apical infarction. Note the large (3.8 cm) thrombus of the left ventricular apex (arrows).

the presence of thrombi in these patients (Figure 12-21). In patients with congestive cardiomyopathy the apical location is also the most common site of thrombus formation (Figure 12-22).[49,51] Recent thrombi appear more shaggy and irregular in configuration and have marked mobility, whereas chronic thrombi are more circumscribed and immobile in presentation.[49]

In patients with transient ischemic attacks the two-dimensional echocardiogram may be helpful in identifying a cardiovascular source. Lovett et al[52] studied patients with one or more recent episodes of cerebral ischemic heart disease and found intracardiac thrombus in 6.5 percent. Cardiac disorders probably related to ischemia

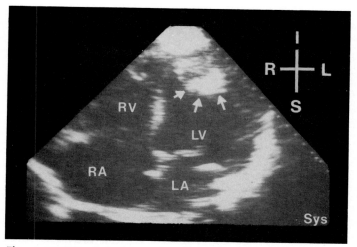

Figure 12-20B. Apical four-chamber view of the same patient. Note the localization of the thrombus at the apex.

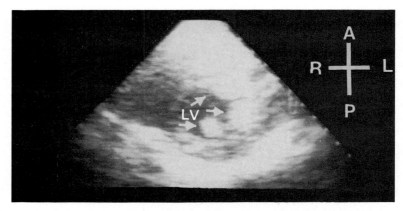

Figure 12-21. Short-axis view at the apex of a patient with multiple apical thrombi following an acute myocardial infarction. Note the multiple thrombi at the apex (arrows).

were found in 23 percent, while 70 percent had normal or near-normal two-dimensional studies. These researchers concluded that the overall low yield of positive findings does not warrant routine use of two-dimensional echocardiography in all patients with transient cerebral ischemia.[52] In selected high-risk patients—i.e. those with cardiomyopathy or evidence of recent or previous transmural myocardial infarction—in whom systemic embolization occurs, two-dimensional echocardiographic evaluation does appear warranted.

Tumors

Tumors found within the heart are usually myxomas,[53] myxosarcomas, hemangiomas, fibromas, and rhabdomyosarcomas.[55] Extracardiac tumors include mediastinal cysts,[56] thymomas,[57] and teratomas.[58] The tumors will be discussed with respect to the cardiac chambers and structures they commonly invade.

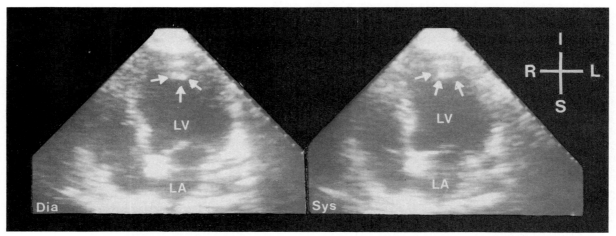

Figure 12-22. Apical four-chamber view of a patient with a congestive cardiomyopathy in diastole and systole. Note the thrombus (arrows) at the ventricular apex. The thrombus appears to be well circumscribed and immobile.

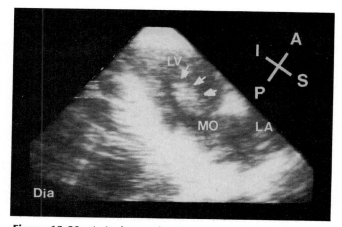

Figure 12-23. Apical two-chamber view of a patient with a left atrial myxoma. Note the tumor (arrows) within the left ventricular inflow tract in diastole. MO, mitral orifice.

Left Atrium

By far the most common left atrial tumor is the atrial myxoma (Figure 12-23). The tumor is frequently pedunculated and usually arises from the interatrial septum. Because of its structure, the myxoma is mobile and moves into the left ventricular inflow tract during diastole (Figure 12-24). During ventricular systole, it prolapses back into the left atrium. The most common presentation for left atrial myxoma, in order of frequency, is congestive heart failure, suspected mitral stenosis, chest pain, pulmonary edema, and systemic embolization.[53,59,60] Occasionally atrial myxoma will be found after sudden death of previously asymptomatic patients. This tumor has a smooth surface, is polypoid, and histologically shows abundant amorphous interstitial ground substance scattered among undifferentiated mesenchymal cells.[59]

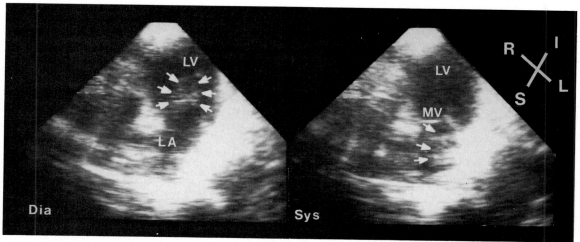

Figure 12-24. Modified apical four-chamber view in diastole and systole of a patient with a left atrial myxoma. Note the tumor within the left ventricle in diastole (arrows). During systole the tumor is seen within the left atrium (arrow). Most atrial myxomas attach to the interatrial septum, are within the left atrium in systole, and are within the left ventricle in diastole.

Although each case has been isolated there are now at least six reported cases of familial myxomas.[60] There appears to be an association of right atrial myxoma with atrial septal defect[61,62] and mitral valve prolapse.[63–65]

M-mode echocardiography has proven quite useful in the diagnosis of myxoma except when the mass is located superiorly in the left atrium and is nonpedunculated.[66,67] Occasionally when the tumor mass does not fall into the left ventricular inflow tract, the M-mode study may be negative unless careful scanning of the left atrium has taken place from a higher intercostal space or from the suprasternal notch.[67–69]

Two-dimensional study has improved the sensitivity and specificity of echocardiography in the diagnosis of myxoma by providing qualitative and relatively quantitative information regarding size, shape, and mobility of the tumor.[70–74] M-mode echocardiography may sometimes not be helpful in distinguishing a left atrial from an extracardiac tumor. In contrast, two-dimensional echocardiography allows direct visualization of the location, size, and motion of the tumor.[71] In the studies to date[70–75] two-dimensional echocardiography is more accurate than M-mode in making the diagnosis of atrial myxoma. In fact, the reliability of two-dimensional echocardiography in the diagnosis of myxoma permits referral of the patient to surgery without confirmatory heart catheterization.[75]

One case of atrial myxoma in which M-mode echocardiography gave false-negative results was attributed to the highly vascular nature of the tumor. But in this case and other false-negative studies excessive damping or reject setting was more likely the cause for the error. Isolated myxomas and fibroadenomas of the mitral valve have also been recognized. Their clinical and angiographic appearance may be quite similar to atrial myxoma. Echocardiographically they appear as a tumor mass attached to the mitral leaflets.[77,78]

Right Atrium

Right atrial myxomas occur at a lower frequency than left atrial myxomas.[60] These tumors are usually diagnosed by M-mode and two-dimensional echocardiography as a mass of abnormal echoes behind the tricuspid valve (Figure 12-25).[79–86] Tricuspid regurgitation may be induced where the tumor mass interferes with tricuspid closure; therefore, there are right ventricular and right atrial enlargement with a right ventricular volume overload pattern. Occasionally, abnormal masses from the tricuspid valve, such as vegetations, will mimic the M-mode echocardiographic findings of myxoma.[81] Right atrial myxoma has been associated with atrial septal defects[61,62] and mitral valve prolapse.[63–65]

Biatrial myxomas have also been reported.[87–89] In these cases the classic M-mode appearance of a left atrial myxoma is apparent behind the anterior mitral leaflet. The echoes from the right atrial tumor are seen in the right ventricle behind the anterior tricuspid leaflet. Frequently both tumors are visualized in the same M-mode plane. Complete examination of all four chambers and valves is warranted in each patient in whom a myxoma is suspected.[87]

Left Ventricle

Numerous left ventricular tumors have been described echocardiographically and include myxomas,[90,91] fibromas,[92,93] rhabdomyomas, and rhabdomyosarcomas (Figure 12–26).[55] Echocardiographically they can be lamellar or oval, mobile or immobile. Two-dimensional echocardiography is quite helpful in differentiating these

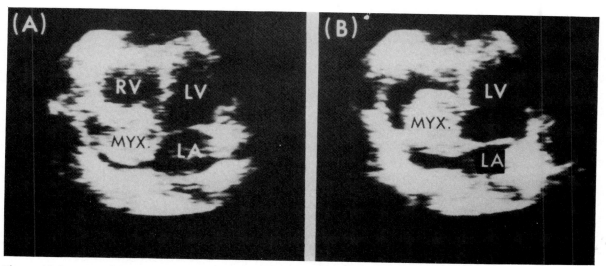

Figure 12-25. Apical four-chamber view of a right atrial myxoma (MYX). The tumor is an echo-dense mass within the right atrium in systole (A) and in the right ventricle in diastole (B). (From Weyman AE: Clinical Application of Cross-Sectional Echocardiography. Philadelphia, Lea & Febiger, 1982. With permission.)

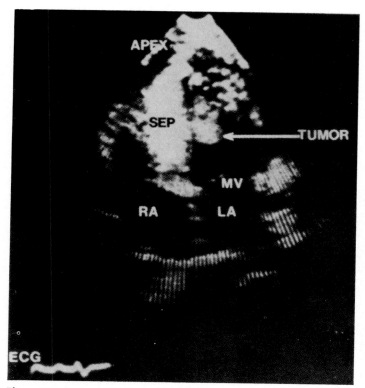

Figure 12-26. Modified apical four-chamber view of a metastatic malignant melanoma within the left ventricle that appears as an intracavitary mass of echoes. SEP denotes septum. (From Ports TA, Cogan J, Schiller NB, et al: Echocardiography of left ventricular masses. Circulation 58:528, 1978. By permission of the American Heart Association, Inc.)

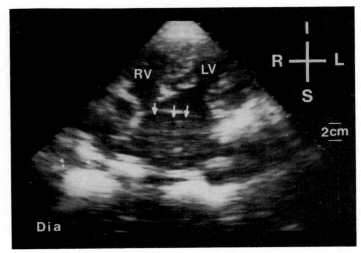

Figure 12-27. Apical four-chamber view of a patient with a mediastinal angiosarcoma. Note complete compression of the left atrium by the tumor (arrows). At surgery the tumor was found also compressing the left pulmonary vein.

tumors from apical thrombi or from normal structures imaged from an atypical M-mode imaging plane.

Right Ventricle

Several types of right ventricular tumors have been diagnosed echocardiographically.[94-100] These include fibromas, myxomas,[94,100] metastatic melanoma,[96] and osteogenic sarcoma.[99] The tumors are frequently seen within the right ventricular cavity; however, not infrequently, they are observed prolapsing into the right ventricular outflow tract[99] or even obstructing the pulmonary valve.[97] Myxomas, which are pedunculated and mobile, are by far the most common.[97,100]

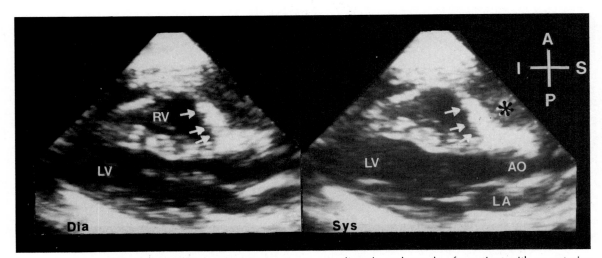

Figure 12-28. Parasternal long-axis view in diastole and systole of a patient with an anterior mediastinal mass. The mass was rigid (asterisk) and compressed the right ventricular outflow tract (arrows). The patient had a testicular tumor with anterior mediastinal metastasis.

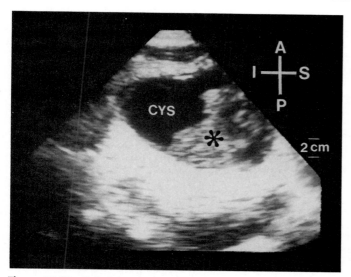

Figure 12-29. Subxiphoid view of a hepatic mass in the region of the inferior vena cava. The hepatic mass (asterisk) was a hepatic metastasis with a cystic component (CYS).

Pericardial or Mediastinal Tumors

Extracardiac tumors that have been diagnosed by echocardiography include mediastinal or pericardial cyst,[56] thymoma,[57] intrapericardial teratoma,[58] and pericardial angiosarcoma (Figure 12-27). These tumors are imaged anterior to the right ventricular free wall (Figure 12-28) or posterior to the left ventricular posterior wall. Two-dimensional echocardiography has been quite helpful in diagnosing these extracardiac tumors[101] (Figure 12-29).

Pseudotumors

Pseudotumors are not infrequently misdiagnosed as right atrial myxoma or left atrial myxoma. A Swan-Ganz catheter across the tricuspid valve or a large tricuspid valve vegetation may mimic a right atrial myxoma.[33–35] Also, not infrequently, a myxomatous mitral valve imaged in long axis or from an apical position can give the false impression of an atrial myxoma.[102]

REFERENCES

1. Spangler RD, Johnson MJ, Holmes HJ, et al: Echocardiographic demonstration of bacterial vegetations in active infective endocarditis. JCU I:126–132, 1973
2. Dillon JC, Feigenbaum H, Konecke LL: Echocardiographic manifestations of valvular vegetations. Am Heart J 86:698–705, 1973
3. Roy P, Tajik AJ, Guiliani ER, et al: Spectrum of echocardiographic findings in bacterial endocarditis. Circulation 53:474–482, 1976
4. Wann LS, Dillon JC, Weyman AE, et al: Echocardiography in bacterial endocarditis. N Engl J Med 295:135–139, 1979
5. Berger M, Delfin LA, Jelveh M, et al: Two-dimensional echocardiographic findings in right-sided infective endocarditis. Circulation 61:855–861, 1980
6. Ginzton LE, Siegel RJ, Criley M: Natural history of tricuspid valve endocarditis: A two-dimensional echocardiographic study. Am J Cardiol 49:1853–1859, 1982
7. Mintz GS, Kotler MN, Segal BL, et al: Comparison of two-dimensional and M-mode echocardiography in the evaluation of patients with infective endocarditis. Am J Cardiol 43:738–744, 1979

8. Wann LS, Hallam CC, Dillon JC, et al: Comparison of M-mode and cross-sectional echocardiography in infective endocarditis. Circulation 60:728–733, 1979

9. Martin RP, Meltzer RS, Chia BL, et al: Clinical utility of two-dimensional echocardiography in infective endocarditis. Am J Cardiol 46:379–385, 1980

10. Stewart JA, Silimperi D, Harris P, et al: Echocardiographic documentation of vegetative lesions in infective endocarditis. Circulation 61:374–380, 1980

11. Mintz GS, Kotler MN, Segal BL, et al: Survival of patients with aortic valve endocarditis. The prognostic implication of the echocardiogram. Arch Intern Med 139:862–866, 1979

12. Pratt C, Whitecomb C, Neuman A, et al: Relationship of vegetations on echocardiography to the clinical course and systemic emboli in bacterial endocarditis (Abstract). Am J Cardiol 41:384, 1978

13. Weinstein L, Schlesinger JJ: Pathoanatomic, pathophysiologic and clinical correlations in endocarditis. N Engl J Med 219:832–839, 1974

14. Roberts WC, Buckbinder NA: Healed left-sided endocarditis: A clinicopathologic study. Am J Cardiol 40:876–888, 1977

15. Davis RS, Strom JA, Frishman W, et al: The demonstration of vegetations by echocardiography in bacterial endocarditis. Am J Med 69:57–63, 1980

16. Bardy G, Talano JV, Reisberg B, et al: Sensitivity and specificity of combined M-mode and two-dimensional echocardiography in infective endocarditis. J Cardiovasc Ultrasound (in press)

17. Takeda P, Skalsky L, Bommer WJ, et al: Two-dimensional echocardiography in infective endocarditis: Early and late diagnosis, therapeutic and prognostic implications (Abstract). Circulation 62:(Suppl III):III-98, 1980

18. DeMaria AN, King JF, Salel AF, Echography and phonography of acute aortic regurgitation in bacterial endocarditis. Ann Intern Med 82:329–334, 1975

19. Melvin M, Berger M, Lutzker P, et al: Noninvasive methods for detection of valve vegetations in infective endocarditis. Am J Cardiol 47:271–278, 1981

20. Berger M, Gallerstein PE, Benhur P, et al: Evaluation of aortic valve endocarditis by two-dimensional echocardiography. Chest 80:61–67, 1981

21. Lundstrom N-R, Bjorkhem G: Mitral and tricuspid valve vegetations in infancy diagnosed by echocardiography. Acta Paediatr Scand 68:345–350, 1979

22. Bamrah VS, Williams GW, Hughes CV, et al: Haemophilus parainfluenza mitral valve vegetation without hemodynamic abnormality. Am J Med 66:543–546, 1979

23. Kisslo J, von Ramm OT, Haney R, et al: Echocardiographic evaluation of tricuspid valve endocarditis. Am J Cardiol 38:502–507, 1976

24. Chandraratna PAN, Aronow WS: Spectrum of echocardiographic findings in tricuspid valve endocarditis. Br Heart J 42:528–534, 1979

25. Jemsek JC, Greenberg SB, Gentry LJ, et al: Haemophilus parainfluenza endocarditis. Repeat of two cases and review of the literature. Am J Med 66:51–55, 1979

26. Ward C, Naik DR, Johnstone MC: Tricuspid endocarditis complicating pacemaker implantation demonstrated by echocardiography. Br J Radiol 52:501–502, 1979

27. Chiang C-W, Lee Y-S, Chang C-H, et al: Preoperative and postoperative echocardiographic studies of pulmonic valvular endocarditis. Chest 80:232–234, 1981

28. Kramer NE, Sukjhit SG, Ramesh P, et al: Pulmonary valve vegetation detected with echocardiography. Am J Cardiol 39:1064–1075, 1977

29. Dzindzio BS, Meyer L, Osterholm R, et al: Isolated gonococcal pulmonary valve endocarditis: diagnosis by echocardiography. Circulation 59:1319–1324, 1979

30. Bain RC, Edwards JE, Scheifley CH, et al: Right-sided bacterial endocarditis and endarteritis: a clinical and pathologic study. Am J Med 24:98–104, 1958

31. Donham WH, Rhoades ER: Endocarditis associated with porcine valve xenografts. Arch Intern Med 139:1350–1352, 1979

32. Kendrick MH, Harrington JJ, Sharma GVRK, et al: Ventricular pacemaker wire simulating a right atrial mass. Chest 72:649–650, 1977

33. Silverman B, Kozma G, Silverman M, et al: Echocardiographic manifestations of postinfarction ventricular septal rupture. Chest 68:778–780, 1975

34. Charuzi Y, Kraus R, Swan HJC: Echocardiographic interpretation in the presence of Swan-Ganz intracardiac catheters. Am J Cardiol 40:989–994, 1977

35. Yarnal JR, Smiley WH: Right atrial mass simulated echocardiographically by a Swan-Ganz catheter. Chest 74:478, 1978

36. Reeves WC, Nanda NC, Barold SS: Echocardiographic evaluation of intracardiac pacing catheters: M-mode and two-dimensional studies. Circulation 58:1049–1056, 1978

37. Gondi B, Nanda NC: Real-time, two-dimensional echocardiographic features of pacemaker perforation. Circulation 64:97–106, 1981
38. Nasser WK, Davis RH, Dillon JC, et al: Atrial myxoma. II. Phonocardiographic, echocardiographic, hemodynamic and angiographic features in nine cases. Am Heart J 83:810–817, 1972
39. Spangler RD, Okin JT: Echocardiographic demonstration of a left atrial thrombus. Chest 67:716–719, 1975
40. Seward JB, Gura M, Haler DJ, et al: Evaluation of M-mode echocardiography and wide angle two-dimensional sector echocardiography in the diagnosis of intracardiac masses (Abstract). Circulation 58 (Suppl II):II-234, 1978
41. Mikell FL, Asinger RW, Rourke T, et al: Detection of intracardiac thrombi by two-dimensional echocardiography (Abstract). Circulation 48 (Suppl II):II-43, 1978
42. Mikell FL, Asinger RW, Rourke T, et al: Two-dimensional echocardiographic demonstration of left atrial thrombi in patients with prosthetic mitral valves. Circulation 60:1183–1190, 1979
43. Sunagawa K, Orita Y, Tanaka S, et al: Left atrial ball thrombus diagnosed by two-dimensional echocardiography. Am Heart J 100:89–94, 1980
44. Asinger RW, Mikell FL, Sharma B, et al: Observations on detecting left ventricular thrombus with two-dimensional echocardiography: emphasis on avoidance of false positive diagnoses. Am J Cardiol 47:145–156, 1981
45. Asinger RW, Mikell FL, Elsperger KJ, et al: Incidence of left ventricular thrombosis after acute transmural myocardial infarction. N Engl J Med 305:297–302, 1981
46. Meltzer RS, Guthaner D, Rakowski H, et al: Diagnosis of left ventricular thrombi by two-dimensional echocardiography. Br Heart J 42:261–265, 1979
47. Mikell FL, Asinger RW, Elsperger KJ, et al: Tissue acoustic properties of fresh left ventricular thrombi and visualization by two-dimensional echocardiography: experimental observations. Am J Cardiol 49:1157–1165, 1982
48. Quinones MA, Nelson JG, Winters WL, et al: Clinical spectrum of left ventricular mural thrombi in a large cardiac population: assessment by two-dimensional echocardiography (Abstract). Am J Cardiol 45:435, 1980
49. DeMaria AN, Bommer W, Neumann A, et al: Left ventricular thrombi identified by cross-sectional echocardiography. Ann Intern Med 90:14–18, 1979
50. Ports TA, Cogan J, Schiller NB, et al: Echocardiography of left ventricular masses. Circulation 48:528–536, 1978
51. Kramer NE, Rathod R, Chawla KK, et al: Echocardiographic diagnosis of left ventricular mural thrombi occurring in cardiomyopathy. Am Heart J 96:381–383, 1978
52. Lovett JL, Sandok BA, Giuliani ER, et al: Two-dimensional echocardiography in patients with focal cerebral ischemia. Ann Intern Med 95:1–4, 1981
53. Nasser WK, et al: Atrial myxoma. I. Clinical and pathologic features in nine cases. Am Heart J 83:694–699, 1972
54. Winer HE, Kronzon I, Fox A, et al: Primary cardiac chondromyxosarcoma—clinical and echocardiographic manifestations: a case report. J Thorac Cardiovasc Surg 74:567–572, 1977
55. Farooki ZQ, Henry JG, Arciniegas E, et al: Ultrasonic pattern of ventricular rhabdomyoma in two infants. Am J Cardiol 34:842–847, 1974
56. Koch PC, Kronzon I, Winer HE, et al: Displacement of the heart by a giant mediastinal cyst. Am J Cardiol 40:445–451, 1977
57. Canedo MI, Otken L, Stefadouros MA: Echocardiographic features of cardiac compression by a thymoma simulating cardiac tamponade and obstruction of the superior vena cava. Br Heart J 39:1038–1043, 1977
58. Farooki ZQ, Hakimi N, Arciniegas E, et al: Echocardiographic features in a case of intrapericardial teratoma. JCU 6:108–112, 1978
59. Bulkley BH, Hutchins GM: Atrial myxomas: a fifty year review. Am Heart J 97:639–643, 1979
60. Powers JC, Falkoff M, Heinle RA, et al: Familial cardiac myxoma. Emphasis on unusual clinical manifestations. J Thorac Cardiovasc Surg 77:782–788, 1979
61. Marpole DGF, Kloster FE, Bristow JD, et al: Atrial myxoma. A continuing diagnostic challenge. Am J Cardiol 23:597–602, 1969
62. Symbas PN, Abbott OA, Logan WD, et al: Atrial myxomas. Special emphasis on unusual manifestations. Chest 59:504–510, 1970
63. Meyers SN, Shapiro JE, Barresi V, et al: Right atrial myxoma with right to left shunting and mitral valve prolapse. Am J Med 62:308–314, 1977
64. DeMaria AN, Vismara LA, Miller RR, et al: Unusual echocardiographic manifestations of right and left heart myxomas. Am J Med 59:713–720, 1975

65. Sharratt GP, Grover ML, Monro JL: Calcified left atrial myxoma with floppy mitral valve. Br Heart J 42:608–610, 1979

66. Millman AE, Federici EE, Miskovits C: Left atrial myxoma: Two-dimensional echocardiographic, angiographic, and pathological correlations. J Med Soc NJ 76:749–753, 1979

67. Petsas AA, Gottlieb S, Kingsley B, et al: Echocardiographic diagnosis of left atrial myxoma. Br Heart J 38:627–632, 1976

68. Lee Y-C, Magram MY: Nonprolapsing left atrial tumor: the M-mode echocardiographic diagnosis. Chest 78:332–333, 1980

69. Kostis JB, Moghadam AN: Echocardiographic diagnosis of left atrial myxoma. Chest 58:550–558, 1970

70. Lappe DL, Bulkley BH, Weiss JL: Two-dimensional echocardiographic diagnosis of left atrial myxoma. Chest 74:55–58, 1978

71. Yoshikawa J, Sabah I, Yanagihara K, et al: Cross-sectional echocardiographic diagnosis of large left atrial tumor and extracardiac tumor compressing the left atrium. Limitation of M-mode echocardiography in distinguishing the two lesions. Am J Cardiol 42:853–857, 1978

72. Sonotani N: Conventional and two-dimensional real-time echocardiographic diagnoses of left heart tumors: three cases of left atrial myxoma. Bull Osaka Med Sch 25:128–138, 1979

73. Bulkley BH, Weiss JL: Atrial myxomas. Triumph of machine over man (Editorial). Chest 75:537–538, 1979

74. Moses HW, Nanda NC: Real time two-dimensional echocardiography in the diagnosis of left atrial myxoma. Chest 78:788–791, 1980

75. Donahoo JS, Weiss JL, Gardner TJ, et al: Current management of atrial myxoma with emphasis on a new diagnostic technique. Ann Surg 189:763–768, 1979

76. Stewart JA, Warnica JW, Kirk ME, et al: Left atrial myxoma: false negative echocardiographic findings in a tumor demonstrated by coronary arteriography. Am Heart J 98:228–232, 1979

77. Sandrasagra FA, Oliver WA, English TAH: Myxoma of the mitral valve. Br Heart J 42:221–223, 1979

78. Read RC, White HJ, Murphy ML, et al: The malignant potentiality of left atrial myxoma. J Thorac Cardiovasc Surg 68:857–868, 1974

79. Pernod J, Piwnica A, Duret JC: Right atrial myxoma: an echocardiographic study. Br Heart J 40:201–203, 1978

80. Yuste P, Asin E, Cerdan FJ, et al: Echocardiogram in right atrial myxoma. Chest 69:94–96, 1976

81. Come PC, Kurland GS, Vine HS: Two-dimensional echocardiography in differentiating right atrial and tricuspid valve mass lesions. Am J Cardiol 44:1207–1212, 1979

82. Seward JB, Gura GM, Hagler DJ, et al: Evaluation of M-mode echocardiography and wide-angle two-dimensional sector echocardiography in the diagnosis of intracardiac masses (Abstract). Circulation 58(Suppl II):II-234, 1978

83. Harbold NB Jr, Gau GT: Echocardiographic diagnosis of right atrial myxoma. Mayo Clin Proc 48:284–291, 1973

84. Farooki ZQ, Green EW, Arciniegas E: Echocardiographic pattern of right atrial tumour motion. Br Heart J 38:580–588, 1976

85. Perod J, Piwnca A, Duret JC: Right atrial myxoma: an echocardiographic study. Br Heart J 40:201, 1978

86. Frishman W, Factor S, Jordon A, et al: Right atrial myxoma: unusual clinical presentation and atypical glandular histology. Circulation 59:1070–1074, 1979

87. Fitterer JD, Spicer MJ, Nelson WP: Echocardiographic demonstration of bilateral atrial myxomas. Chest 70:282–284, 1976

88. Nicholson KG, Prior AL, Norman AG, et al: Bilateral atrial myxomas diagnosed preoperatively and successfully removed. Br Med J 2(6084):440–449, 1977

89. Gustafson AG, Edler IG, Dahlback OK: Bilateral atrial myxomas diagnosed by echocardiography. Acta Med Scand 201:391–397, 1977

90. Meller J, Teichholz LE, Pichard AO, et al: Left ventricular myxoma: echocardiographic diagnosis and review of the literature. Am J Med 63:816–822, 1977

91. Morgan DI, Palazola J, Reed W, et al: Left heart myxomas. Am J Cardiol 40:611–619, 1977

92. Oliva PB, Breckinridge JC, Johnson ML, et al: Left ventricular outflow obstruction produced by a pedunculated fibroma in a newborn. Chest 74:590–591, 1978

93. Levisman JA, MacAlpin RN, Abbasi AS, et al: Echocardiographic diagnosis of a mobile, pedunculated tumor in the left ventricular cavity. Am J Cardiol 36:957–964, 1975

94. Asayama J, Kunishige H, Katsume H, et al: The ultrasound cardiographic findings of myxoma in the right ventricular wall. Cardiovasc Sound Bull 5:129, 1975

95. Nanda NC, Barold SS, Gramiak R, et al: Echocardiographic features of right ventricular outflow tumor prolapsing into the pulmonary artery. Am J Cardiol 40:272–274, 1977

96. Ports TA, Schiller NB, Strunk BL: Echocardiography of right ventricular tumors. Circulation 56:439–444, 1977

97. Chandraratna PAN, Pedro S, Elkins RC, et al: Echocardiographic, angiocardiographic, and surgical correlations in right ventricular myxoma simulating valvar pulmonic stenosis. Circulation 55:619–676, 1977

98. Roelandt J, Bletter WB, Leuftink EW, et al: Ultrasonic demonstration of right ventricular myxoma. JCU 5:191–201, 1977

99. Jaffe CC, Kelley MJ, Taunt KA: Two-dimensional echocardiographic identification of a right ventricle tumor. Radiology 129:471–478, 1978

100. Melendez LJ, Sears GA, Coles JC: Right ventricular tumour demonstrated by echocardiography. CMA Journal 118:62–63, 1978

101. Yoshikawa J, Sabah I, Yanagihara K, et al: Cross-sectional echocardiographic diagnosis of large left atrial tumor and extracardiac tumor compressing the left atrium. Am J Cardiol 42:853–859, 1978

102. Liedtke AJ, Babb JD, DeJoseph RL: Mitral valve echoes in patients with mitral valve prolapse syndrome. Am Heart J 97:286–290, 1979

CHAPTER 13

Congenital Heart Disease

Elizabeth A. Fisher

Two-dimensional echocardiography has contributed significantly to the noninvasive evaluation of congenital heart defects, often providing a definitive anatomic diagnosis. It improves spatial orientation over M-mode echocardiography. This is of particular value in defining septal defects and positional anomalies of the great vessels and atrioventricular valves. Structures such as coronary arteries, the interatrial septum, the aortic arch, the pulmonary artery bifurcation, vena cavae, and pulmonary veins, not easily recognized by other noninvasive means, can often be demonstrated. It visualizes structures from positions other than the precordium, which is especially helpful in anomalies of the right side of the heart frequently encountered in congenital heart disease.

In this chapter emphasis is placed on the two-dimensional echocardiographic diagnosis of those congenital heart defects which may be encountered in adolescents and adults. The defects are classified according to their echocardiographic—rather than hemodynamic—features, since the latter may have little relevance to the echocardiographic interpretation. This approach provides a basis for the systematic analysis of two-dimensional echocardiograms by pattern recognition. For example, the major echocardiographic features of atrial septal defect and total anomalous pulmonary venous drainage are very similar, since both have right ventricular dilatation. Hemodynamically, however, they belong to different groups of acyanotic and cyanotic heart disease. Further echocardiographic analysis should identify distinguishing features that allow a definitive diagnosis.

Some forms of congenital heart disease are characterized by a spectrum of anatomic features. This can result in different echocardiographic patterns in patients with the same congenital defect. In tricuspid atresia some patients may have two clearly demonstrable ventricles and a pattern of left ventricular dilatation; in some patients there may be only one demonstrable ventricle and therefore a pattern of single ventricle.

Eight major echocardiographic patterns in congenital heart disease have been defined; these are:

- Right ventricular dilatation
- Left ventricular dilatation
- Left atrial dilatation
- Right ventricular hypertrophy
- Left ventricular hypertrophy

- Loss of anatomic continuity
- Great artery malpositions
- Single ventricular chamber

I will discuss the echocardiographic features of the congenital defects that present with each pattern.

RIGHT VENTRICULAR DILATATION

The nonspecific echocardiographic pattern of dilatation of the right ventricle is present in many forms of congenital heart disease, primarily those with right ventricular volume overload. In the presence of right ventricular dilatation, right ventricular wall thickness is usually normal. The left ventricle may appear small in its anteroposterior dimension because of compression of that chamber by the enlarged right ventricle. In massive right heart dilatation, the interventricular septum is displaced posterior to the anterior wall of the aorta, giving the impression of an overriding aorta. Except where noted, reversed (paradoxical) or flat septal motion is commonly associated with right ventricular dilatation.

Atrial Septal Defect

The interatrial septum can be visualized by two-dimensional echocardiography from the parasternal, apical, and subcostal views. The diagnosis of atrial septal defect is made by direct visualization of the defect.[1-6] The diagnosis is most reliably made from the subcostal four-chamber view.[2-6] The interatrial septum is oriented parallel to the ultrasound beam in the apical four-chamber and parasternal short-axis views; therefore, drop-out of echoes from the fossa ovalis cannot be differentiated from a secundum atrial septal defect[1-6] (Figure 13-1), and may give an erroneous impression of the size of a primum atrial septal defect.[3] The sensitivity specificity of the echocardiographic diagnosis of atrial septal defect approaches 100 percent in patients in whom an adequate subcostal examination can be obtained.[4,5]

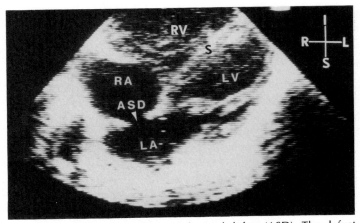

Figure 13-1. Subcostal four-chamber view, secundum atrial septal defect (ASD). The defect is in the midportion of the septum. LA denotes left atrium; LV, left ventricle, RA, right atrium, RV, right ventricle, S, interventricular septum.

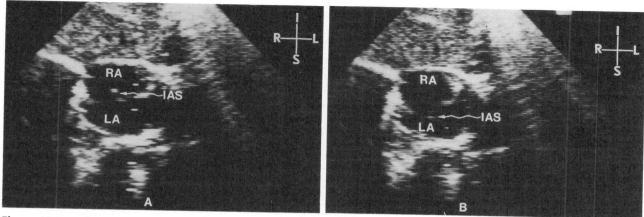

Figure 13-2. Subcostal four-chamber view, complete D-transposition of the great arteries, one day after balloon atrial septostomy. The torn flap of the interatrial septum (IAS) can be seen in the right atrium and the left atrium in different phases of the cardiac cycle (A and B, respectively).

The defect of secundum atrial septal defect is in the midportion of the interatrial septum in the region of the fossa ovalis[4,5] (Figures 13-1 and 13-2). Some authors report a high incidence of anterior mitral valve prolapse in secundum atrial septal defect,[2] but this finding is disputed by others.[7]

A primum atrial septal defect is situated low in the interatrial septum contiguous with the atrioventricular valve rings[1,4,5,8] (Figure 13-3). Its superior margin generally produces a bright linear echo.[3,6] A cleft in the anterior leaflet of the mitral valve is present in most patients with primum atrial septal defect.[2,6,9] This is best seen in a somewhat oblique plane between the parasternal long-axis and short-axis views that transversely cuts through the anterior leaflet.[8] The superior and inferior portions of the cleft anterior leaflet separate in diastole, the superior portion narrowing the left

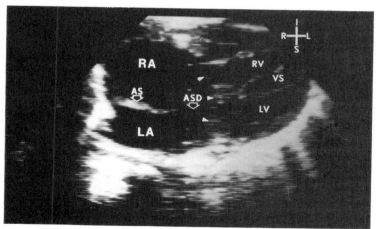

Figure 13-3. Subcostal four-chamber view, primum atrial septal defect (ASD). The defect is in the lower atrial septum (AS), confluent with the atrioventricular valve rings (arrowheads). Note the dilatation of the right ventricle. VS denotes interventricular septum.

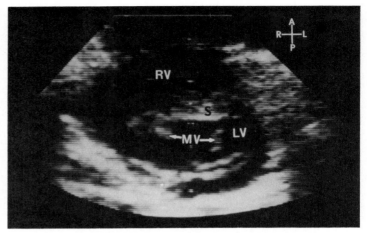

Figure 13-4. Parasternal view, between long- and short-axis views, of cleft mitral valve (MV). The cleft of the anterior leaflet and the abnormal positions of the portions of the leaflet in diastole are evident.

ventricular outflow tract (Figure 13-4). The encroachment of the anterior leaflet on the left ventricular outflow tract can also be appreciated in the parasternal or sub-costal views.[10] The division of the anterior leaflet is evident in the parasternal short-axis view,[6] but the abnormal motion is not as well appreciated. A malpositioned tricuspid valve or malpositioned papillary muscles should not be misinterpreted as a cleft mitral valve.[11]

Common atrium has been diagnosed from the apical four-chamber view by failure to visualize any atrial septal echoes.[6] The diagnosis is best reserved, however, for those patients in whom this finding is confirmed from the subcostal four-chamber view, since drop-out from the fossa ovalis in the apical four-chamber view may lead to a false diagnosis in patients with primum atrial septal defect[3] (Figure 13-5).

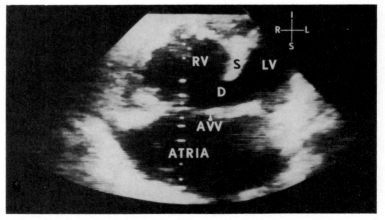

Figure 13-5. Apical four-chamber view, complete atrioventricular canal (Type C). No atrial septal echoes were seen, even though the patient did not have a common atrium. There is a large posterior ventricular septal defect (D) and an undivided anterior leaflet of the common atrioventricular valve (AVV).

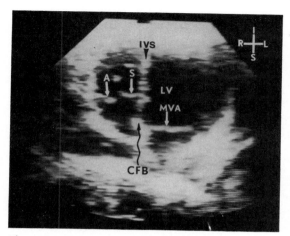

Figure 13-6. Apical four-chamber view, Ebstein's anomaly of the tricuspid valve. The septal (S) leaflet of the tricuspid valve is displaced inferiorly from the central fibrous body (CFB) into the right ventricle. A denotes anterior leaflet of the tricuspid valve; IVS, interventricular septum; MVA, mitral valve annulus.

Ebstein's Anomaly of the Tricuspid Valve

There are no definitive diagnostic features of Ebstein's anomaly by M-mode echo-cardiography,[12,13] whereas there are by two-dimensional echocardiography. The attachments of the atrioventricular valves to the central fibrous body are best seen from a four-chamber apical or subcostal view. In Ebstein's anomaly the two-dimensional echocardiographic diagnosis is based on demonstrating the displacement of the small septal and the large anterior leaflets of the tricuspid valve inferiorly into the right ventricle[3,12–16] (Figure 13-6). The septal leaflet hinge point with the septum is displaced inferiorly from the central fibrous body and ranges from 1.4 to 3.2 cm in one series[16] and from 2 to 7 cm in another.[12] This displacement of even a few millimeters beyond normal appears to be a sensitive sign for Ebstein's anomaly. However, this measurement is not a good index of severity in the absence of normal values for age. Atrial septal defect, patent foramen ovale, and pulmonary valvular stenosis are commonly associated lesions.

Anomalous Pulmonary Venous Drainage

Partial anomalous pulmonary venous drainage is indistinguishable from atrial septal defect by M-mode and two-dimensional echocardiography[17] because the majority of patients with partial anomalous pulmonary venous drainage have an associated secundum atrial septal defect. It is also not always possible to visualize normally each of the pulmonary veins as they enter the left atrium.[3,18] Total anomalous pulmonary venous drainage can be excluded by recording at least one pulmonary vein entering the left atrium[18] from the apical or subcostal four-chamber view.

Separation of all the pulmonary veins from the left atrium and mitral valve is characteristic of total anomalous pulmonary venous drainage.[18,19,21,22] In total anomalous pulmonary venous drainage to the coronary sinus, the dilated coronary sinus appears as an oval or circular echo-free structure just posterior to the mitral valve

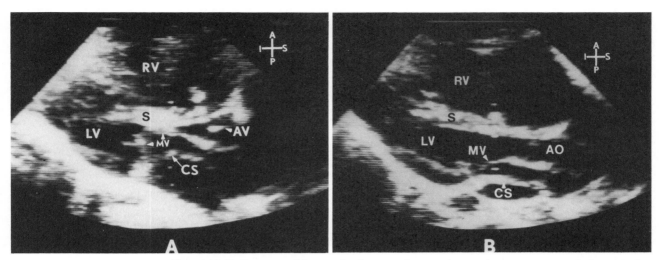

Figure 13-7. Parasternal long-axis view, total anomalous pulmonary venous drainage to the coronary sinus (CS). In diastole (A), the dilated coronary sinus bulges toward the mitral valve (MV) annulus. In systole (B), the coronary sinus appears as an oval echo-free space behind the mitral valve annulus. Note the marked dilatation of the right ventricle and the small left ventricle. AO, aorta; AV, aortic valve; S, interventricular septum.

annulus in the parasternal long-axis view[18,19] (Figure 13-7). Locating the pulmonary veins entering the coronary sinus is diagnostic of this type of total anomalous pulmonary venous drainage.[19] From the apical four-chamber view this lesion may be indistinguishable from a congenital left atrial membrane.[23]

In total anomalous pulmonary venous drainage to the left superior vena cava or left vertical vein, the suprasternal short-axis view shows a vascular collar surrounding the transverse aorta.[20] It is comprised of the dilated left and right superior vena cavae laterally and the left innominate vein superiorly (Figure 13-8). This is the echocar-

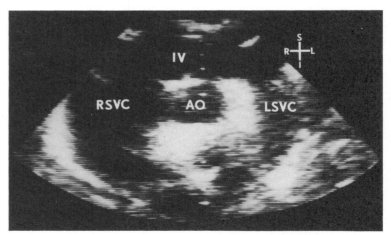

Figure 13-8. Suprasternal notch short-axis view, total anomalous venous drainage. The dilated right superior vena cava (RSVC), left superior vena cava (LSVC), and innominate vein (IV) surround the aorta in a vascular collar.

diographic equivalent of the classic "snowman" appearance of the frontal chest x-ray in this variant of total anomalous pulmonary venous drainage. In still-frame, the dilated great veins resemble the aortic arch, but in real-time the smaller, pulsatile aorta is easily differentiated.

Although findings in other forms of total anomalous pulmonary venous drainage have been described, they are less definitive.[18,21] Reports of 100 percent sensitivity and specificity of the echocardiographic diagnosis have appeared,[18,21] but this experience must yet be confirmed.

In isolated persistence of the left superior vena cava, there are features which are similar to those of total anomalous pulmonary venous drainage; however, the left innominate vein is not demonstrated. The coronary sinus, which receives the left superior caval blood flow, is prominent.[19,24,25] In the absence of other defects, the right and left superior vena cavae and right ventricle are normal in size.

Hypoplastic Left Ventricle

The hypoplastic left ventricle syndrome with aortic valve atresia and a slitlike, nonfunctional left ventricle is never encountered beyond early infancy (Figure 13-9). Severe obstruction at or near the left ventricular inflow tract associated with right-to-left shunting distal to the obstruction may result in a form of hypoplastic left ventricle compatible with survival into early adulthood. Double outlet right ventricle with mitral stenosis or atresia is one such lesion. Massive right ventricular volume overload may simulate hypoplastic left ventricle syndrome, especially in the long-axis view, as the dilated right ventricle compresses the left ventricle.

Other

Right ventricular dilatation is a prominent feature of several other forms of congenital heart disease to be discussed later. These include forms of left heart obstruction with secondary pulmonary hypertension, such as mitral stenosis and related lesions (see section on Left Atrial Dilatation), infantile forms of aortic stenosis and coarctation of the aorta (see section on Left Ventricular Hypertrophy), and complete

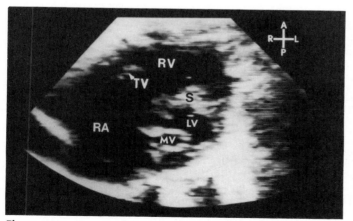

Figure 13-9. Parasternal short-axis view, hypoplastic left ventricle. The stenotic mitral valve is seen in cross-section within the hypoplastic left ventricle. TV denotes tricuspid valve.

or D-transposition of the great arteries (see section on Great Artery Malpositions). In left heart obstruction with pulmonary hypertension, interventricular septal motion is normal.

LEFT VENTRICULAR DILATATION

Dilatation of the left ventricule and the left atrium is a nonspecific echocardiographic feature most commonly present in left heart volume overload. In such cases interventricular septal motion is normal in direction but is usually exaggerated or hyperdynamic. Left ventricular fractional shortening and mitral valve excursion are often increased. Left ventricular posterior wall thickness and interventricular septal thickness are normal. The right ventricular dimensions tend to be small in long-axis views. The interventricular septum is displaced anteriorly by the large left ventricle and may be difficult to visualize from the precordium.

Ventricular Septal Defect

Defects in the interventricular septum may occur in several locations. Which transducer position best demonstrates the defect will depend on the defect's location and size, as well as the characteristics of the instrument used. The large subaortic malalignment type of ventricular septal defect present in tetralogy of Fallot, truncus arteriosus, and some forms of double outlet right ventricle is easily imaged from most transducer positions with sensitivity approaching 100 percent[3,26] (Figure 13-10). Membranous or subaortic ventricular septal defects (best seen from the parasternal and subcostal long-axis and subcostal short-axis positions) are confluent with the aortic root (Figure 13-11). In diastole the defect is often obscured by the tricuspid valve[26] (Figure 13-12A). Although some authors indicate that the diagnosis of aneurysm of the membranous septum can be made by two-dimensional echocardiography,[27] others feel that it cannot be differentiated from tricuspid valve tissue adjacent to the septal defect (Figure 13-12B).[26]

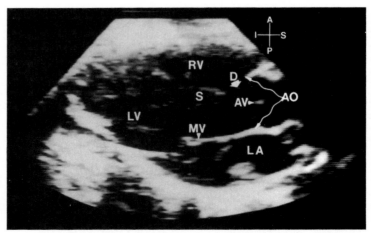

Figure 13-10. Parasternal long-axis view, tetralogy of Fallot. The large subaortic malalignment ventricular septal defect (D) and overriding aorta (AO) are shown. AO–MV (mitral valve) continuity is present.

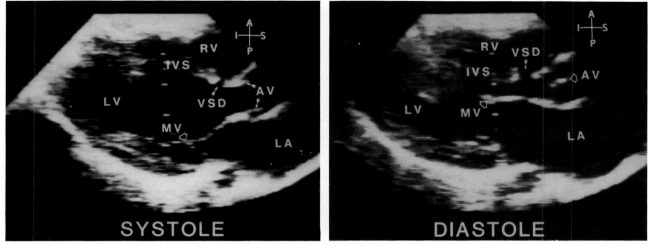

Figure 13-11. Parasternal long-axis view, subaortic (membranous) ventricular septal defect (VSD). The defect, located just inferior to the aorta, is smaller in size in systole than in diastole. Note the dilatation of the left ventricle and left atrium and the bright echoes at the edges of the defect.

The location of the posterior ventricular septal defect is best appreciated in the apical four-chamber view.[28] Scanning anteriorly to the aortic root shows an intact septum, whereas in scanning posteriorly to the plane of the atrioventricular valves, the defect is seen (Figure 13-13). The large posterior defect of a complete atrioventricular canal is easily seen from most transducer positions.[3,6,27] Subpulmonic defects can be imaged from the parasternal long-axis position by shifting the plane of imaging clockwise from the long axis of the left ventricular to an oblique view through the superior, anterior aspect of the interventricular septum immediately inferior to the

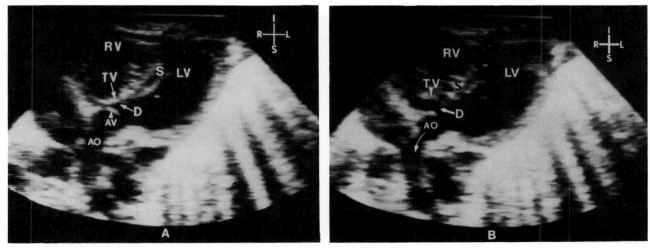

Figure 13-12. Subcostal long-axis view, subaortic (membranous) ventricular septal defect (D). The defect is obscured by the septal leaflet of the tricuspid valve in diastole (A). In systole (B) the tricuspid valve moves away from the defect. Note the normal origin of the arching aorta (AO) from the left ventricle.

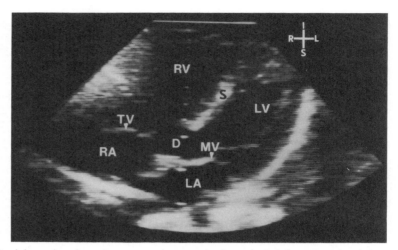

Figure 13-13. Apical four-chamber view, posterior ventricular septal defect (D). The defect is in the posterior interventricular septum (S), in confluence with the mitral and tricuspid valves. The atrioventricular valves are normal, excluding the diagnosis of complete atrioventricular canal.

pulmonic valve (Figure 13-14). These defects may also be imaged from the subcostal short-axis view.[26]

Muscular ventricular septal defects (Figure 13-15) are the most difficult to image because of their often circuitous course through the septum or because of the presence of multiple small defects whose size is below the resolution of the technique.[26] A false-positive or false-negative diagnosis of muscular defects may be caused by large trabeculations in the lower portion of the right ventricular septum.[26] Drop-out of echoes from the superior septum may lead to a false-positive diagnosis of subaortic ventricular septal defect, particularly from the apical four-chamber view.[29] Visual-

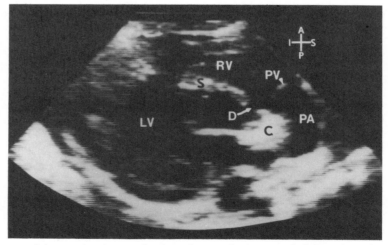

Figure 13-14. Parasternal long-axis view, subpulmonic ventricular septal defect (D). The defect is immediately below the pulmonic valve (PV). Note the dilated left ventricle. C denotes subpulmonic conus; PA, pulmonary artery.

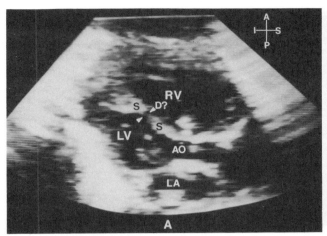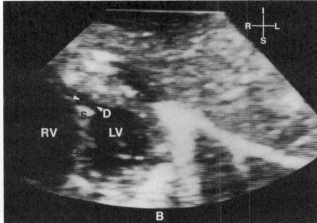

Figure 13-15. Parasternal long-axis view (A) and subcostal four-chamber view (B) of muscular ventricular septal defect (D). There is thinning of the midportion of the interventricular septum, suggesting a muscular defect (arrowheads), in A. The patient also had coarctation of the aorta and pulmonary hypertension, which explains the pattern of right ventricular dilatation observed.

ization of a defect from two or more positions and presence of broadening echoes at the edges of the defect (the "T" artifact) (see Figures 13-12B and 13-13) add considerable weight to the echocardiographic diagnosis of ventricular septal defect.[30]

The smallest ventricular septal defect that can be imaged by two-dimensional echocardiography has been estimated at 2 mm by ultrasound measurement[30] and 4 mm by angiographic measurement.[29] This measurement will vary with the type of instrument and transducer used. Various studies of the echocardiographic diagnosis of ventricular septal defect have estimated the sensitivity at 74 to 94 percent and specificity at 88 to 91 percent[26,29,30] in patients undergoing diagnostic cardiac catheterization who have membranous, malalignment, or posterior defects. In muscular and subpulmonic defects sensitivity is reported at 36 and 67 percent, respectively.[26]

Patent Ductus Arteriosus

A patent ductus arteriosus, which can be imaged from parasternal, subcostal, and suprasternal positions, appears as a curving, superior, rightward extension of the main pulmonary artery (Figure 13-16). Thereafter it becomes confluent with the descending aorta.[31-33] The position and orientation of the ductus is variable, and the particular view which best demonstrates it in an individual patient is unpredictable. Although one group[31] has reported 100 percent sensitivity and 98 percent specificity in the echocardiographic diagnosis of patent ductus arteriosus, further experience is needed to confirm the reliability of this technique. The smallest patent ductus arteriosus imaged in that study measured 1.5 mm in diameter.[31]

Complete Atrioventricular Canal

The diagnosis of complete atrioventricular canal can be made by two-dimensional echocardiography in 96 percent of cases.[6] In complete atrioventricular canal, the diagnostic features include a primum atrial septal defect (see section on Right Ven-

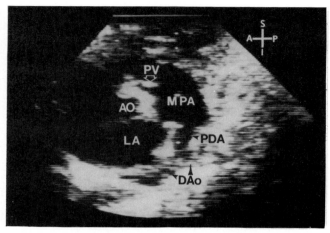

Figure 13-16. Suprasternal short-axis view of the main pulmonary artery (MPA), showing a large patent ductus arteriosus (PDA). The caliber of the patent ductus arteriosus is approximately the same as that of the descending aorta (DA).

tricular Dilatation), a large posterior ventricular septal defect (see section on Left Ventricular Dilatation), and markedly abnormal atrioventricular valves.[3,4,6] The atrial septal defect is usually, but not invariably, large. The anterior leaflet encroaches upon the left ventricular outflow tract, resulting in a narrowing corresponding to the "goose-neck" deformity[10] seen by angiography (Figure 13-17). Rotation of the transducer about 30° clockwise from the parasternal short axis shows the common anterior leaflet crossing the interventricular septum into the right ventricle.[6]

In the parasternal or subcostal short-axis view, scanning from the ventricular apex up to the level of the atrioventricular valve shows the common valve opening into both ventricles, with the anterior leaflet bridging the ventricular septal defect (Figure 13-18A). The atrioventricular valve attachments are best demonstrated from the

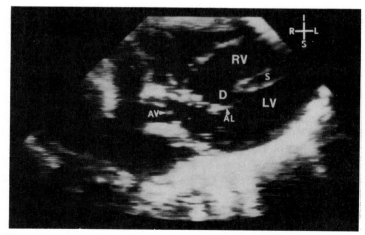

Figure 13-17. Subcostal long-axis view, complete atrioventricular canal. The anterior leaflet (AL) of the common atrioventricular valve opens into the left ventricular outflow tract, giving a picture similar to the "goose-neck" deformity seen by contrast angiography in this lesion.

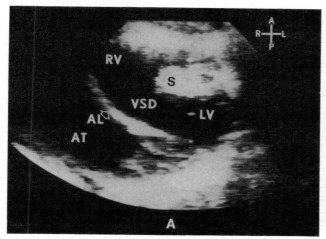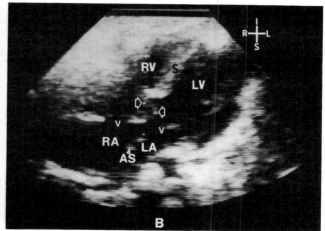

Figure 13-18. A: Parasternal short-axis view, complete atrioventricular canal (Type C). The anterior leaflet of the common atrioventricular valve and large ventricular septal defect (VSD) are noted. B: Apical four-chamber view, complete atrioventricular canal (Type A). The attachments (open arrows) of the atrioventricular valve (V) are to the crest of the interventricular septum.

apical or subcostal four-chamber views. This defect has three subtypes. In Type A (Figure 13-18B), there is a divided anterior leaflet with attachments from both the right and left sides to the crest of the interventricular septum.[4,6] In Type B, chordae tendineae attach from the right- and left-sided portions of the common atrioventricular valve to the right septal surface.[6] In Type C, the large, undivided anterior leaflet bridges the atrioventricular ring and does not attach to the septum[4,6] (see Figures 13-5 and 13-18A).

In incomplete and partial forms of atrioventricular canal, there is a primum atrial septal defect and various atrioventricular valve deformities. The ventricular septal defect (which is distinctly smaller than that seen in complete atrioventricular canal) may be obscured by atrioventricular valve tissue or chordal attachments to the septum.[6]

Anomalous Origin of the Left Coronary Artery from the Pulmonary Artery

This form of congenital heart disease has nonspecific echocardiographic features of left heart dilatation and decreased interventricular septal and posterior wall motion characteristic of a dilated cardiomyopathy. In patients with normal coronary arteries the left coronary artery can usually be visualized from the parasternal or suprasternal short-axis views as a linear echo-free structure just lateral to the left, inferior aspect of the aortic root[34-37] (Figure 13-19). Visualizing the left coronary artery from its aortic confluence to its bifurcation may be difficult in normal patients, since the vigorous contraction of the heart moves the coronary artery in and out of the imaging plane. In patients with cardiomyopathy or anomalous left coronary artery, the markedly diminished heart contraction makes it far easier to visualize the left coronary artery for a long distance, often well beyond the bifurcation.

A slight clockwise rotation from a parasternal short-axis view through the great

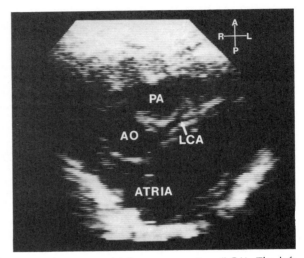

Figure 13-19. Suprasternal notch short-axis view, normal left coronary artery (LCA). The left coronary artery appears as a linear, branching, echo-free space (arrow) in a cloud of echoes related to the left aspect of the aortic root (AO). The confluence of the left coronary artery and the aortic root is shown. PA denotes pulmonary artery.

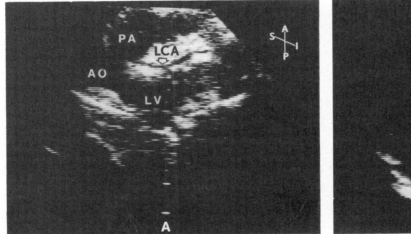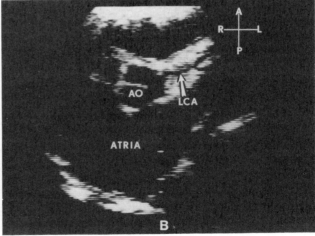

Figure 13-20. Parasternal short-axis view, great artery level, anomalous origin of the left coronary artery from the pulmonary artery. Preoperatively (A), the left coronary artery is in confluence with the posterior aspect of the pulmonary artery. Following surgical reimplantation (B), the left coronary artery is in confluence with the aorta. (From Fisher E, Sepehri B, Lendrum B, et al: Two-dimensional echocardiographic visualization of the left coronary artery in anomalous origin of the left coronary artery from the pulmonary artery. Circulation 63:698, 1981. By permission of the American Heart Association, Inc.)

arteries will usually visualize the confluence of the left coronary artery with the posterior pulmonary artery in patients with anomalous origin of this vessel from the pulmonary artery[37] (Figure 13-20A). It is vital to visualize the confluence, as the left coronary artery occupies a normal position for most of its course even in patients with anomalous origin from the pulmonary artery. The reimplanted left coronary artery and its aortic confluence can be demonstrated after surgical correction[37] (Figure 13-20B).

Hypoplastic Right Ventricle

In tricuspid atresia or pulmonary atresia with intact interventricular septum, the long axis view is similar to left heart volume overload—i.e., a dilated left ventricle and left atrium and a small right ventricle. In left heart volume overload, however, a four-chamber view demonstrates a normal-size right ventricle and the tricuspid and pulmonary valves are easily identifiable. In some patients with tricuspid atresia it is possible to demonstrate a ventricular septal defect or pulmonic valve. From a parasternal short-axis[38] or apical or subcostal four-chamber view, the tricuspid valve area appears as a dense band of immobile echoes[3,38] (Figure 13-21A). The definitive diagnosis of tricuspid atresia rests on demonstration of two ventricles and an atretic tricuspid valve, with the only right atrial outlet through an atrial septal defect or foramen ovale. Care must be taken to avoid mistaking the band of echoes often produced by a normal valve annulus for an atretic valve.[39]

In pulmonary atresia with intact interventricular septum, a small, opening tricuspid valve can be recorded.[38] A pulmonary artery, without a pulmonic valve, is seen from the parasternal or suprasternal views in both pulmonary atresia and in tricuspid atresia. If the small right ventricle is not demonstrable, the differential echocardiographic diagnosis of hypoplastic right ventricle includes single ventricle with atresia

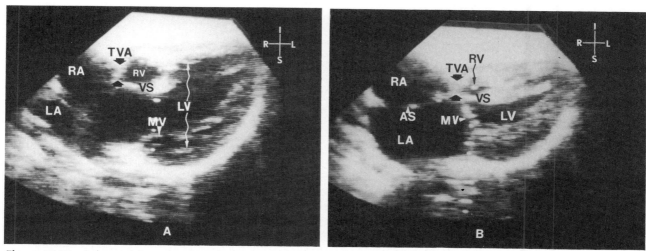

Figure 13-21. Subcostal four-chamber view, tricuspid atresia. In the diastolic frame (A), the small right ventricle and dilated left ventricle are well seen. In the systolic frame (B) the right ventricle is barely perceptible. There is a dense band of echoes in the tricuspid valve area (TVA).

of one atrioventricular valve or a common atrioventricular valve. For further discussion of hypoplastic right ventricle, see the section on Single Ventricular Chamber.

LEFT ATRIAL DILATATION

Left atrial dilatation without left ventricular dilatation or hypertrophy should strongly suggest the presence of obstruction at or near the mitral valve. Its prominent features include secondary pulmonary hypertension, which results in right ventricular and pulmonary artery dilatation, and normal septal motion.

Mitral Stenosis

Because of the rarity and varied anatomy of congenital mitral stenosis, few two-dimensional echocardiographic reports have appeared. The disease is characterized by thick, stiff mitral valve leaflets with limited diastolic excursion (Figure 13-22) and small mitral valve area[22,40] (Figure 13-23). Mitral valve motion may be similar in any patient with left heart dysfunction; however, in those patients the left ventricle is dilated. In parachute mitral valve only a single papillary muscle is present at the left ventricular apex[22,40] (Figure 13-24). We have also noted this finding in a patient with complete atrioventricular canal, where the attachments of the left atrioventricular valve were to a single left ventricular papillary muscle.

Left Atrial Membrane

In cor triatriatum and supravalvar stenosing mitral ring, there is a linear echo just superior to the mitral annulus[3,22,40] best seen from the apical four-chamber view. The two conditions cannot be reliably differentiated by two-dimensional echocardiography,[22,40] nor can the diagnosis of total anomalous pulmonary venous drainage to the coronary sinus be excluded on the basis of the apical four-chamber view.[23] The mitral valve, however, is more likely to be normal in cor triatriatum.[22,24] In the

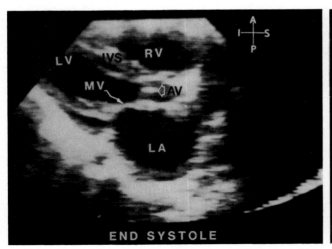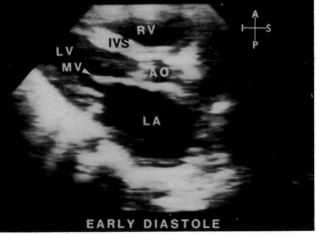

Figure 13-22. Parasternal long-axis view, congenital valvular mitral stenosis. The thick mitral valve leaflets have a very limited excursion in diastole. Note the marked dilatation of the left atrium but the normal left ventricle.

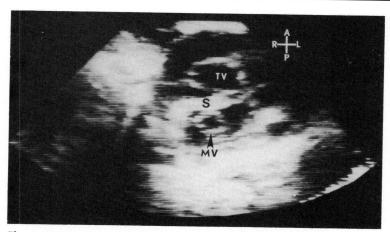

Figure 13-23. Parasternal short-axis view, congenital mitral stenosis. Note the large cross-sectional area of the tricuspid valve and the small cross-sectional area of the stenotic mitral valve.

parasternal long-axis view, the dilated coronary sinus in total anomalous pulmonary venous drainage to the coronary sinus should be easily identified. With nonstenotic left atrial membrane, the membrane is linear rather than circular and extends obliquely across the left atrium from the posterior atrial wall to the posterior aortic root; this is best seen in the parasternal long-axis view.[40]

RIGHT VENTRICULAR HYPERTROPHY

Increased thickness of the right ventricular wall is a prominent feature of right ventricular pressure overload states. Interventricular septal thickness may be increased as well. In right ventricular pressure overload, the right ventricular dimension is normal or smaller than normal.

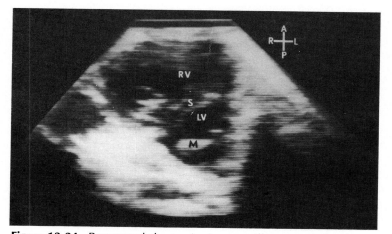

Figure 13-24. Parasternal short-axis view, papillary muscle level, congenital mitral stenosis. A single large papillary muscle (M) is seen in the left ventricular apex. The patient had a parachute mitral valve at autopsy (same patient as in Figures 13-22 and 13-23).

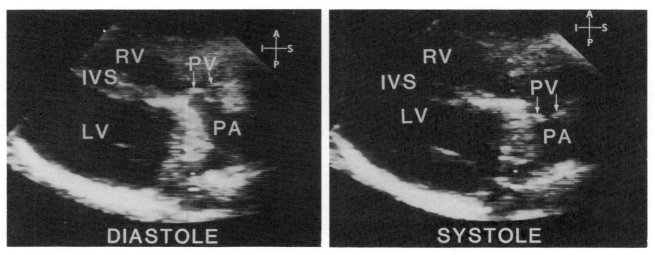

Figure 13-25. Parasternal long-axis view, valvular pulmonary stenosis. In diastole the two leaflets of the pulmonic valve are seen in coaptation. In systole the leaflets have moved several millimeters posteriorly, but the leaflets maintain a curve or dome toward the center of the pulmonary artery and there is only slight separation of the free edges. The patient had tetralogy of Fallot with subvalvular and supravalvular pulmonary stenosis as well, explaining the lack of pulmonary artery dilatation usually seen in valvular pulmonary stenosis.

Pulmonary Stenosis

The anterior position of the pulmonic valve makes imaging, particularly from the precordium, difficult. Often only the posterior cusp is seen throughout the cardiac cycle[41]; the anterior cusp is usually seen only in diastole. Two-dimensional echocardiography is superior to M-mode in visualization of the pulmonic valve[41,42] and diagnosis of pulmonic valvular stenosis.[41] In valvular stenosis the cusps are thickened and domed, maintaining an inward curve toward the center of the pulmonary artery root during systole[41] (Figure 13-25). Systolic doming is the hallmark of semilunar

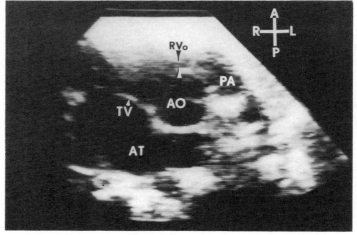

Figure 13-26. Parasternal short-axis view, great artery level, tetralogy of Fallot. The large aorta and small pulmonary artery are in normal position. The small right ventricular outflow tract (RVo) is anterior to the aorta. AT denotes atria.

valve stenosis.[41-43] As in many patients only the posterior cusp is seen, maximum pulmonic cusp separation is not helpful in estimating the severity of pulmonary stenosis.[43]

Infundibular or subvalvular pulmonary stenosis is most often associated with a large subaortic ventricular septal defect and an overriding aorta, i.e., tetralogy of Fallot (see section on Loss of Continuity). The right ventricular outflow tract lies anterior to the aorta and can be visualized from the parasternal short-axis position as a curving, echo-free space between the chest wall and the aortic root. In subvalvular stenosis the dimensions of this space are distinctly reduced, which relates well to the severity of stenosis as assessed by contrast angiography[44] (Figure 13-26).

Other

Right ventricular hypertrophy is a prominent feature of any lesion with a large ventricular communciation and systemic right ventricular pressure, such as large ventricular septal defect, tetralogy of Fallot, and complete atrioventricular canal. Right ventricular dimensions are normal or smaller than normal in these lesions.

In pulmonary hypertension, right ventricular volume overload, and transposition of the great arteries, right ventricular wall thickness may be normal because of right ventricular dilatation.

LEFT VENTRICULAR HYPERTROPHY

Thickening of the left ventricular posterior wall and interventricular septum is typically found in left ventricular pressure overload. The left ventricular cavity is normal or small in size, but the left atrium may be dilated due to increased resistance to emptying presented by the hypertrophied left ventricle.

Aortic Stenosis

Two-dimensional echocardiography has been shown to be far superior to M-mode in assessing the presence and severity of valvular aortic stenosis.[43] The thickened leaflets dome—i.e., maintain an inward curve toward the center of the aortic root in systole (Figure 13-27B)—rather than lie parallel to the long axis of the root as in normals. Measurement of maximum aortic cusp separation (MACS) at the free edges is not a reliable index of severity.[43,45] Expressing MACS as a percentage of aortic root diameter (AOD), however, increases its usefulness.[43] In patients with severe stenosis—i.e., with measured peak systolic gradients across the aortic valve of greater than 50 mm Hg—MACS/AOD was 20 to 35 percent. In moderate stenosis (gradient less than 50 mm Hg) the ratio ranged from 42 to 62 percent. In normal patients, the ratio was 63 to 92 percent.[43]

In discrete membranous subvalvular aortic stenosis the left ventricular outflow tract below the aortic annulus is narrowed. The anterior portion of the membrane encircling the outflow tract is seen as a distinct linear echo arising from the left septal surface[42,46,57] (Figure 13-28). There is often a second linear echo or thickening of the mitral valve annulus on the opposite side of the outflow tract.[42,46,47] The apparent linear echo is in reality a thin membrane that appears thicker due to beam width artifact.[46] Two-dimensional echocardiography poses less of a problem than M-mode, for in the latter technique a rapid scan from left ventricle to aorta could greatly

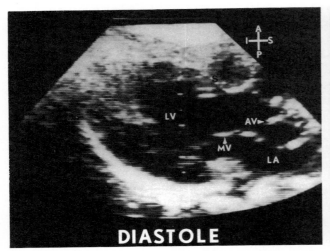
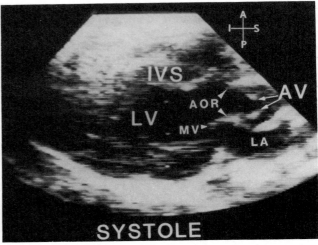

Figure 13-27. Parasternal long-axis view, valvular aortic stenosis. In systole the aortic valve domes—i.e., the leaflets curve toward the center of the aortic root (AOR), showing little separation of the free edges. S and IVS denote interventricular septum.

exaggerate or completely obscure the narrowing.[48] The echocardiographic differentiation between discrete and diffuse subaortic stenosis is primarily one of degree or length of the subvalvular narrowing[42,46,47] (Figure 13-29).

Supravalvular aortic stenosis is very difficult to evaluate by M-mode echocardiography, as the lack of spatial orientation makes artifacts from poor transducer positioning difficult to avoid.[51] By two-dimensional echocardiography, however, a large portion of the ascending aorta can be visualized in a single field (Figure 13-30). Despite the capability, it is reported that two-dimensional echocardiography underestimates the severity of supravalvular stenosis.[47]

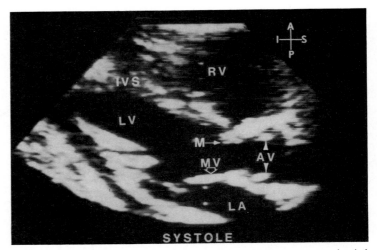

Figure 13-28. Parasternal long-axis view, membranous subvalvular aortic stenosis. The left ventricular outflow tract is narrowed by a linear echo produced by the membrane (M) beneath the left septal surface. There is also thickening of the mitral valve annulus. The aortic valve opens normally.

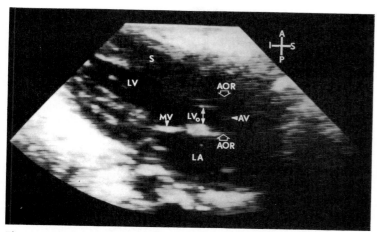

Figure 13-29. Parasternal long-axis view, diffuse subvalvular aortic stenosis. The left ventricular outflow tract (LVo) is narrowed by thick echoes in the area of the mitral valve annulus and beneath the left septal (S) surface. There is severe left ventricular hypertrophy. This patient was shown to have diffuse subaortic stenosis, or fibromuscular tunnel, at contrast angiography.

Coarctation of the Aorta

Although the sensitivity of two-dimensional echocardiography is yet to be established, the diagnosis of coarctation of the aorta can be made with a high degree of specificity[20,49,50] when a good image of the aortic arch and descending thoracic aorta can be obtained from the suprasternal view. Care must be taken to image the aortic lumen distal to the obstruction in order to avoid misinterpreting an oblique image of the vessel as evidence for luminal narrowing. The presence of bright echoes from the area of a discrete coarctation, similar to the "T" artifact seen at the edge of a ventricular septal defect, is helpful in avoiding overdiagnosis due to poor imaging[49]

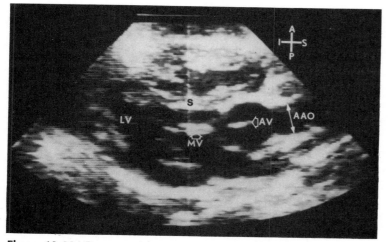

Figure 13-30. Parasternal long-axis view, supravalvular aortic stenosis. The aortic valve is normal. There is a diffuse narrowing of the ascending aorta (AAO) just above the aortic sinuses.

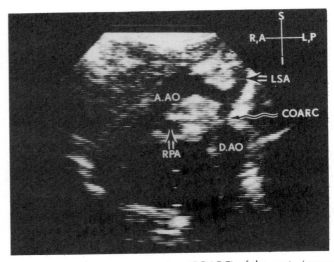

Figure 13-31. Suprasternal long-axis view, discrete coarctation (COARC) of the aorta (wavy arrow). Note the dilated descending aorta (D.AO) distal to the coarctation. A.AO denotes ascending aorta; LSA, left subclavian artery; RPA, right pulmonary artery.

(Figure 13-31 and 13-32). Marked pulsation of the aorta proximal to the obstruction is usually observed. It has been our experience that a normal descending aorta can be imaged in most patients, but we are less frequently able to obtain a diagnostic image of the descending aorta in patients with coarctation of the aorta.

Hypoplasia of the transverse aortic arch (fetal coarctation), which may occur in conjunction with discrete coarctation of the aorta or as an isolated lesion, appears from the suprasternal view as a diffuse narrowing of the arch[49,50] (Figure 13-32).

Bicuspid aortic valve, aortic stenosis, mitral stenosis or insufficiency, and ventricular septal defect are commonly associated with coarctation and hypoplasia of the aorta.

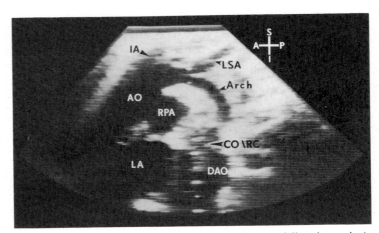

Figure 13-32. Suprasternal notch long-axis view of the aortic arch. There is diffuse hypoplasia of the arch, as well as a discrete coarctation of the aorta. Note the dilated descending aorta distal to the coarctation. IA denotes innominate artery.

────────────────────────── **LOSS OF ANATOMIC CONTINUITY**

The normal structural continuity of the anterior wall of the posterior great artery to the interventricular septum is lost in lesions in which there is a large subaortic malalignment ventricular septal defect. This results in a gap between the superior portion of the septum and the anterior wall of the posterior great artery (aorta). The anterior wall of the posterior great artery is usually dilated and lies anterior to the plane and overrides the interventricular septum. Continuity is also lost when both great arteries arise primarily from the right ventricle (double-outlet right ventricle), regardless of the type of ventricular septal defect present.

Tetralogy of Fallot

The large subaortic malalignment ventricular septal defect present in tetralogy of Fallot is easily imaged from most transducer positions.[3,26] The relation of the anterior aortic wall to the interventricular septum is best appreciated from the parasternal long-axis view (see Figure 13-10). The parasternal short-axis view superimposing the great arteries and the ventricles,[50] or a scan from one plane to the other, shows the larger posterior great artery overriding the septal defect. The aorta is dextroposed but maintains normal position with respect to the pulmonary artery.[51–53] The great artery positions are more easily demonstrated with two-dimensional than with M-mode echocardiography because it is frequently difficult to record the pulmonic valve.[44] Subvalvular pulmonary stenosis in tetralogy of Fallot has been discussed (see section on Right Ventricular Hypertrophy and Figure 13-26). In tetralogy of Fallot with pulmonary atresia, a small right ventricular outflow tract without a pulmonic valve is present; only a single great artery is seen.[52]

Truncus Arteriosus

The appearance of truncus arteriosus is similar to that of tetralogy of Fallot,[44,54] except that the right ventricular outflow tract and pulmonic valve are absent.[52,53] In tetralogy of Fallot with pulmonary atresia it is not always possible to clearly demonstrate the right ventricular outflow tract because of its proximity to the chest wall. In this instance the two lesions may be indistinguishable. The size of the left ventricle tends to be large in truncus and normal or small in tetralogy; the great artery tends to be larger in truncus. These features, however, do not provide a definitive diagnosis. In some patients with truncus, the origin of the pulmonary artery from the left lateral or posterior aspect of the arterial root is demonstrable from the suprasternal notch or high parasternal position (Figure 13-33), making a definitive diagnosis of truncus possible. Demonstration of two sets of semilunar valves excludes the diagnosis of truncus arteriosus.

Double Outlet Right Ventricle

In double outlet right ventricle with subaortic or subpulmonic ventricular septal defect, the echocardiographic features from the parasternal long-axis views may be similar to that of tetralogy of Fallot and truncus arteriosus. In addition, however, there is loss of the posterior great artery–mitral valve continuity due to the presence of a muscular conus seen as a bright, thick echo separating the posterior wall of the

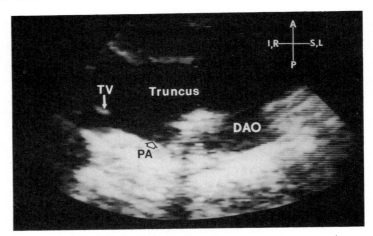

Figure 13-33. High parasternal view, between long- and short-axis views, truncus arteriosus. The large truncus is seen in long axis. The pulmonary artery arises from the posterior aspect of the truncus, well above the truncal valve (TV). This patient had pulmonary artery banding as an infant, and the hypoplastic distal branches of the pulmonary artery were not seen.

posterior artery and the anterior leaflet of the mitral valve[28,53] (Figure 13-34). Pulmonic valve stenosis is common, most often occurring when the aorta is situated anteriorly.[28] The great arteries may be normally related, but malpositions are frequent.

GREAT ARTERY MALPOSITIONS

Two-dimensional echocardiography is particularly useful in evaluating those lesions in which the normal position of the great arteries is altered with respect to each other and/or to the atrioventricular valves and the ventricles when both are present.

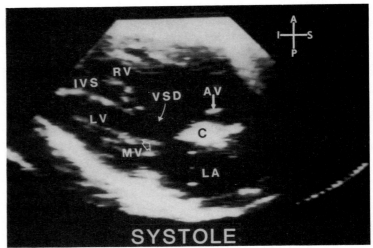

Figure 13-34. Parasternal long-axis view, double outlet right ventricle. There is a large sub-aortic ventricular septal defect. The aortic valve is separated from the mitral valve by a large subaortic conus (C).

Other echocardiographic features depend on the particular malposition and associated lesions.

Complete or D-Transposition of the Great Arteries

Demonstrating an anterior great artery on the right and a posterior great artery on the left is suggestive of complete (dextro-) transposition of the great arteries.[51–53] This relationship is best demonstrated in the parasternal as well as the suprasternal short-axis view. Imaging of the bifurcation of the left-sided posterior great artery into right and left pulmonary arteries serves to identify it as the pulmonary artery (Figure 13-35B). From the parasternal long-axis view, the posterior left ventricle is seen to give rise to a great artery that turns abruptly posterior, a characteristic of the pul-

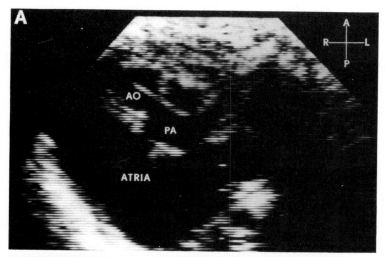

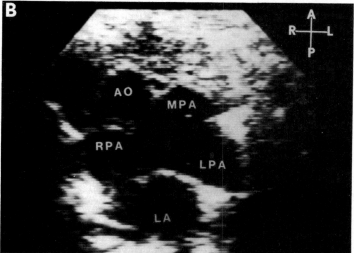

Figure 13-35. Parasternal short-axis view, D-transposition of the great arteries. The anterior great artery is to the right in A. In B the bifurcation of the left-sided artery identifies it as the main pulmonary artery.

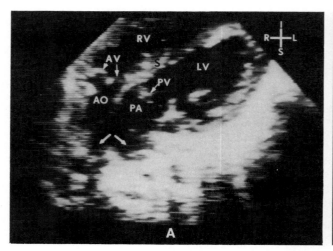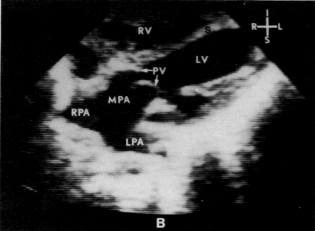

Figure 13-36. Subcostal long-axis view, D-transposition of the great arteries. The two great arteries have a parallel origin from the base of the heart (A). The artery arising from the left ventricle is seen to bifurcate early (B) and thus is identified as the pulmonary artery. The origin of the aorta from the right ventricle is also shown.

monary artery.[52,57,58,60,61] The retrosternal position of the aorta and the parallel course of the great arteries is often appreciable in this view as well.[52,57,58] In the parasternal short-axis view the parallel course of the great arteries is suggested by the circular appearance of both roots[52,53] (Figure 13-35A). In the subcostal long-axis view the posterior great artery arises from the left ventricle and bifurcates into right and left pulmonary arteries, thus demonstrating the origin of the pulmonary artery from the left ventricle[33] (Figure 13-36A). The origin of the curved, nonbifurcating aorta from the right ventricle is often visualized from the subcostal position as well[33] (Figure 13-36B). Occasionally the great arteries are directly aligned one in front of the other with the aorta being anterior. Rarely, the aorta lies anterior and to the left.[53] In the latter case, demonstrating the abnormal connections of the great arteries to the ventricles is essential to confirm the diagnosis of complete transposition of the great arteries.

Most patients with uncomplicated transposition have right ventricular dilatation with normal or reversed septal motion. Commonly associated lesions are atrial and ventricular septal defects and pulmonary stenosis. With the development of pulmonary hypertension, the left ventricle and pulmonary artery dilate. D-Transposition of the great arteries can also be found in some forms of double outlet right ventricle and single ventricle.

Corrected or L-Transposition of the Great Arteries

In corrected transposition the great artery position may appear normal,[59] but more often they take on a side-by-side position[53] (Figure 13-37). The roots are viewed as circular in cross-section, suggesting their parallel origin from the heart.[52] The bifurcation of the right-sided great artery into right and left pulmonary arteries identifies it as the pulmonary artery; the aorta is to the left in L-transposition of the great arteries. The ventricles are inverted or reversed in position; the interventricular

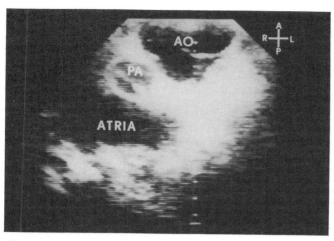

Figure 13-37. Parasternal short-axis view, great artery level, L-transposition of the great arteries. The large anterior great artery is to the left. The patient has severe valvular pulmonary stenosis.

septum is oriented in an anteroposterior position, often parallel to the echo beam, making it difficult to demonstrate. In the parasternal or subcostal short-axis view, the anatomic right ventricle is identified by its heavy trabeculations, while the left septal surface is smoothwalled (Figure 13-38). An example of normally positioned ventricles is shown for comparison (Figure 13-39).

The left-sided tricuspid valve, related to the right ventricle, is identified by inferior displacement of its hinge point relative to the right-sided mitral valve (four-chamber view). In the short-axis view the left-sided tricuspid valve has three leaflets, giving it a triangular appearance in diastole[60]; the bicuspid mitral valve has a "fish-mouth" appearance. The origin of the great arteries from the ventricles is very difficult to demonstrate in this lesion due to the inability to visualize the interventricular septum

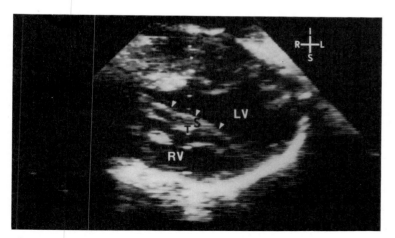

Figure 13-38. Subcostal short axis view, L-transposition of the great arteries. In this patient the interventricular septum is in a nearly horizontal position, so that the anatomic left ventricle, identified by its smooth septal surface (arrowheads), is inferior and slightly to the left of the anatomic right ventricle, identified by its trabeculated septal surface.

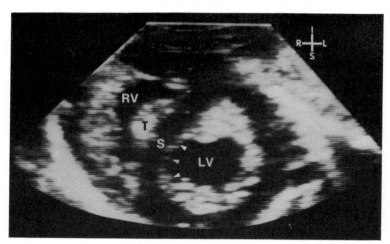

Figure 13-39. Subcostal short-axis view, normally positioned ventricles. Note the smooth left septal surface (arrowheads), in contrast to the trabeculated (T) right septal surface. The left ventricle is slightly superior and to the left of the right ventricle.

and the superior and anterior position of the left-sided aorta. The long-axis plane showing the left-sided ventricle and atrioventricular valve is posterior to the plane of the aorta. There is lack of continuity of the left-sided atrioventricular valve and the aorta due to the presence of the subaortic conus.[53] The interventricular septum intervenes between the left-sided atrioventricular valve and the posterior, inferior pulmonary artery, which arises from the right-sided ventricle. In the presence of an associated subpulmonic ventricular septal defect, the proximity of these structures may be demonstrated. In patients with corrected transposition of the great arteries, an Ebstein's-like deformity of the left-sided atrioventricular valve is not uncommon. Pulmonary stenosis and ventricular septal defect are also commonly associated. L-Transposition of the great arteries is common in single ventricle (see section on Single Ventricular Chamber).

Double Outlet Right Ventricle

In double outlet right ventricle the great arteries may be side by side (Figure 13-40) or transposed (D-transposition). As mentioned earlier, both arteries arise primarily from the right ventricle, so that there is loss of the normal aortoseptal and aorto-atrioventricular valve continuity (see also section on Loss of Anatomic Continuity).

SINGLE VENTRICULAR CHAMBER

The interventricular septum may be difficult to image from the standard precordial positions in some patients due to an unusual orientation of the ventricles or to the presence of a large septal defect. Before making a diagnosis of single ventricle, therefore, it is important to utilize all available transducer positions in an attempt to demonstrate the septum. A large muscle bundle or papillary muscle may be mistaken for the septum in long-axis views, but on short axis it should appear as a discrete circular mass. The interventricular septum should have length as well as

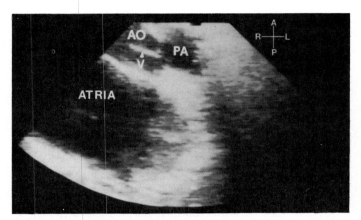

Figure 13-40. Parasternal short axis view, great artery level, double outlet right ventricle. The great arteries are side by side. V denotes semilunar valve.

width and divide the ventricular cavity into two chambers, each receiving an atrioventricular valve. If no interventricular septum is demonstrated, two forms of congenital heart disease should be considered: single ventricle and hypoplastic right ventricle. The form of hypoplastic left ventricle found in early infancy may also appear as a single ventricle from long-axis views, but in short axis it is generally possible to demonstrate the small left ventricle.

Single Ventricle

Demonstration of a single ventricular chamber receiving two atrioventricular valves is diagnostic of single ventricle (primitive ventricle, double inlet left ventricle) (Figure 13-41A). The outlet chamber, which is present below the anterior great artery frequently in single ventricle, may be demonstrated from a high parasternal or subcostal position (Figure 13-41B). It appears as a ridge of muscle separating the main ventricular chamber from a chamber beneath the anterior semilunar valve. This muscular ridge should not be confused with an interventricular septum because both atrioventricular valves are located posterior and inferior to it[61] (Figure 13-41A). In most patients with single ventricle there is malposition of the great arteries, most commonly L-transposition but occasionally D-transposition. In both, the outlet chamber is anterior, beneath the aorta. In L-transposition the outlet chamber is situated to the left; in D-transposition it is to the right. In patients with normally related great arteries, no outflow chamber is present (Figure 13-41A). Pulmonary stenosis or atresia is a commonly associated lesion. In the latter, only a single anterior great artery root is demonstrable.

Atrioventricular valve abnormalities are not uncommon. Left-sided Ebstein's anomaly may occur in those patients with L-transposition of the great arteries. Common atrioventricular valve or atresia of the right- or the left-sided atrioventricular valve may also occur and make a definitive diagnosis more difficult.

In single ventricle with common atrioventricular valve there is an associated primum atrial septal defect or common atrium with a communication between the atria and the single ventricle, best demonstrated from a four-chamber view. With single ventricle and atresia of an atrioventricular valve, there is no communication between

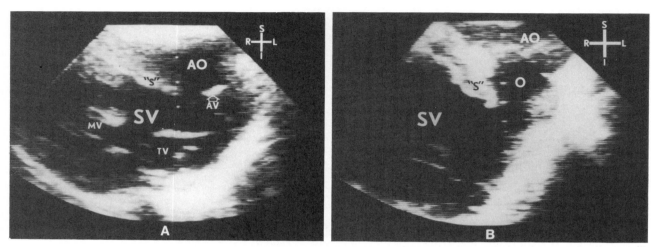

Figure 13-41. A: High parasternal view, between long and short axis, of single ventricle (SV). The reversed atrioventricular valves are related to the single ventricle. Note the fish-mouth appearance of the right-sided mitral valve and the triangular appearance of the left-sided tricuspid valve in this diastolic frame. The very small outflow chamber beneath the aorta is separated from the single ventricle and the atrioventricular valves by a "septum" ("S") or muscular ridge. B: Parasternal long-axis view, single ventricle. The aorta is seen to originate from an outflow chamber (O). There is a ridge of muscle ("S") separating the single ventricular chamber from the outflow chamber.

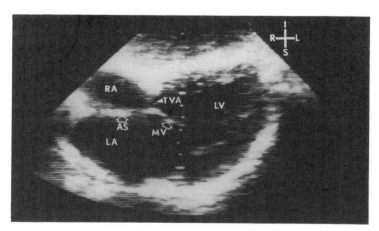

Figure 13-42. Subcostal four-chamber view, hypoplastic right ventricle. Only a single ventricular chamber is evident. No tricuspid valve motion was seen in real time. The study suggests tricuspid atresia (TVA) or pulmonary atresia with intact ventricular septum, although single ventricle with an atretic right-sided atrioventricular valve cannot be ruled out.

300

the atrium on that side and the single ventricle. When the atretic valve is right-sided this form of single ventricle may be impossible to distinguish from tricuspid atresia. The presence of great artery malposition favors a diagnosis of single ventricle. Demonstrating an outlet chamber is definitive evidence for single ventricle.

Hypoplastic Right Ventricle

In many patients with tricuspid atresia or pulmonary atresia with intact interventricular septum, the hypoplastic right ventricle is so small as to be unrecognizable. The cardiac image then is composed of a single ventricular chamber from the apical and subcostal four-chamber views[3] (Figure 13-42). This is in contrast to some patients with hypoplastic right ventricle who may have two demonstrable ventricles and a pattern of left ventricular dilatation. In the latter a definitive diagnosis of tricuspid atresia is possible (see section on Left Ventricular Dilatation). It may not be possible, however, to differentiate between tricuspid atresia without a right ventricle and single ventricle with atresia of the right-sided atrioventricular valve if an outlet chamber or great artery malposition is not present.

————————————————————— REFERENCES

1. Dillon JC, Weyman AE, Feigenbaum H, et al: Cross-sectional echocardiographic examination of the interatrial septum. Circulation 55:115, 1977
2. Lieppe W, Scallion R, Behar VS, et al: Two-dimensional echocardiographic findings in atrial septal defect. Circulation 56:447, 1977
3. Silverman NH, Schiller NB: Apex echocardiography. A two-dimensional technique for evaluating congenital heart disease. Circulation 57:503, 1978
4. Lange LW, Sahn DJ, Allen HD, et al: Subxiphoid cross-sectional echocardiography in infants and children with congenital heart disease. Circulation 59:513, 1979
5. Bierman FZ, Williams RG: Subxiphoid two-dimensional imaging of the interatrial septum in infants and neonates with congenital heart disease. Circulation 60:80, 1979
6. Hagler DJ, Tajik AJ, Seward JB, et al: Real-time wide-angle sector echocardiography: atrioventricular canal defects. Circulation 59:140, 1979
7. Schreiber TL, Feigenbaum H, Weyman AE: Effect of atrial septal defect repair on left ventricular geometry and degree of mitral valve prolapse. Circulation 61:888, 1980
8. Beppu S, Nimura Y, Nagata S, et al: Diagnosis of endocardial cushion defect with cross-sectional and M-mode scanning echocardiography: differentiation from secundum atrial septal defect. Br Heart J 38:911, 1976
9. Beppu S, Nimura Y, Sakakibara H, et al: Mitral cleft in ostium primum atrial septal defect assessed by cross-sectional echocardiography. Circulation 62:1099, 1980
10. Yoshida H, Funabashi T, Nagata S, et al: Subxiphoid cross-sectional echocardiographic imaging of the "goose-neck" deformity in endocardial cushion defect. Circulation 62:1319, 1980
11. Feigenbaum H: Congenital heart disease, in Echocardiography (ed 3). Philadelphia, Lea & Febiger, 1981, p 352
12. Ports TA, Silverman NH, Schiller NB: Two-dimensional echocardiographic assessment of Ebstein's anomaly. Circulation 58:336, 1978
13. Gussenhoven WJ, Spitaels SEC, Bom N, et al: Echocardiographic criteria for Ebstein's anomaly of the tricuspid valve. Br Heart J 43:31, 1980
14. Hirschklau MJ, Sahn DJ, Hagan AD, et al: Cross-sectional echocardiographic features of Ebstein's anomaly of the tricuspid valve. Am J Cardiol 40:400, 1977
15. Matsumoto M, Matsuo H, Nagata S, et al: Visualization of Ebstein's anomaly of the tricuspid valve by two-dimensional and standard echocardiography. Circulation 53:69, 1976
16. Kambe T, Ichimiya S, Toguchji M, et al: Cross-sectional echocardiographic study of Ebstein's anomaly using electronic sector scan. J Cardiogr 9:269, 1979

17. Feigenbaum H: Congenital heart disease, in Echocardiography (ed 3). Philadelphia, Lea & Febiger, 1981, pp 371–372

18. Sahn DJ, Allen HD, Lange LW, et al: Cross-sectional echocardiographic diagnosis of the sites of total anomalous pulmonary venous drainage. Circulation 60:1317, 1979

19. Snider AR, Ports TA, Silverman NH: Venous anomalies of the coronary sinus: detection by M-mode, two-dimensional and contrast echocardiography. Circulation 60:721, 1979

20. Snider AR, Silverman NH: Suprasternal notch echocardiography: a two-dimensional technique for evaluating congenital heart disease. Circulation 63:165, 1981

21. Bierman FZ, Williams RG: Subxiphoid two-dimensional echocardiographic diagnosis of total anomalous pulmonary venous return in infants (Abstract). Am J Cardiol 43:401, 1979

22. Snider AR, Roge CL, Schiller NB, et al: Congenital left ventricular inflow obstruction evaluated by two-dimensional echocardiography. Circulation 61:848, 1980

23. Feigenbaum H: Congenital heart disease, in Echocardiography (ed 3). Philadelphia, Lea & Febiger, 1981, p 373

24. Cohen BE, Winer HE, Kronzon I: Echocardiographic findings in patients with left superior vena cava and dilated coronary sinus. Am J Cardiol 44:158, 1979

25. Stewart JA, Fraker TD, Slosky DA, et al: Detection of persistent left superior vena cava by two-dimensional contrast echocardiography. JCU 7:357, 1979

26. Bierman FZ, Fellows K, Williams RG: Prospective identification of ventricular septal defects in infancy using subxiphoid two-dimensional echocardiography. Circulation 62:807, 1980

27. Fast JH, Moene RJ: Echocardiographic diagnosis of an aneurysm of the membranous ventricular septum. Acta Paediatr Scand 66:521, 1977

28. Hagler DJ, Tajik AJ, Seward JB, et al: Double-outlet right ventricle: wide-angle two-dimensional echocardiographic observations. Circulation 63:419, 1981

29. Cheatham JP, Latson LA, Gutgesell HP: Ventricular septal defect in infancy: detection with two-dimensional echocardiography. Am J Cardiol 47:85, 1981

30. Canale JM, Sahn DJ, Allen HD, et al: Factors affecting real-time, cross-sectional echocardiographic imaging of perimembranous ventricular septal defects. Circulation 63:689, 1981

31. Sahn DJ, Allen HD: Real-time, cross-sectional echocardiographic imaging and measurement of the patent ductus arteriosus in infants and children. Circulation 48:343, 1978

32. Baba K, Kohata T, Tanimoto T, et al: Identification of the great artery relations in infants by real-time two-dimensional echocardiography. J Cardiogr 9:159, 1979

33. Bierman FZ, Williams RG: Prospective diagnosis of D-transposition of the great arteries in neonates by subxiphoid, two-dimensional echocardiography. Circulation 60:1496, 1979

34. Weyman AE, Feigenbaum H, Dillon JC, et al: Noninvasive visualization of the left main coronary artery by cross-sectional echocardiography. Circulation 54:169, 1976

35. Yoshikawa J, Yanagihara K, Owaki T, et al: Cross-sectional echocardiographic diagnosis of coronary artery aneurysms in patients with the mucocutaneous lymph node syndrome. Circulation 59:133, 1979

36. Hiraishi S, Hashiro K, Kusano S: Noninvasive visualization of coronary arterial aneurysm in infants and young children with mucocutaneous lymph node syndrome with two-dimensional echocardiography. Am J Cardiol 43:1225, 1979

37. Fisher EA, Sepehri B, Lendrum B, et al: Two-dimensional echocardiographic visualization of the left coronary artery in anomalous origin of the left coronary artery from the pulmonary artery, pre- and post-operative studies. Circulation 63:698, 1981

38. Beppu S, Nimura Y, Tamai M, et al: Two-dimensional echocardiography in diagnosing tricuspid atresia: differentiation from other hypoplastic right heart syndromes and common atrioventricular canal. Br Heart J 40:1174, 1978

39. Feigenbaum H: Congenital heart disease, in Echocardiography (ed 3). Philadelphia, Lea & Febiger, 1981, p 350

40. Rogé C, Snider R, Silverman N: Echocardiography evaluation of left ventricle inflow obstruction in children using an 80 degree two-dimensional sector scanner, in Lancee CT (ed): Echocardiography. The Hague, Martinus Nijhoff, 1979, pp 342–344

41. Weyman AE, Hurwitz RA, Girod DA, et al: Cross-sectional echocardiographic visualization of the stenotic pulmonary valve. Circulation 56:769, 1977

42. Weyman AE, Feigenbaum H, Hurwitz RA, et al: Localization of left ventricular outflow tract obstruction by cross-sectional echocardiography. Am J Med 60:33, 1976

43. Weyman AE, Feigenbaum H, Hurwitz RA, et al: Cross-sectional echocardiographic assessment of the severity of aortic stenosis in children. Circulation 55:773, 1977

44. Caldwell RL, Weyman AE, Hurwitz RA, et al: Right ventricular outflow tract assessment by cross-sectional echocardiography in tetralogy of Fallot. Circulation 59:395, 1979

45. DeMaria AN, Bommer W, Joye J, et al: Value and limitations of cross-sectional echocardiography of the aortic valve in the diagnosis and quantification of valvular aortic stenosis. Circulation 62:304, 1980

46. Weyman AE, Feigenbaum H, Hurwitz, RA, et al: Cross-sectional echocardiography in evaluating patients with discrete subaortic stenosis. Am J Cardiol 37:358, 1976

47. Williams DE, Sahn DJ, Friedman WF: Cross-sectional echocardiographic localization of sites of left ventricular outflow tract obstruction. Am J Cardiol 37:250, 1976

48. Feigenbaum H: Congenital heart disease, in Echocardiography (ed 3). Philadelphia, Lea & Febiger, 1981, pp 335–337

49. Sahn DJ, Allen HD, McDonald G, et al: Real-time cross-sectional echocardiographic diagnosis of coarctation of the aorta. Circulation 56:762, 1977

50. Weyman AE, Caldwell RL, Hurwitz RA, et al: Cross-sectional echocardiographic detection of aortic obstruction. 2. Coarctation of the aorta. Circulation 57:498, 1978

51. Henry WL, Maron BJ, Griffith JM: Cross-sectional echocardiography in the diagnosis of congenital heart disease. Circulation 56:267, 1977

52. Henry WL, Maron BJ, Griffith JM, et al: Differential diagnosis of anomalies of the great arteries by real-time two-dimensional echocardiography. Circulation 51:283, 1975

53. DiSessa TG, Hagan AD, Pope C, et al: Two-dimensional echocardiographic characteristics of double outlet right ventricle. Am J Cardiol 44:1146, 1979

54. Feigenbaum H: Congenital heart disease, in Echocardiography (ed 3). Philadelphia, Lea & Febiger, 1981, p 383

55. Hagler DJ, Tajik AJ, Seward JB, et al: Wide-angle two-dimensional echocardiographic profiles of conotruncal abnormalities. Mayo Clin Proc 55:73, 1980

56. Aziz KU, Paul MH, Muster AJ, et al: Positional abnormalities of atrioventricular valves in transposition of the great arteries including double outlet right ventricle, atrioventricular straddling and malattachment. Am J Cardiol 44:1135, 1979

57. Sahn DJ, Terry R, O'Rourke R, et al: Multiple crystal cross-sectional echocardiography in the diagnosis of cyanotic congenital heart disease. Circulation 50:230, 1974

58. Houston AB, Gregory NL, Coleman EN: Echocardiographic identification of aorta and main pulmonary artery in complete transposition. Br Heart J 40:377, 1978

59. Houston AB, Gregory NL, Coleman EN: Two-dimensional sector scanner echocardiography in cyanotic congenital heart disease. Br Heart J 39:1076, 1977

60. Feigenbaum H: Congenital heart disease, in Echocardiography (ed 3). Philadelphia, Lea & Febiger, 1981, p 387

61. Seward JB, Tajik AJ, Hagler DJ, et al: Cross-sectional echocardiography in common ventricle utilizing 80 degree phased-array sector scanner (Abstract). Circulation 56(Suppl III):III-41, 1977

CHAPTER 14

Two-Dimensional Contrast Echocardiography

William J. Bommer, Harsha Gandhi, Mark Keown, Thomas Jackson, Randall Mapes, Dean T. Mason, and Anthony DeMaria

During a routine cardiac catheterization in 1966 Claude Joyner noticed that the first injection produced a mass of echoes, a discovery that originated what is now called contrast echocardiography. From that beginning until the present, contrast echocardiography has provided a useful and stimulating contribution to diagnostic echocardiography.

ECHOCONTRAST EFFECT AND TECHNIQUE

What Joyner had injected was radiographic dye. Subsequent investigators were to inject saline, blood, indocyanine green dye, and glucose in water to obtain the same effect. Gramiak and coworkers[1] postulated that the mass of echoes was caused either by the presence of miniature bubbles or by cavitation. Although cavitation vapor bubbles can be seen with very high-velocity injections, these velocities are not achieved during routine hand injections. Recent studies have shown that the predominant echocardiographic contrast effect is caused by echoes from small air bubbles in the injectate.[2,3]

Nearly any liquid will produce an echocontrast effect when injected in a manner that introduces gas bubbles. Even careful handling of closed intravenous lines will produce some echocontrast effect; the addition of small amounts of gas to the liquid prior to injection will provide a maximal contrast effect. The initial flow through an intravenous line introduces small, nearly invisible bubbles that adhere to the walls of the tubing. Rapid intravenous flushing then displaces these nearly invisible microbubbles into the liquid, and they are washed into the circulation to produce a contrast effect. Additional contrast can be achieved by first agitating a liquid–gas mixture and then eliminating the larger visible bubbles prior to the injection. Special caution must be exercised when performing these techniques. At one extreme is the introduction of small, visually undetectable microbubbles that are probably injected routinely during cardiac catheterization procedures and during intravenous infusions. Such injections appear to be safe, based on the previous lack of complications during

We would like to thank Mrs. Hatie Ellingburg for her secretarial help.

routine cardiac catheterization and intravenous infusion procedures. At the other extreme, the introduction of large amounts of gas can produce gas embolization with significant symptoms or complications, especially when injected systemically or in patients with right-to-left shunts.[4] For this reason it is safest to follow guidelines that have been previously established for safe catheterization and IV infusion.

Although contrast echocardiography was extensively used in early echocardiographic investigations, it was some time until a more comprehensive understanding of its effects developed. A large number of contrast agents have been proposed; however, almost all of the effective agents have been shown to contain gas bubbles, which is understandable, as the strength of the ultrasound reflection is related to acoustic impedance difference between interfaces. The great difference in densities at a gas–liquid interface produces a tremendous acoustic impedance difference; this interface shows an extremely strong echocontrast effect.

As the time from the injection increases and the gas is gradually absorbed into the blood, the contrast effect diminishes.[5–10] It further dwindles as the gas is absorbed

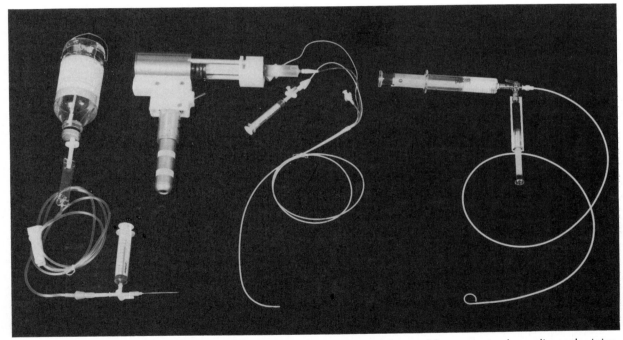

Figure 14-1. Equipment and materials that can be used for contrast echocardiography injections. On the left an intravenous bottle of dextrose and water saline is connected to IV tubing that runs to a three-way stopcock. The stopcock is connected to a plastic syringe and an angiocath, which is inserted into a peripheral vein. During injections, solution is rapidly drawn up into the syringe and then rapidly injected through the angiocath into the peripheral vein. If green dye is to be injected, it can be drawn up separately in the syringe, then injected into the IV line, and finally followed by an intravenous flush of IV solution. In the center a pressurized CO_2 cartridge injector is seen attached to the proximal part of a Swan-Ganz catheter. This injector provides a reasonably fast injection rate with a uniform speed, which may be advantageous when performing quantitative analysis studies. On the right a standard indocyanine green dye syringe and flush syringe are hooked up to a pigtail catheter for left heart opacification. Routine catheterization injections often produce echocontrast images.

during passage through the pulmonary and systemic capillary systems, which act as filters. Any bubbles sufficiently small to pass through the lungs are quickly collapsed by surface tension and thus never imaged in the left side of the heart.

Figure 14-1 illustrates some of the equipment and materials used in contrast echocardiography. We prefer to use a syringe, stopcock, and IV solution, as this arrangement facilitates repeated injections. If the contrast effect of a dextrose and water or saline injection is inadequate, an injection of green dye followed by a flush will usually suffice. In neonates the aspiration of blood followed by its reinjection usually produces a contrast effect without altering the blood volume. A more uniform injection speed can be obtained by using the carbon dioxide–pressurized syringe system. In addition to peripheral venous injections, both left and right heart catheter-injections can be made to detail specific areas or chambers.

Verification of Anatomy

The development of echocardiography was to some extent dependent on the fortuitous discovery and use of contrast echoes in identifying M-mode echo patterns. Prior to contrast echocardiography, verification required either a hazardous guess or a postmortem examination. However, Gramiak and Shah, in their first articles on M-mode echocardiography of the aorta and cardiac chambers, were able to verify these structures with echocontrast injections.[1,11] Subsequently, all of the major echo patterns were confirmed by contrast echocardiography.[12]

In Figure 14-2 contrast echoes can be seen in the anterior chamber following a peripheral intravenous injection, which confirms identification of the anterior right ventricular cavity. In Figure 14-3 a catheter injection into the aortic root outlines the "boxcar" shape of the aortic valve leaflets surrounding the nonopacified blood ejected from the ventricle.

With the added spatial resolution of two-dimensional echocardiography, identi-

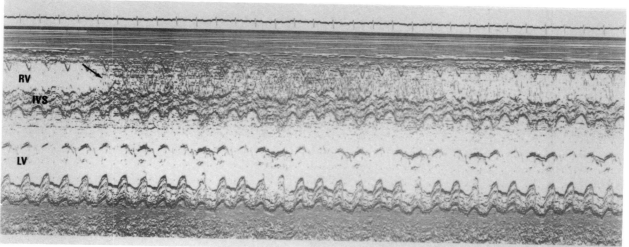

Figure 14-2. M-mode echocardiogram performed during an echocontrast injection. The arrow indicates the beginning of the contrast effect, seen here as multiple linear echoes in the right ventricular chamber. RV denotes right ventricle; IVS, interventricular septum; LV, left ventricle.

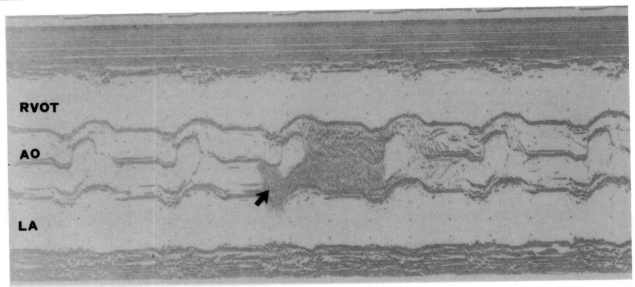

Figure 14-3. M-mode echocardiogram of the right ventricular outflow tract (RVOT), aorta (AO), and left atrium (LA). A contrast injection was performed in the aortic root. The arrow illustrates the beginning of the contrast effect, which is seen as a densely packed group of echoes in the aorta surrounding the aortic valve leaflets.

fying basic anatomic structures using contrast injections is no longer required. In the evaluation of newly discovered or complex congenital anomalies, and especially in verification of two-dimensional echocardiographic images, however, contrast echography continues to play a major role.[13–26]

Figure 14-4 is a long-axis view of the left atrium in which echocontrast is seen in

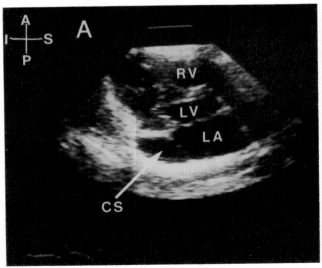
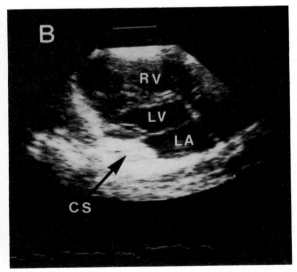

Figure 14-4. A: Parasternal long-axis view of the heart in persistent left superior vena cava. B: Following the injection of contrast into a peripheral left arm vein, the area of the coronary sinus (CS) becomes brightly opacified with contrast. With short-axis views this coronary sinus contrast could be seen to drain into the right atrium.

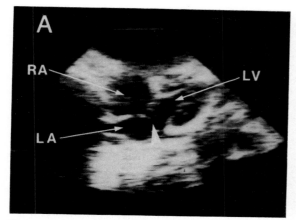
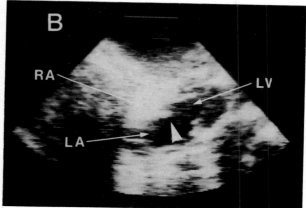

Figure 14-5. A: Two-dimensional echocardiogram recorded in a four-chamber orientation from a subcostal window. The large arrow points to a thin aneurysmal bulging of the interatrial septum. B: Following the peripheral injection of echocontrast, the right atrium becomes densely opacified, filling out the localized aneurysm of the interatrial septum. Additional contrast also flows through a right-to-left shunt into the left ventricle.

a chamber posterior to the left atrium following a left arm venous injection. The appearance of contrast following the left arm injection and the absence of contrast following a right arm venous injection strongly supports a diagnosis of persistent left superior vena cava draining into the coronary sinus and subsequently into the right atrium.[14] Figure 14-5 shows a thin, localized outpouching of the interatrial septum. Following a peripheral venous injection, contrast echoes fill this structure and then flow into the left atrium, delineating a localized atrial septal aneurysm with a right-to-left shunt.[16] Additional verification of the following abnormalities has been recently made with the contrast echocardiography: left main coronary artery,[24] coronary artery fistula,[17] eustachian valves,[25] and diverticuli.[26]

Contrast echocardiography is especially useful in defining endocardial boundaries to determine exact wall or chamber dimensions. The right septal surface is often especially irregular and produces multiple echo lines: contrast may define the precise right septal border and confirm the presence of septal hypertrophy. In complex congenital heart disease, a major benefit of peripheral contrast is in verifying the venous receiving, venous pumping, and outflow structures both before and after surgery.

Detection of Blood Flow Patterns: Shunt Flow

Perhaps the widest use of contrast echo is in the evaluation of blood flow patterns. Once injected, echocontrast microbubbles flow with the blood and serve as an easily imageable marker. In addition, complete echocontrast absorption in the lungs makes it a unique indicator. As echocontrast bubbles do not pass through the lungs, the appearance of contrast echoes in a left heart chamber following a peripheral venous injection confirms the presence of an abnormal right-to-left shunt. As it requires only a few microbubbles, of the millions injected, to cross the defect and to confirm the diagnosis, this technique is potentially an extremely sensitive test for a shunt.

Figure 14-6 shows a patient with an atrial septal defect and a significant right-to-left shunt. Initially the chambers are clear (Figure 14-6A). Following a peripheral injection, contrast appears first in the right atrium (Figure 14-6B) and then in the

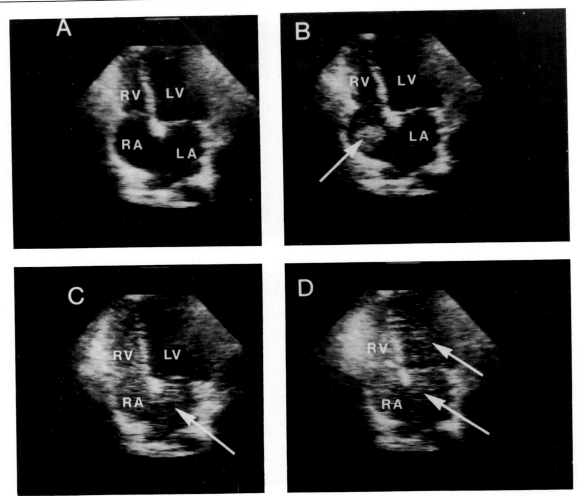

Figure 14-6. A: Two-dimensional echocardiogram obtained from the apical four-chamber view. B: The arrow points to the initial appearance of a contrast echo in the right atrium. C: The echocontrast effect now fills the right ventricle, right atrium, and left atrium (shown by the arrow). D: All four chambers of the heart contain echocontrast; the arrows point to the contrast echoes in the left atrium and left ventricle.

right ventricle (Figure 14-6C). In Figure 14-6C, contrast has also crossed the interatrial septum and appears in the left atrium. During diastole the contrast that has crossed into the left atrium moves into the left ventricle (Figure 14-6D). Not only can the right-to-left shunt and atrial septal defect be diagnosed, but the pattern of interatrial shunt flow can also be studied by evaluating sequential frames.

In evaluating right-to-left shunts, most authors have found contrast echocardiography to be highly sensitive and specific.[27–29] Contrast echocardiography appears to be more sensitive than oximetry and at least as sensitive as dye dilution techniques in detecting right-to-left shunts as small as 3 percent. It is thus often sufficiently sensitive to disclose small right-to-left shunts in patients with a patent foramen ovale or a surgically repaired atrial septal defect when other techniques show no such abnormality.[30]

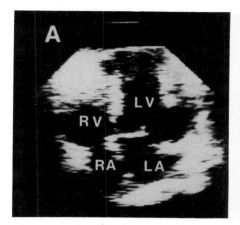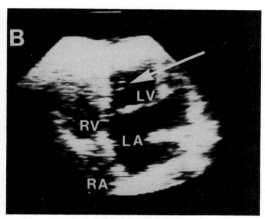

Figure 14-7. A: Two-dimensional echocardiogram obtained from the apical window in a four-chamber view. B: Following the injection of contrast, only two contrast echoes are identified in the left ventricle, as indicated by the arrow. The mitral valve in this patient is abnormal as well.

Figure 14-7 is an apical four-chamber view of a contrast injection in a patient with an insignificant right-to-left shunt following repair of an atrial septal defect. Following a peripheral venous injection, a two-dimensional echocardiogram in this patient showed only two contrast echoes in the left ventricle. There was a small tear in an atrial septal patch, and the shunt was too small to be demonstrated by oxygen saturation determinations.

Right-to-left shunting at the ventricular level can also be identified. Figure 14-8 is an apical four-chamber view with echoes absent in the area of the interventricular septum. The diagnosis of a ventricular septal defect was determined in this patient by following the flow of echocontrast. Initially, the right atrial and the right ventricular chambers filled (Figures 14-8B, C). Subsequently, contrast moved through the defect in the interventricular septum into the left ventricle (Figure 14-8D), confirming a ventricular septal defect with right-to-left shunt. Numerous studies have confirmed the high sensitivity and specificity of contrast echocardiography in the detection of right-to-left ventricular shunts.[27–31]

In addition to the detection of right-to-left shunting at atrial and ventricular levels, contrast echocardiography has also been used to reveal right-to-left shunting in patients with patent ductus ateriosus[20] and aortopulmonary windows.[15] Although only a small number of these patients have been reported, it would be expected that a reasonable sensitivity and specificity could be achieved in detecting right-to-left shunts at these levels if the aorta could be successfully visualized.

In addition to disclosing right-to-left shunts, it would be extremely useful to demonstrate predominantly left-to-right shunts as well. A catheter-injection of echocontrast into the left atrium demonstrates all four cardiac chambers in Figure 14-9. In this patient, following the injection of contrast into the left atrium, contrast flows into the left ventricle and also crosses the interatrial septum to fill the right atrium and right ventricle, thus confirming the presence of an atrial septal defect with a left-to-right shunt. This catheter-injection technique has applications in individuals for whom radiation or radiographic contrast injections are contraindicated. In addition, echocontrast is a portable technique; it can be safely repeated; and it provides a tomographic image of several chambers at one time. In many such instances

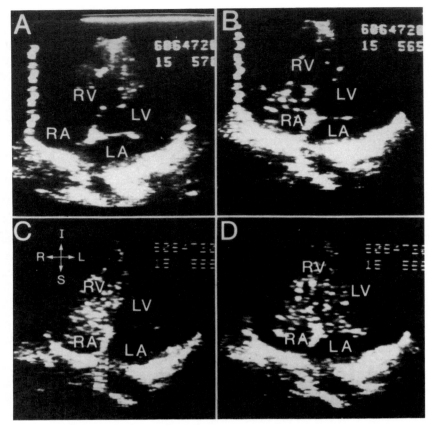

Figure 14-8. A: Two-dimensional echocardiogram obtained in the apical four-chamber view. Just inferior to the tricuspid and mitral valves there is an echo-free space between the right ventricle and the left ventricle. B: Following a peripheral injection of contrast, bright contrast echoes can be seen in the right atrium. C: Contrast echoes have now filled the right atrium and right ventricle. D: Contrast echoes, having filled the right atrium and right ventricle, are now appearing in the left ventricle.

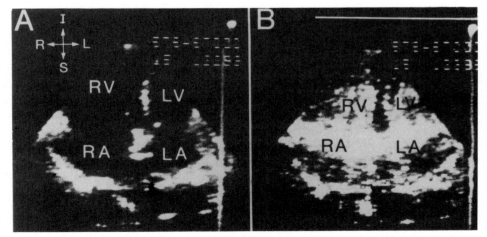

Figure 14-9. A: Two-dimensional echocardiogram recorded in the apical view. The linear echo crossing the area of the interatrial septum represents a catheter. B: Following injection of contrast into the left atrium, all four chambers of the heart become opacified, confirming the presence of a left-to-right shunt.

contrast echocardiography can be superior to standard angiography.[32] Even more advantages would accrue if a less invasive diagnostic procedure could provide the same information.

As contrast echocardiography has progressed, it has been found that the majority of patients with predominantly left-to-right shunts through an atrial septal defect have small transient right-to-left shunts as well.[33–38] Although the diagnosis of minor right-to-left shunt may not be vital, it does signify an atrial septal defect and, therefore, the potential for a significant left-to-right shunt as well. These transient right-to-left shunts can often be evoked by having the patient perform a number of vasoactive maneuvers. Both the Valsalva and Mueller maneuvers may alter intrathoracic and cardiac pressures sufficiently to cause some blood and, therefore, contrast to cross an atrial septal defect in a right-to-left direction.

Patients with predominantly left-to-right ventricular shunts may also demonstrate a small right-to-left shunt. It appears in early diastole and is seen in patients who have a right ventricular pressure that approaches two-thirds of the left ventricular pressure.[31] Right-to-left shunting does not appear to occur in patients with small ventricular septal defects. Thus, this technique may identify patients with more significant ventricular septal defects.

In addition to large as well as small right-to-left shunts in the presence of a predominantly left-to-right shunt, a number of investigators have reported a "negative-contrast effect" that is seen exclusively in patients with left-to-right shunts.[39–41] By injecting the right side of the heart with a large amount of contrast, the entire chamber can be opacified. Thus, if a left-to-right shunt exists, nonopacified blood from the left atrium, left ventricle, or aorta will wash contrast away from the interatrial,[40] interventricular,[41] or periaortic area,[42] yielding a negative-contrast effect. Although this may require a large amount of contrast and special views, some

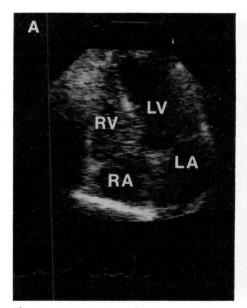 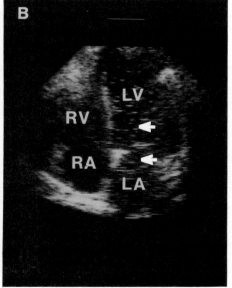

Figure 14-10. A: Two-dimensional echocardiogram obtained from the cardiac apex in a four-chamber view. Contrast is present in the right atrial and right ventricular chambers but is absent from the left side. B: After a 6-second delay, contrast echoes appear in the left atrium and left ventricle (arrows).

investigators have reported very good results. At the present time, it appears easier to demonstrate the negative-contrast effect in the atrium than in the ventricle.

Echocontrast can also be used to detect ductal[43,44] and pulmonary shunting.[45] In Figure 14-10A, the right atrium and right ventricle were seen to be opacified during a peripheral venous injection. Six seconds later, after the contrast had completely cleared from the right side of the heart, multiple echoes were seen in the left atrium and left ventricle (Figure 14-10B). The 6-second delay was explained by an abnormal "short circuit," a shunt through the lungs that did not block the microbubbles or allow them to be absorbed. This diagnosis of an anomalous right-to-left intrapulmonary shunt was additionally confirmed at cardiac catheterization and by pulmonary angiograms demonstrating multiple pulmonary arteriovenous fistulas that were sufficiently large to allow the microbubbles to pass through unimpeded.

Although a qualitative estimate of the severity of the shunt can often be made with contrast echocardiography, more refined estimations may require additional instrumentation.[46–48]

Valvular Regurgitation

Valvular regurgitation can be directly demonstrated by contrast echocardiography using catheter-injections. Figure 14-11A shows a parasternal long-axis view of a patient with aortic regurgitation. Following catheter-injection, contrast appears in the left ventricle (Figure 14-11B). Although the extent of contrast-revealed regurgitation is greater in more severe valvular regurgitations, an exact quantitation is not yet available. Again, however, this technique may be of diagnostic value when x-irradiation or radiographic iodine is contraindicated or simultaneous multichamber tomographic viewing is advantageous.[32] Other regurgitant lesions have also been directly demonstrated with downstream catheter-injections. It appears that contrast echocardiography has a reasonably high sensitivity in detecting regurgitant lesions and is capable of demonstrating regurgitant flows as small as 10 percent.[49]

Indirect evidence of regurgitation can be obtained with upstream injections as

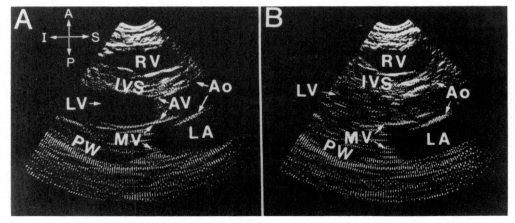

Figure 14-11. A: Two-dimensional echocardiogram obtained from the parasternal long-axis view, aortic regurgitation. AV denotes aortic valve; MV, mitral valve; PW, posterior wall. B: Following a catheter-injection into the aorta, multiple echoes are seen in the left ventricular chamber.

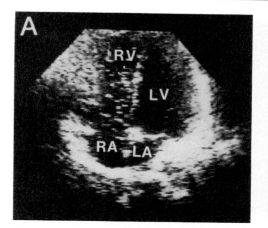
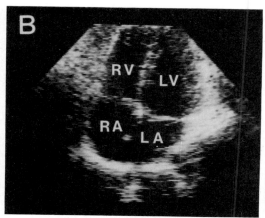

Figure 14-12. A: Two-dimensional echocardiogram obtained from the apex in a four-chamber view. Contrast is seen in the normal right atrial and right ventricular chambers. B: After 3 to 4 seconds, echocontrast is no longer visible.

well. This technique has been applied mainly in the evaluation of tricuspid regurgitation with peripheral venous injections. Figure 14-12 shows a normal right heart contrast sequence. The contrast appears in the right atrium and then the right ventricle and washes out after 3 to 4 seconds (Figure 14-12B). A similar contrast injection in a patient with tricuspid regurgitation is shown for comparison in Figure 14-13. Here the contrast remains in the chambers considerably longer and is still apparent (Figure 14-13B) 10 seconds after its initial appearance. Occasionally, individual contrast bubbles can also be tracked crossing the valve in a retrograde direction, lending support to the diagnosis of regurgitation.

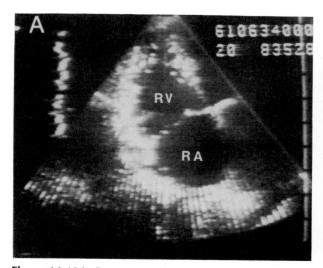
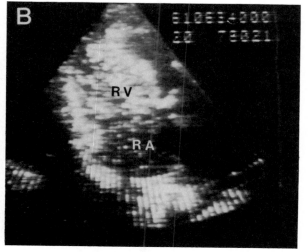

Figure 14-13A, B. A: Apical two-chamber view prior to echocontrast injection in a patient with tricuspid regurgitation. B: Ten seconds after the initial injection, a considerable amount of echocontrast remains in the right heart chambers. In addition to a slow disappearance rate, individual contrast echoes could be occasionally seen to cross from the right ventricle into the right atrium.

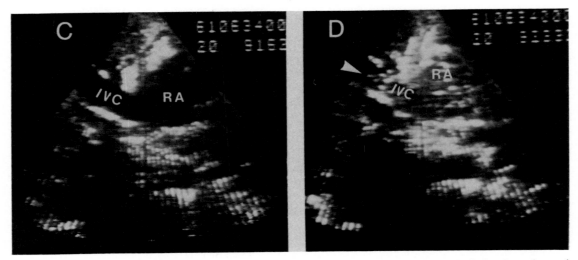

Figure 14-13C, D. C: The inferior vena cava (IVC) and right atrium are labeled in this subcostal short-axis view of the same patient as in Figures 14-13A and B. D: Following the arrival of echocontrast in the right atrium, contrast echoes can be seen to proceed down into the inferior vena cava and hepatic veins as indicated by the arrow.

Considerable attention has been focused on the inferior vena cava and hepatic veins during contrast injections. Figure 14-13C shows a short-axis subcostal view of the inferior vena cava and right atrium. Following the injection of contrast in a peripheral arm vein, echocontrast flows into the right atrium and partly into the inferior vena cava and hepatic veins in a retrograde manner (Figure 14-13D). Persistent inferior vena cava reflux has been associated with tricuspid regurgitation in several studies and thus provides indirect evidence of tricuspid regurgitation.[50–52]

Cardiac Output

The quick passage of blood and indicators through the heart has been associated with normal or increased cardiac output. Since contrast microbubbles behave in much the same manner as other indicators, echocontrast studies can be used to measure cardiac output. A simple way to monitor this contrast is by placing a photocell on the echo screen. Figure 14-14 shows the right atrium and right ventricle before and following a peripheral venous contrast injection. The circled area outlines the region monitored by the photocell. The echocardiographic brightness curves produced by the photocell in patients with three different levels of cardiac output are illustrated in Figure 14-15. In this figure the upper illustrations reflect the photo intensity at two different gain settings in patients with cardiac outputs of 7, 5, and 2.7 liters/minute, respectively. As the cardiac output declines, the washout of echocardiographic brightness takes longer. The lower tracings represent the thermal indicator curves obtained with a Swan-Ganz catheter. With the thermal curves there is a similar prolongation of the washout of the indicator as the cardiac output declines. Although a number of variables are ignored in this procedure and the correlation is not exact, this technique can provide an estimation of cardiac output with an intravenous contrast injection.[53–55]

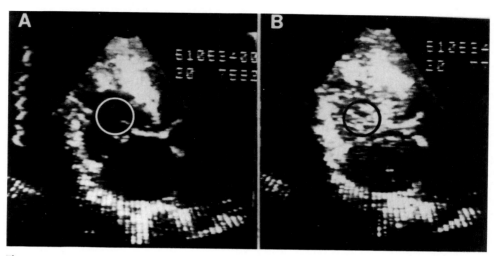

Figure 14-14. A: Apical four-chamber view of the right atrium and right ventricle. The white circle outlines an area of the right ventricle. B: Contrast now fills the right ventricle and is monitored within the black circle by the external photocell.

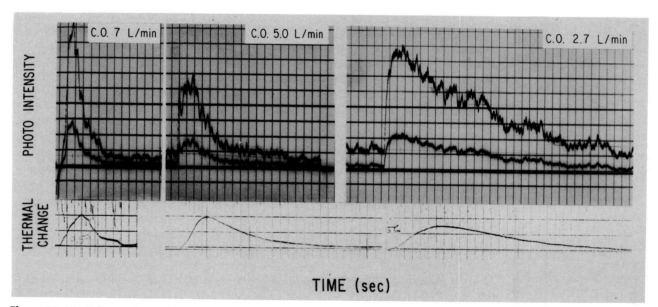

Figure 14-15. Echocardiographic contrast curves and Swan-Ganz thermodilution curves from three patients with cardiac outputs of 7, 5, and 2.7 liters/minute. The upper curves represent the DC output from the digital photocell recorded in foot-lamberts on the vertical scale and time in seconds on the horizontal scale. The upper curves of photo intensity show the unattenuated echocontrast brightness and can be compared with the thermodilution curves in the lower graphs.

Limited blood velocity measurements can also be obtained from contrast echocardiography. While an individual bubble is within the transducer field its motion can be followed either with M-mode or two-dimensional echo. Although absolute calculations are difficult, relative velocity changes following interventions may be appreciated.[56]

NEW INJECTION TECHNIQUES

Although standard contrast microbubbles are too large to pass through the lungs, a forced injection with a catheter in the pulmonary artery wedge position will drive standard contrast microbubbles through to the left side.[57,58] This technique can be used to visualize left-to-right shunts or produce left-sided echocontrast angiograms when only a right heart catheterization is possible. Although limited experience with these and similar pulmonary artery wedge radiographic injections has not shown complications in humans, the exact safety of this technique cannot be determined until wider experience is obtained.

INVESTIGATIVE CONTRAST ECHOCARDIOGRAPHY

Early studies showed that a variety of agents produced echocontrast effects. Several solids and liquids have different acoustic impedance properties from blood[59] and therefore produce an echocontrast effect; the greatest difference in acoustic impedance, and thus the greatest contrast effect, is seen with gas microbubbles in the blood stream. It is for this reason that the newer contrast agents either contain gas or produce gas following injection. Gases that have been injected directly or in a fluid carrier have included carbon dioxide, oxygen, nitrogen, hydrogen, and air.[57,60–63] Since large injections of any of these gases have been reported to cause gas emboli with complications, most studies have employed extremely small amounts of gas; usually patients with right-to-left shunts have been excluded. At present, the maximum amount of gas or microbubbles that can be safely tolerated is unknown.

Gas-producing liquids that have been injected include solutions of supersaturated carbon dioxide,[57] supersaturated nitrogen, hydrogen peroxide,[64,65] and ether.[66] These agents produce superb echocontrast effects, but their safety remains to be proven.

Gas-containing microbubbles can also be designed and produced for specific purposes. Gelatin-coated microbubbles of a uniform size have lent themselves to quantitative studies of blood flow and cardiac output.[57,67] Collagen has also been used as a coating material. Although these protein shells are fairly soft and flexible, the newer saccharide coatings are very hard and designed to protect the inner bubble. Since these hard-shell microbubbles can be made small enough to pass through capillaries, they can cross the pulmonary and systemic capillary system to produce left heart and tissue perfusion images.[68–70]

Figure 14-16A shows the initial appearance of echocontrast from saccharide-coated microbubbles in the right ventricle. In Figure 14-16B some of the contrast has passed through the lungs and appears in the left ventricle. Following pulmonary transmission, this left heart contrast can aid in the diagnosis of abnormal blood flow patterns in the left ventricle and in the diagnosis of left-to-right shunts.

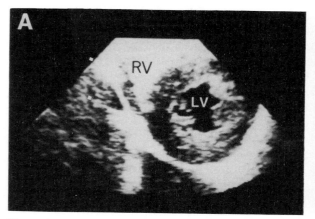
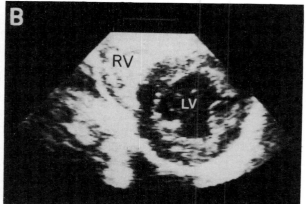

Figure 14-16. A: Two-dimensional echocardiogram obtained in parasternal short-axis view. Contrast echoes completely fill the right ventricular chamber. B: Following pulmonary transmission, fainter contrast echoes now appear in the left ventricular chamber as well.

Figure 14-17A shows a short-axis view of the heart in which the myocardium of the left ventricle is very echolucent. Following the injection of saccharide-coated microbubbles into the coronary arteries, the entire myocardium becomes brightly opacified. This echocontrast then disappears, giving the effect of an echocontrast myocardial perfusion scan. Since this perfusion scan can be viewed in real-time at multiple tomographic levels, it may offer substantial advantages over currently available radionuclide perfusion images.

In addition to imaging applications, microbubbles can also be used to estimate intracardiac pressures.[71] One technique utilizes microbubbles that contain a pressurized gas and are encapsulated with a hard saccharide shell. Once injected, the shell dissolves and the gas explodes outward to create a vibrating bubble. This bubble

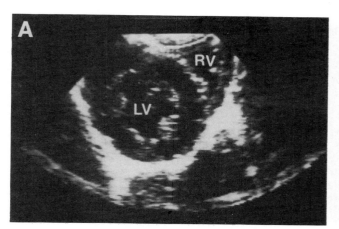
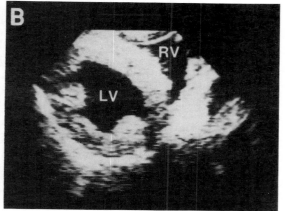

Figure 14-17. A: Two-dimensional echocardiogram obtained in a reversed short-axis view. The left ventricular myocardium is dark, with few echoes seen. B: Following the injection of contrast, the entire left ventricular myocardium becomes brightly echo-dense. This bright contrast appearance then gradually disappears, giving the appearance of an echocontrast myocardial perfusion scan.

oscillates at a frequency proportional to its size, which is in turn proportional to the pressure within the chamber. Recording the frequency of the radiating sonic waves permits the pressures within the right side of the heart to be calculated.[72–74] If the initial pressurized microbubbles can be made small enough to pass through the lungs, left heart pressures may be obtained as well.

The potential of these carefully designed new agents goes far beyond standard physiologic measurement and imaging purposes. Theoretically, these new agents could be designed for pharmaceutical drug delivery and activation, blood component absorption and therapy, and blood function replacement, just to name a few. If the technical and safety questions can be answered, the only real limits on use of these agents will be the limits of our imagination.

CONCLUSIONS

From its very beginning, contrast echocardiography has played a vital role in the development of echocardiography. At present it continues to play a useful part in the evaluation of congenital and valvular heart disease. It is likely that as new techniques and agents are developed, contrast echocardiography will continue to play an even larger part in the diagnosis and perhaps even the therapy of cardiovascular disease.

REFERENCES

1. Gramiak R, Shah PM, Kramer DH: Ultrasound cardiography. Contrast studies in anatomy and function. Radiology 92:939–948, 1969
2. Barrera JG, Fulkerson PK, Rittgers SE, et al: The nature of contrast echocardiographic "targets." Circulation 58(Suppl II):II-233, 1978
3. Meltzer R, Tickner EG, Sahines TP, et al: The source of ultrasonic contrast effect. JCU 8:121–127, 1980
4. Stauffer HM, Durant TM, Oppenheimer MJ: Gas embolism: Roentgenologic considerations, including the experimental use of carbon dioxide as an intracardiac contrast material. Radiology 66:686–692, 1956
5. Yang W-J: Dynamics of gas bubbles in whole blood and plasma. J Biomech 4:119–125, 1971
6. Epstein PS, Plesset MS: On the stability of gas bubbles in liquid–gas solutions. J Chem Phys 18:1505–1509, 1950
7. Ward CA, Tucker AS: Thermodynamic theory of diffusion-controlled bubble growth or dissolution and experimental examination of the predictions. J Appl Phys 46:233–238, 1975
8. Plesset MS, Prosperetti A: Bubble dynamics and cavitation. Annu Rev Fluid Mech 9:145–185, 1977
9. Yang WS, Echigo R, Wotton R, et al: Experimental studies of the dissolution of gas bubbles in whole blood and plasma. I. Stationary bubbles. J Biomech 3:275–281, 1971
10. Yang WS, Echigo R, Wotton R, et al: Experimental studies of the dissolution of gas bubbles in whole blood and plasma. II. Moving bubbles or liquids. J Biomech 4:283–288, 1971
11. Gramiak R, Shah PM: Echocardiography of the aortic root. Invest Radiol 3:356–388, 1968
12. Feigenbaum H, Stone JM, Lee DA, et al: Identification of ultrasound echoes from the left ventricle by use of intracardiac injections of indocyanine green. Circulation 41:614–621, 1970
13. Sahn DJ, Williams DE, Shackelton S, et al: The validity of structure identification for cross-sectional echocardiography. JCU 2:201–216, 1974
14. Snider AR, Ports TA, Silverman NH: Venous anomalies of coronary sinus: Detection by M-mode and two-dimensional and contrast echocardiography. Circulation 60:721–727, 1979
15. Satomi G, Nakamura K, Imai Y, et al: Two-dimensional echocardiographic diagnosis of aortico-pulmonary window. Br Heart J 43:351–356, 1980
16. Gondi B, Nanda NC: Two-dimensional echocardiographic features of atrial septal aneurysms. Circulation 63:452–457, 1981

17. Reeder GS, Tajik AJ, Smith HC: Visualization of coronary artery fistula by two-dimensional echocardiography. Mayo Clin Proc 55:185–189, 1980

18. Truman AT, Syamasundar Rao P, Kulangara RJ: Use of contrast echocardiography in diagnosis of anomalous connection of right superior vena cava to left atrium. Br Heart J 44:718–723, 1980

19. Silverman NH, Snider AR, Colo J, et al: Superior vena caval obstruction after Mustard's operation: Detection by two-dimensional contrast echocardiography. Circulation 64:392–396, 1981

20. Mortera C, Leon G: Detection of persistent ductus in hypoplastic left heart syndrome by contrast echocardiography. Br Heart J 44:596–598, 1980

21. Koiwaya Y, Watanabe K, Orita Y, et al: Contrast two-dimensional echocardiography in diagnosis of tricuspid atresia. Am Heart J 101:507–510, 1981

22. Aziz KU, Paul MH, Bharati S, et al: Echocardiographic features of total anomalous pulmonary venous drainage into the coronary sinus. Am J Cardiol 42:108–113, 1978

23. Tomoe A, Yoshida Y, Ogata H, et al: Peripheral contrast echocardiographic findings of anomalous drainage of the right superior vena cava into the left atrium. Tohoku J Exp Med 130:353–358, 1980

24. Weyman AE, Feigenbaum H, Dillon JC, et al: Noninvasive visualization of the left main coronary artery by cross-sectional echocardiography. Circulation 54:169–174, 1976

25. Bommer WJ, Kwan OL, Mason DT, et al: Identification of prominent eustachian valves by M-mode and two-dimensional echocardiography: Differentiation from right atrial masses (Abstract) Am J Cardiol 45:402, 1980

26. Minami Y, Iwasa M, Takahashi Y, et al: Two-dimensional echocardiographic findings of a right ventricular diverticulum: A case report. J Cardiogr 11:289–296, 1981

27. Seward JB, Tajik AJ, Hagler DJ, et al: Peripheral venous contrast echocardiography. Am J Cardiol 39:202–212, 1977

28. Valdes-Cruz LM, Pieroni DR, Roland JMA, et al: Echocardiographic detection of intracardiac right-to-left shunts following peripheral vein injections. Circulation 54:558–562, 1976

29. Pieroni DR, Varghese PJ, Freedom RM, et al: The sensitivity of contrast echocardiography in detecting intracardiac shunts. Cathet Cardiovasc Diagn 5:19–29, 1979

30. Valdes-Cruz LM, Pieroni DR, Roland J-MA, et al: Recognition of residual postoperative shunts by contrast echocardiographic techniques. Circulation 55:148–152, 1977

31. Serwer GA, Armstrong BE, Anderson AW, et al: Use of contrast echocardiography for evaluation of right ventricular hemodynamics in the presence of ventricular septal defects. Circulation 58:327–336, 1978

32. Waldman JD, Rummerfield PS, Gilpin EA, et al: Radiation exposure to the child during cardiac catheterization. Circulation 64:158–163, 1981

33. Swan HJC, Burchell HB, Wood EH: The presence of venoarterial shunts in patients with interarterial communications. Circulation 10:705–713, 1954

34. Levin AR, Spach MS, Boineau JP, et al: Atrial pressure–flow dynamics in atrial septal defects (secundum type). Circulation 37:476–488, 1968

35. Bourdillon DV, Foale RA, Rickards AF: Identification of atrial septal defects by cross-sectional contrast echocardiography. Br Heart J 44:401–405, 1980

36. Kronik G, Slany J, Moesslacher H: Contrast M-mode echocardiography in diagnosis of atrial septal defect in acyanotic patients. Circulation 59:372–378, 1979

37. Fraker TD, Harris PJ, Behar VS, et al: Detection and exclusion of interatrial shunts by two-dimensional echocardiography and peripheral venous injection. Circulation 59:379–384, 1979

38. Serruys PW, Ligtvoet CM, Hagemeijer F, et al: Intracardiac shunts in adults studied with bidimensional ultrasonic contrast techniques after peripheral intravenous injections. (Abstract). Circulation 56(Suppl III):III-26, 1977

39. Weyman AE, Wann LS, Hurwitz, RA, et al: Negative contrast echocardiography: A new technique for detecting left-to-right shunts. (Abstract). Circulation 56 (Suppl III):III-26, 1977

40. Weyman AE, Wann LS, Caldwell RL, et al: Negative contrast echocardiography: A new method for detecting left-to-right shunts. Circulation 59:498–505, 1979

41. Farcot JC, Boisante L, Rigaud M, et al: Two-dimensional echocardiographic visualization of ventricular septal rupture after acute anterior myocardial infarction. Am J Cardiol 45:370–377, 1980

42. Nakamura K, Suzuki S, Satomi G: Detection of ruptured aneurysm of sinus of Valsalva by contrast two-dimensional echocardiography. Br Heart J 45:219–221, 1981

43. Sahn DJ, Allen HD, Goldberg S: A serial contrast echo study of cardiac shunts in newborns with heart and lung disease (Abstract). Circulation 54(Suppl II):II-89, 1976

44. Valdes-Cruz LM, Dudell GG: Specificity and accuracy of echocardiographic and clinical criteria for diagnosis of patent ductus arteriosus in fluid-restricted infants. J Pediatr 98:298–305, 1981

45. Lewis AB, Gates GF, Stanley P: Echocardiography and perfusion scintigraphy in the diagnosis of pulmonary arteriovenous fistula. Chest 73:675–677, 1978
46. Gilbert BW, Drobac M, Rakowski H: Contrast two-dimensional echocardiography in inter-atrial shunts (Abstract). Am J Cardiol 45:402, 1980
47. Seward JB, Tajik AJ, Spangler JG, et al: Echocardiographic contrast studies. Mayo Clin Proc 50:163–169, 1975
48. Kronik G, Hutterer B, Moesslacher H: Diagnosis of atrial left-to-right shunts by cross-sectional contrast echocardiography. Z Kardiol 70:138–145, 1981
49. Kerber RE, Kioscho JM, Lauer RM: Use of an ultrasonic contrast method in the diagnosis of valvular regurgitation and intracardiac shunts. Am J Cardiol 34:722–727, 1974
50. Lieppe W, Behar VS, Scallion R, et al: Detection of tricuspid regurgitation with two-dimensional echocardiography and peripheral vein injections. Circulation 57:128–132, 1978
51. Reeves WC, Leaman DM, Buonocore E, et al: Detection of tricuspid regurgitation and estimation of central venous pressure by two-dimensional contrast echocardiography of the right superior hepatic vein. Am Heart J 102:374–377, 1981
52. Chen CC, Morganroth J, Mardelli TJ, et al: Tricuspid regurgitation in tricuspid valve prolapse demonstrated with contrast cross-sectional echocardiography. Am J Cardiol 46:983–987, 1980
53. Bommer WJ, Neef J, Neumann A, et al: Indicator-dilution curves obtained by photometric analysis of two-dimensional echo-contrast studies (Abstract). Am J Cardiol 41:370, 1978
54. Bommer WJ, Lantz B, Miller L, et al: Advances in quantitative contrast echocardiography: Recording and calibration of linear time-concentration curves by video densitometry (Abstract). Circulation 60(Suppl II):II-18, 1979
55. DeMaria AN, Bommer W, Riggs K, et al: In vivo correlation of cardiac output and densitometric dilution curves obtained by contrast two-dimensional echocardiography (Abstract). Circulation 62(Suppl III):III-101, 1980
56. Shiina A, Kondo K, Nakasone Y, et al: Contrast echocardiographic evaluation of changes in flow velocity in the right side of the heart. Circulation 63:1408–1416, 1981
57. Bommer WJ, Mason D, DeMaria A: Studies in contrast echocardiography: Development of new agents with superior reproducibility and transmission through lungs (Abstract). Circulation 60(Suppl II):II-17, 1979
58. Reale A, Pizzuto F, Gioffre PA, et al: Contrast echocardiography: Transmission of echoes to the left heart across the pulmonary vascular bed. Eur Heart J I:101–106, 1980
59. Ophir J, McWhirt RE, Maklad NF: Aqueous solutions as potential ultrasonic contrast agents. Ultrasonic Imaging I:265–279, 1979
60. Phillips JH, Burch GE, Hellinger R: The use of intracardiac carbon dioxide in the diagnosis of pericardial disease. Am Heart J 61:748–755, 1961
61. Turner AF, Meyers HI, Jacobson G, et al: Carbon dioxide cineangiography in the diagnosis of pericardial disease. Am J Roent Rad Ther 97:342–349, 1966
62. Oppenheimer MJ, Durant TM, Stauffer HM, et al: In vivo visualization of intracardiac structures with gaseous carbon dioxide: Cardiovascular-respiratory effects and associated changes in blood chemistry. Am J Physiol 186:325, 1956
63. Scatliff JH, Kummer AJ, Janzen AH: The diagnosis of pericardial effusion with intracardiac carbon dioxide. Radiology 73:871–883, 1979
64. Xinfang W, Jiaen W, Youzhen H, et al: Contrast echocardiography with hydrogen peroxide. I. Experimental study. Chin Med J (Engl) 92(9):595–599, 1979
65. Xinfang W, Jiaen W, Hanrong C, et al: Contrast echocardiography with hydrogen peroxide. II. Clinical application. Chin Med J (Engl) 92(10):693–702, 1979
66. Ziskin MC, Bonakdarpour A, Weinstein DP, et al: Contrast agents for diagnostic ultrasound. Invest Radiol 7:500–505, 1972
67. Carroll BA, Turner RJ, Tickner EG, et al: Gelatin encapsulated nitrogen microbubbles as ultrasonic contrast agents. Invest Radiol 15:260–266, 1980
68. Bommer WJ, Tickner G, Rasor J, et al: Development of a new echocardiographic contrast agent capable of pulmonary transmission and left heart opacification following peripheral venous injection (Abstract). Circulation 62(Suppl III):III-34, 1980
69. Bommer WJ, Rasor J, Tickner G, et al: Quantitative regional myocardial perfusion scanning with contrast echocardiography (Abstract). Am J Cardiol 47:403, 1981
70. DeMaria AN, Bommer W, Rasor J, et al: Visualization of myocardial perfusion by contrast two-dimensional echocardiography: Quantitative videodensitometric comparison of contrast agents and injection sites (Abstract). Clin Res 29:186A, 1981

71. Fairbank WM, Scully MO: A new noninvasive technique for cardiac pressure measurement: Resonant scattering of ultrasound from bubbles. IEEE Trans Biomed Eng 24:107–110, 1977

72. Tickner EG, Rasor NS: Noninvasive assessment of pulmonary hypertension using bubble ultrasonic resonance pressure (BURP) method. NIH report HF-62917-1A. Bethesda, National Institutes of Health, Apr 1977

73. Tickner EG, Rasor NS: Noninvasive assessment of pulmonary hypertension using bubble ultrasonic resonance pressure (BURP) method. NIH report HR-62917-2A. Bethesda, National Institutes of Health, June 1978

74. Tucker C, Sahines T, Rasor J, et al: Non-invasive right ventricular pressure measurement by microbubble oscillation, (Abstract). Circulation 64(Suppl IV):IV-65, 1981

CHAPTER 15

Doppler Echocardiography

Julius M. Gardin

Doppler echocardiography provides a research and clinical tool to study valvular and congenital heart lesions and to quantitate cardiac function. The technique has also been used to detect flow in native coronary arteries and coronary bypass grafts, explain physiologic and pathophysiologic phenomena by recording Doppler flow in the heart and great arteries, and display simultaneous flow velocities and echocardiographic images from multiple cardiac regions. Although many of these applications of the Doppler technique are still in the investigative stage, several have demonstrated clinical utility. In this chapter an overview of the basic principles as well as the current research and clinical applications of Doppler echocardiography are provided.

PRINCIPLES AND THEORY OF DOPPLER ULTRASOUND

The Doppler principle states that an emitted ultrasound pulse has its frequency "shifted" by moving targets in direct proportion to the velocities of these targets along the ultrasound axis. Red blood cells act as ultrasound targets that reflect and shift the frequency of ultrasound in direct proportion to their velocities. The Doppler principle can thus be used to estimate cardiac blood flow velocity. Note in Figure 15-1 that as the target (red blood cell) moves toward the reference point (e.g., a transducer) the reflected ultrasound has less distance to travel. Consequently, the wavelength of the reflected ultrasound diminishes and the frequency increases. Conversely, as the target moves away from the reference point the reflected ultrasound has a longer distance to travel, which results in a decrease in frequency. Doppler frequency shifts from individual blood cells can be analyzed for velocity, direction, and other characteristics—e.g., relative laminarity or turbulence of blood flow.

The Doppler equation relates the flow velocity (V) in cm/second of red blood cells, in the direction parallel to the long axis of blood flow, directly to the Doppler frequency shift (Δf) in hertz, and inversely to the fundamental frequency of the emitted ultrasound (f_o) in hertz (Hz):

$$V = \frac{\Delta f c}{2 f_o \cos \theta} \tag{1}$$

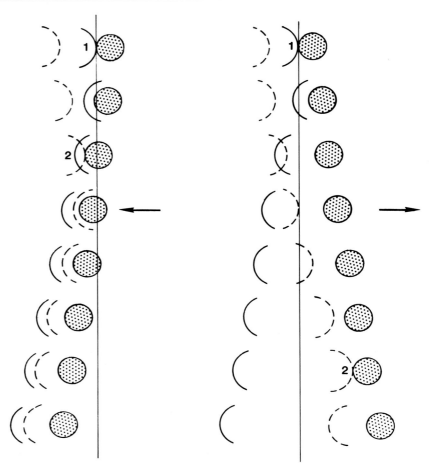

Figure 15-1. The Doppler principle. The panel on the left depicts the origin of the shift in frequency of ultrasound reflected from a red blood cell moving toward the transducer. The panel on the right illustrates the shift in frequency arising from a red blood cell moving away from the transducer. The numbers 1 and 2 denote the times the first and second ultrasound waves, respectively, make contact with the red blood cell (see text for further details).

where c equals the velocity of sound in tissue (1540 m/second), and θ is the angle between the emitted ultrasound and the long axis of blood flow (flow velocity vector).[1-3]

Continuous Wave Versus Pulsed Doppler

Two basic Doppler modalities have been employed in cardiac diagnosis: continuous wave and pulsed (range-gated). The continuous wave (CW) technique employs two transducers: a transmitter that emits ultrasound continuously at a constant frequency, and a receiver that detects the frequency shifts of reflected ultrasound.[4-7] The continuous wave modality has the advantage of detecting high flow velocities—over 4 m/second—important in estimating peak flow velocity in a jet stream, e.g., in a stenotic orifice or in a chamber receiving regurgitant blood. The disadvantage of continuous wave Doppler is shown in Figure 15-2. Although it is quite useful in peripheral vessels for detecting blood flow in a single direction, it has distinct dif-

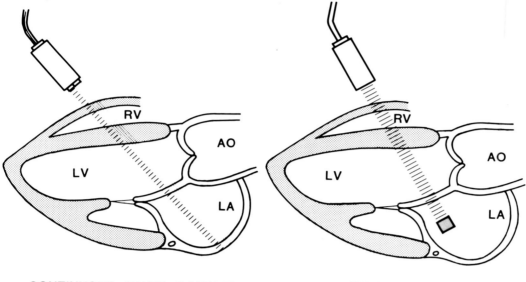

CONTINUOUS   WAVE   DOPPLER   **PULSED   DOPPLER**

Figure 15-2. Diagrams of the heart in the parasternal long-axis view with an ultrasound beam shown traversing a series of intracardiac structures in its path from the front to the back of the heart. Note that in the continuous wave Doppler technique, one transducer emits ultrasound essentially continuously while a second transducer receives the reflected ultrasound waves. Frequency shifts from red blood cells and structures along the entire beam path are recorded. On the other hand, in the pulsed Doppler technique, frequency shifts from a specific region (or sample volume), such as the left atrium or left ventricular outflow tract, can be selectively recorded. In this illustration, the sample volume is positioned in the left atrium. LA denotes left atrium; LV, left ventricle; RA, right atrium; RV, right ventricle.

ficulties in differentiating intracardiac flow in more than one direction—e.g., flow in the left atrium from flow in the left ventricular outflow tract. The ability to detect blood flow in specific cardiac chambers or vessels is particularly useful in various cardiac lesions, e.g., in differentiating mitral regurgitation from hypertrophic obstructive cardiomyopathy, tricuspid regurgitation, or ventricular septal defect.

The pulsed Doppler technique utilizes a "range-gating" mechanism featuring a time delay which allows a time sampling "window" to be electronically entered into the pulsed Doppler instrument (Figure 15-2). Only the frequency shifts from signals reflected from this "window," or sample volume, are recorded by the system.[8-14] The trade-off for utilizing pulsed Doppler rather than the continuous wave technique is that the range–velocity product (see following definition) limits the utility of pulsed Doppler in measuring higher flow velocities (higher frequency shifts) at greater depths from the transducer.

The range–velocity product is derived from the Nyquist equation (sampling rate theorem), which states that the pulse repetition frequency (PRF) of the emitted ultrasound must be at least twice the maximum frequency shift (Δf_{max}) to be sampled. This avoids errors (known as *aliasing errors*) of uncertainty as to the magnitude of the frequency shift[1,2,10-15]:

$$\Delta f_{max} = \frac{PRF}{2} \qquad (2)$$

If one desires to measure flow velocity and range (sample depth) without ambiguity, then the *maximum range* (R_{max} in cm) that can be sampled according to the *sampling rate theorem* is defined by the following equation:

$$R_{max} = \frac{1}{(1.3 \times 10^{-5}) \times PRF} \qquad (3)$$

The number of emitted and received ultrasound cycles per second limits the sampling depth to which the ultrasound beam can travel in a given time period. Therefore, the maximum range at which the pulsed Doppler system can function is inversely proportional to the magnitude of the *pulse repetition frequency*. The maximum Doppler frequency shift (Δf_{max}) that can be detected is related to the maximum depth or range (R_{max}) at which the system can function by the following equation:

$$\Delta f_{max} = \frac{1}{(2.6 \times 10^{-5}) \times R_{max}} \qquad (4)$$

Equation 4 can be combined with equation 1 to give the maximum flow velocity that can be detected for a given range (depth), fundamental emitted frequency (f_o), and angle (θ) between the ultrasound beam and the flow velocity vector:

$$V_{max} = \frac{c}{(5.2 \times 10^{-5}) R_{max} \times f_o \times \cos\theta} \qquad (5)$$

where V_{max} is the maximum detectable velocity at R_{max}.[1] For a 2.25 megahertz (MHz) transducer, and an angle θ of zero degrees, the range–velocity product can be calculated from equation 5 to be approximately 1300 cm²/second.

In our experience, adults exhibit normal resting peak (midspectral) flow velocities up to 120 cm/second.[16] Measuring flow velocities in the ascending aorta with a 2.25 MHz pulsed Doppler transducer in normals may be unreliable at a sample volume depth greater than 10 to 12 cm from the transducer. To measure flow velocity with pulsed Doppler where the velocities (frequency shifts) exceed the range–velocity product limit (equation 5), one must resort to a more sophisticated pulsed Doppler system that is not limited by the sampling rate theorem. Such a system—resorting to methods such as tagging each emitted ultrasound pulse with a decipherable pseudo-random noise code or tolerating some uncertainty as to range information—makes it unnecessary for the reflected ultrasound pulse to reach the transducer before a new Doppler pulse is emitted.[1,17] Another simple approach that may be clinically applicable can be inferred from equation 5. If the other factors are kept constant, a higher maximum velocity (V_{max}) can be detected by using a transducer that emits a lower fundamental frequency (f_o), such as 1.6 MHz. Finally, if one is not concerned about sampling from a particular sample volume, continuous wave Doppler can be used to measure higher flow velocities.

COMPARISON OF ULTRASOUND FOR CARDIAC IMAGING AND FOR DOPPLER FLOW STUDIES

Ultrasound transducers utilized both for echocardiography and for Doppler blood flow studies emit ultrasound of similar fundamental frequency (range 1–10 MHz) and similar pulse repetition frequency (range 2000–10,000 cycles/second, i.e., 2–10 kHz). Consequently, the same ultrasound crystal may be used for imaging as well as for measuring Doppler flow velocity. Simultaneous or near-simultaneous acquisition of imaging and Doppler data is now possible with a number of sector scanners currently in use.

Despite the similarity of the ultrasound energy utilized for imaging and for flow studies, there are a number of differences between the use of ultrasound in echocardiography and in Doppler applications: (1) In cardiac imaging, the ultrasound beam is optimally directed perpendicular to the structures to be evaluated, whereas in sampling Doppler flow velocity characteristics, the ultrasound beam is ideally directed parallel to the long axis of blood flow. (2) In echocardiographic imaging, the depth and intensity of the reflected signals from all targets along the beam path are displayed, whereas with the Doppler technique, the frequency shifts either from along the entire ultrasound beam path (continuous wave mode) or from a specific sample volume (pulsed mode) are detected. (3) The ultrasound beam becomes attenuated as it passes through tissues so that, for a given tissue density, the intensity of the ultrasound signals reflected from deep cardiac structures is less than for shallow structures. The physical principle of ultrasound is more important in imaging than in blood flow measurements. (4) When pulsed Doppler is used to examine flow in deeper structures, the range–velocity product significantly limits the magnitude of the flow velocities (i.e., frequency shifts) that can be sampled. The range–velocity product is not a practical problem in either imaging or continuous wave Doppler modes. (5) Finally, the pulse repetition frequency of ultrasound used in imaging is constant, whereas in pulsed Doppler studies the pulse repetition frequency of the emitted ultrasound beam may be varied in an attempt to maximize the magnitude of the flow velocity recorded at any given depth (equations 2 and 3).

DISPLAY AND ANALYSIS OF DOPPLER DATA

The information from Doppler flow signals can be processed to provide both audio and graphic output. The audio signals reflect the spectrum of Doppler frequency shifts (in the range of 400 Hz to 5 kHz) produced by moving red blood cells. The audio signal sampled from an area of laminar blood flow sounds "tonal" or smooth; it appears graphically as a relatively smooth curve consisting of uniform frequency shifts from the sample volume (Figure 15-3A). The audio signal from an area of disturbed or turbulent blood flow is "noisy" or rough, and appears graphically as a broad spectrum of frequency shifts, or spectral dispersion (Figure 15-3B). A typical "whipping" sound is audible and recordable in the paravalvular region; this corresponds to valve leaflet motion.[11,15] Cardiac chamber and vessel walls also reflect ultrasound and produce Doppler frequency shifts; these relatively low-frequency shifts are intentionally filtered out of the display.

The graphic analysis and display of Doppler signals has been accomplished by several methods.

Zero-Crossing Detection

An early method utilized to graphically analyze Doppler frequency shifts was the zero-crossing detector.[1,2,10–13,15] In zero-crossing detection, a pulse is generated each time that the input signal crosses zero (or a pre-set threshold level) in one direction; it then counts the number of pulses (zero-crossings) that occur per second.

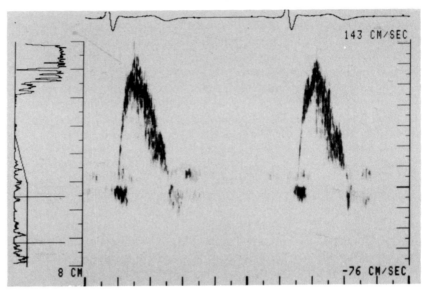

Figure 15-3A. Pulsed Doppler flow velocity recording from the ascending aorta in a normal subject. Note the relatively laminar, or smooth, systolic flow pattern.

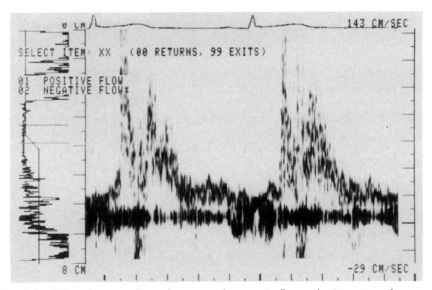

Figure 15-3B. Pulsed Doppler recording of an ascending aortic flow velocity pattern from a patient with aortic stenosis. Note the turbulent systolic flow pattern, exhibiting marked spectral dispersion.

A time interval histogram can then be constructed by plotting a set of points of the reciprocals of the zero-crossing intervals (Figure 15-4). For lower frequency shifts, i.e., longer periods between zero-crossings, a dot on the time interval histogram is printed near the zero-flow line. Conversely, for high-frequency shifts and short intervals between zero-crossings, the dot is recorded further from the zero-flow line. Thus, the distance of a dot from the zero-line on the time interval histogram is directly proportional to the Doppler frequency shift. The initial prototype Duplex scanner designed by Baker and associates[9] employed a zero-crossing detection system to display Doppler data. This instrument featured a mechanical sector scanner for two-dimensional imaging mounted alongside a pulsed Doppler transducer.

The major limitations to the use of zero-crossing detection[2,10,11,15] are that the Doppler signal is composed of a spectrum of frequencies, as opposed to a single frequency shift, which changes with time; furthermore, the Doppler signal is not a perfect sine wave, which results in a spectrum of frequency shifts that cannot be analyzed accurately by zero-crossing detection. Also, the time interval histogram generated by zero-crossing detection is gain- and frequency threshold-dependent; therefore, its output is difficult to calibrate. A threshold arrangement can be utilized to reject low-level noise; however, there may be a problem when high-gain and low-threshold settings are necessary to record weak Doppler signals. This means that electronic "noise" inherent in the Doppler instrument may itself cause a "wide-

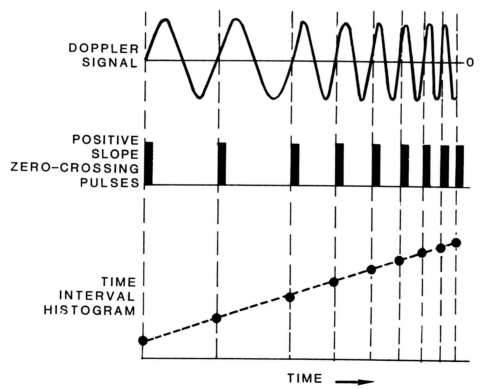

Figure 15-4A. Diagram depicting the construction of a time interval histogram using the zero-crossing detection method. Data points correspond to the reciprocals of the zero-crossing intervals detected by the Doppler velocimeter (see text for details).

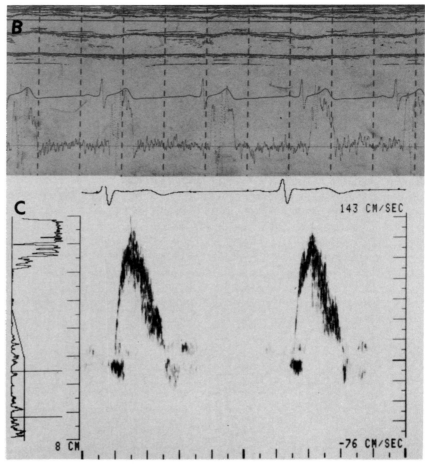

Figure 15-4B, C. Comparison of ascending aortic flow velocity tracings from the same normal subject as in Figure 15-3A recorded utilizing a zero-crossing detector (B) and a spectrum analyzer (C). Note the greater deviations from the mean flow pattern recorded by the zero-crossing method.

band" pattern to appear on the graphic display. This apparent Doppler spectral broadening may be mistaken for disturbed blood flow when, in fact, the blood flow is normal. Another important limitation of this method is that it does not process Doppler signals properly if forward and reverse flow are present simultaneously.

To summarize, the time interval histogram can be used to display relatively homogeneous Doppler recordings (laminar flow), but the technique is not helpful when marked spectral dispersion (turbulent flow) or bidirectional flow is present. Finally, zero-crossing detectors cannot accurately display the flow spectrum when both high- and low-frequency shift signals are present simultaneously.

Spectral Analysis

An important approach to deriving quantitative information from Doppler signals involves analysis of the flow velocity spectrum. Two types of spectral analysis of practical use in Doppler signal analysis are types of discrete Fourier transform—

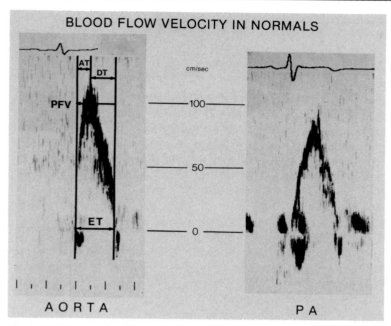

Figure 15-5. Doppler flow velocity tracings from a normal subject recorded in the ascending aorta (left) and the main pulmonary artery (PA, right). The aortic flow tracing is labeled to show how the peak flow velocity (PFV), ejection time (ET), acceleration time (AT), and deceleration time (DT) are measured. Average acceleration and average deceleration can be derived by dividing the peak flow velocity by the acceleration time and deceleration time, respectively. Note that the peak flow velocity is higher, the ejection time is shorter, and the average acceleration is greater in the normal aorta than in the normal pulmonary artery.

namely, the fast Fourier transform (FFT) and the Chirp-Z transform.[15a] The prototype of one ultrasound instrument utilizing a dedicated microprocessor and FFT analysis was designed by Griffith and Henry. This real-time system combines a two-dimensional mechanical sector scanner for imaging with a pulsed Doppler flow velocity meter.[14] A number of commercially available ultrasound systems feature a dual-channel real-time spectrum analyzer which permits the display of pulsed Doppler frequency shift signals at frequent (e. g., 2-millisecond) intervals on a strip chart recorder. In this spectrum analyzer the frequency shifts are intensity-modulated so that the Doppler frequency shift of large amplitudes (reflecting the flow velocity of the greatest number of blood cells during a given sampling interval) is displayed as the darkest spot on the video display monitor or strip chart recorder. Doppler frequency shifts of lower amplitudes—i.e., corresponding to the flow velocity of fewer blood cells—are displayed as less intense signals (spots) on either side of the darkest spot (see Figures 15-3A and 15-5). The ability of the spectrum analyzer to display simultaneously frequency shifts of flow toward and away from the ultrasound transducer (on two separate channels) as well as both high- and low-frequency shift signals overcomes some of the limitations of the zero-crossing detection system.

Other types of commercially available display options include (1) display of maximal and mean spectral frequency shifts or flow velocities, and (2) simultaneous display of frequency shift–flow velocity information from multiple sample volumes ("multi-gate" sampling).

DOPPLER FLOW VELOCITY IN THE GREAT VESSELS

Principles and Measurements

The flow velocity profiles in the thoracic aorta and the main pulmonary artery are similarly "flat" or "blunt" across the entire vessel until just at its periphery.[18,19] A flat velocity profile implies that flow velocity data obtained from any Doppler sample volume taken from any locus in the cross-section of the vessel can be extrapolated to the entire cross-section of the vessel. However, a flat velocity profile is not present in smaller arteries. In the coronary arteries, for example, the flow tends to be more parabolic, with higher flow velocities occurring at the center of the vessel.[13]

Another important characteristic of the normal great vessels is that flow during systole is generally laminar—i.e., there is a fairly narrow spectrum of frequency shifts. A relatively narrow Doppler spectrum exists during the majority of the acceleration phase; however, during peak flow and deceleration there is increased spectral broadening.[20] This degree of turbulence is, however, relatively minor when compared with turbulence recorded distally or proximally to stenotic or regurgitant lesions (see Figures 15-3B, 15-8, and 15-9).

Doppler signals from the heart or great vessels (Figure 15-5) may be displayed as flow velocity in cm/second (vertical axis) versus time in seconds (horizontal axis). In addition, the depth and the axial extent of the sample volume (adjustable in some units) can be easily displayed. It is possible for an ultrasound instrument (with the aid of a microprocessor) to solve the Doppler equation (equation 1) for velocity if the angle between the incident ultrasound beam and the long axis of blood flow is known or is assumed to be zero.

Measurement Parameters

One convention utilized to measure various systolic blood flow velocities in both the ascending aorta and the main pulmonary artery is shown in Figure 15-5. Peak flow velocity (cm/second) is determined by inspection of the midpoint of the Doppler flow spectrum at the time of maximum blood flow velocity. Acceleration time is calculated as the time in milliseconds from the onset of ejection to peak flow velocity. Similarly, deceleration time is measured in milliseconds as the time from peak flow velocity to the end of deceleration. The average acceleration can be calculated in cm/second/second by dividing peak flow velocity by the acceleration time. Average deceleration is calculated in cm/second/second by dividing peak flow velocity by the deceleration time. Ejection time is measured in milliseconds from the onset to the end of systolic ejection. The area under the systolic flow velocity curve, or the flow velocity integral, is expressed in centimeters and can be determined by planimetry.[16,21–23]

Pulmonary Artery Blood Flow

For recording pulmonary artery blood flow, a two-dimensional sector scanner can be utilized to image the main pulmonary artery in the parasternal short-axis view (Figure 15-6A). The sample volume controls are adjusted to place the pulsed Doppler sample volume in the proximal main pulmonary artery with the ultrasound beam parallel to the long axis of pulmonary blood flow. Minor angulations of the ultrasound transducer can then be made in order to maximize the frequency of the audible

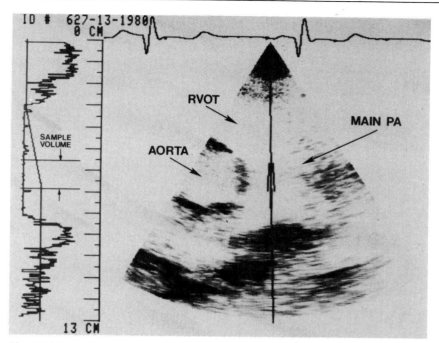

Figure 15-6A. Parasternal short-axis view at the level of the great arteries to show proper positioning of the sample volume relatively parallel to the long axis of blood flow in the main pulmonary artery. RVOT denotes right ventricular outflow tract.

Doppler signal and the peak flow velocity of the recorded Doppler signal. If the cosine of the angle between the ultrasound beam and the long axis of blood flow is 20° or less, the difference between the recorded Doppler flow velocity and the true peak flow velocity is less than 6 percent.[14,24]

Ascending Aortic Flow Velocity

One method of recording ascending aortic blood flow velocity is to utilize a relatively small two-dimensional transducer from the suprasternal notch. A right-angle M-mode transducer has also been utilized to record pulsed Doppler peak ascending aortic flow velocity by "mapping."[16,22] This technique involves adjusting the pulsed Doppler instrument controls so that the sample volume is moved in 1-cm increments from approximately a 3-cm to a 9-cm depth from the transducer. At each depth minor angulations of the transducer are performed until the maximum flow velocity at that depth is obtained (Figure 15-6B). The flow signal with the greatest maximum flow velocity is the one used for analysis. This technique assumes that the greatest blood flow velocity is recorded when the sample volume is approximately parallel to the long axis of blood flow in the ascending aorta. As noted previously, however, if the sample volume and blood flow are parallel or within 20° of each other, the error in recording peak flow velocity would be no greater than 6 percent—acceptable for most analyses.[14,24] In a study measuring suprasternal ascending aortic flow velocity in normal subjects, we noted a less than 5 percent mean difference between Doppler measurements of peak flow velocity, ejection time, and flow velocity integral made by two technicians.[16] Furthermore, we have recently shown that the mean interobserver and day-to-day variability in measure-

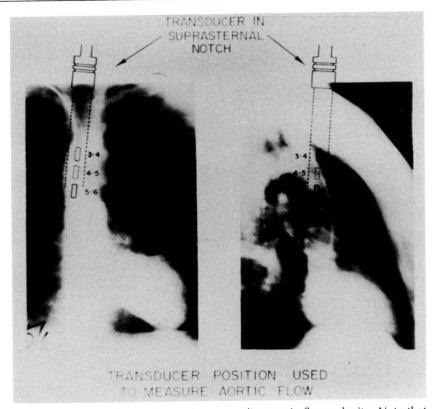

Figure 15-6B. "Mapping" technique for recording ascending aortic flow velocity. Note that in the absence of aortic imaging the sample volume is moved in 1-cm increments and the maximum flow velocity recorded in each sample volume. The peak flow velocity is the highest flow velocity recorded from any sample volume using this technique.

ments for aortic peak flow velocity and ejection time are both 5 percent or less.[22a] Other workers have utilized both continuous wave and pulsed Doppler techniques to record flow velocity patterns in the ascending or transverse aorta.[4-6]

Normal Flow Velocity

A comparison between the ascending aorta and main pulmonary artery (PA) flow velocity recordings in 20 normal subjects revealed significant differences ($p < 0.001$) in the following parameters: peak flow velocity (aorta = 92 cm/second mean, PA = 63 cm/second); acceleration time (aorta = 98 milliseconds, PA = 159 milliseconds), average acceleration (aorta = 940 cm/second/second, PA = 396 cm/second/second; deceleration time (aorta = 197 milliseconds, PA = 172 milliseconds); average deceleration (aorta = 473 cm/second/second, PA = 356 cm/second/second); and ejection time (aorta = 294 milliseconds, PA = 331 milliseconds).[16,22] Despite a four to five times higher arterial resistance in the systemic artery compared to the pulmonary artery, acceleration of blood is two to three times more rapid in the ascending aorta than in the main pulmonary artery. When compared to the pulmonary artery, the aorta exhibits a higher peak flow velocity, which is achieved earlier in systole and with a shorter ejection time (Figure 15-5).

QUANTITATIVE EVALUATION OF
VENTRICULAR FUNCTION

Absolute Stroke Volume and Cardiac Output

Various investigators have evaluated left ventricular stroke volume and cardiac output utilizing Doppler echocardiography.[24–29b] Stroke volume by this technique is estimated from the average velocity of blood flow in the aorta or pulmonary artery and the cross-sectional area of the orifice through which the blood is flowing. In order to calculate average long-axis blood flow velocity two parameters must be known: the area under the flow velocity curve (flow velocity integral), and the angle of incidence between the ultrasound beam and the long axis of flow (velocity vector). Placing the sample volume as parallel as possible to the long axis of flow obviates the necessity for correction for the cosine of the angle θ in the Doppler equation (equation 1).

Various workers have shown that Doppler echocardiography can be utilized to document beat-to-beat variations in stroke volume in dogs.[24,25] In one study utilizing a continuous wave Doppler system for recording flow velocity, 20 closed-and open-chest dogs were studied under the following conditions: (1) resting state, (2) after hemorrhage and reinfusion, (3) after administration of propranolol, and (4) after infusion of dopamine. These investigators reported a close similarity between Doppler and electromagnetic flow wave forms, and a close correlation between Doppler and thermodilution values for cardiac output—except at rates exceeding 160 beats/minute.[25]

A group of patients with acute myocardial infarction and another group undergoing routine cardiac catheterization had Doppler outputs obtained by multiplying the 1-minute sum of the systolic integral of aortic blood flow velocity by the average systolic diameter of the aortic root measured from the M-mode echocardiogram. This study showed excellent correlations ($r = 0.96$ to 0.99) between cardiac outputs obtained with the thermodilution or Fick techniques and Doppler ultrasound cardiac output. At heart rates exceeding 150 beats/minute, however, the correlation between the Doppler and invasive techniques was poor.[26] More recently, other workers have also demonstrated good correlations between cardiac outputs determined by continuous wave Doppler and invasive methods.[26a,26b]

Other workers have evaluated a combined Doppler and phased-array two-dimensional echocardiographic system in estimating cardiac output. Two-dimensional echocardiography was used to determine aortic vessel diameter and a superimposed cursor used to locate the range and angle of the Doppler sample.[27] In 11 patients in whom Fick cardiac outputs were compared with Doppler–phased-array outputs, a correlation of $r = 0.83$ was obtained. Doppler consistently underestimated cardiac this study were that the Fick and Doppler estimates of cardiac output were not obtained simultaneously and the Doppler cardiac output determinations varied considerably when different transducer locations were used in the same patient. The variation between Doppler and Fick cardiac output estimates was largest when the angle between the ultrasound beam and the long axis of blood flow was greater than 65°.

Studies in children have also used the Doppler technique to measure stroke volume. In one report, range-gated pulsed Doppler measurements of flow velocity could be obtained in 15 of 19 children utilizing a combined two-dimensional echocardiographic-Doppler system.[28] For this preliminary study, however, vessel diameter was determined by angiography. Two-dimensional echocardiography was utilized to estimate the angle between the Doppler sample volume and the major axis of blood flow. Eighteen determinations (8 pulmonary and 10 aortic) of cardiac output were made and compared to simultaneous indicator-dilution or angiographic cardiac outputs. An excellent correlation was obtained (r = 0.95), with the slope of the regression line approaching identity.

It should be noted that recording Doppler data from the great arteries adequate for stroke volume determination is not possible in many patients: 34 percent had inadequate data in one study.[28a] The major limitation to the use of Doppler data from the great arteries is the presence of excessive spectral dispersion—e.g., from turbulent aortic flow in patients with aortic valve disease.

Another interesting approach to the estimation of cardiac output is the mitral valve orifice method, which should be particularly useful when there is difficulty obtaining adequate Doppler flow velocity patterns or echocardiographic imaging in the ascending aorta or main pulmonary artery.[29] In an open-chest dog model, mitral valve flows were recorded from an apical four-chamber view with the pulsed Doppler sample volume positioned in the left ventricular inflow area. This approach permitted flow sampling from an incident angle nearly parallel to the flow stream. Maximal mitral orifice area was planimetered in the parasternal short-axis view. However, since mitral orifice size varies during the different diastolic phases, a correction for mean area was calculated by planimetering the mean separation of the valve leaflets from a derived M-mode recording. Comparison of systemic flows determined by this method with simultaneous pump-regulated outputs in the dog model and with thermodilution cardiac outputs obtained in adult patients has yielded an excellent correlation (r = 0.94).[29]

Changes in Stroke Volume and Flow Velocity

Buchtal et al, in a pilot study, demonstrated the clinical utility of Doppler in the assessment of the cardiovascular response to drugs and fluid therapy in critically ill patients.[21] We have similarly evaluated the ability of Doppler to predict the response of patients undergoing vasodilator therapy and intra-aortic balloon counterpulsation. In a series of 13 patients undergoing 18 therapeutic interventions, Doppler aortic flow velocity measurements were compared with simultaneous thermodilution stroke volumes.[23] The correlations between thermodilution stroke volume and Doppler peak aortic flow velocity, ejection time, and flow velocity integral were found to be poor (r < 0.4 in all cases). However, there were better correlations between percentage change in thermodilution stroke volume and percentage change in aortic flow velocity integral (r = 0.88). Furthermore, changes in peak aortic flow velocity following vasodilator therapy correlated well (r = 0.89) with invasively measured changes in systemic vascular resistance. Thus, Doppler echocardiography may be useful in noninvasively evaluating the acute response to afterload reduction.

Exercise Studies

The ability of Doppler echocardiography to estimate changes in stroke volume should, theoretically, add additional hemodynamic data to that which is commonly collected during stress testing (i.e., heart rate, blood pressure, duration of exercise, and electrocardiographic response). In a preliminary study Doppler aortic blood flow velocity was used to noninvasively assess hemodynamic changes during supine bicycle exercise in 10 normal subjects.[30] Doppler peak aortic blood flow velocity, ejection time, and flow velocity integral were measured before, during, and after exercise. At peak exercise an increase in peak flow velocity and marked decreases in ejection time and flow velocity integral were observed. Despite problems relating to aliasing (exceeding the range–velocity product) encountered at peak exercise, it is likely that pulsed and/or continuous wave Doppler exercise studies will be clinically applicable in evaluating patients with known or suspected cardiovascular disease.

EVALUATION OF PRESYSTOLIC FLOW AND SYSTOLIC PRESSURE IN THE PULMONARY ARTERY

Two-dimensional echocardiography combined with Doppler flow velocity measurements has been utilized to demonstrate that the "a" wave present on the pulmonic valve echogram in normal subjects occurs simultaneously with a presystolic flow deflection in the pulmonary artery (see Figure 15-5). Similarly, the absence of the a wave on the pulmonic valve echocardiogram in patients with atrial fibrillation appears to correlate with the absence of Doppler presystolic flow deflections in the pulmonary artery.[31] Measurements made from M-mode and two-dimensional echocardiograms and Doppler flow velocity recordings—both at the level of the main pulmonary artery and at its bifurcation—indicate that the Doppler presystolic deflection recorded in the main pulmonary artery represents an actual displacement of blood (i.e., flow within the pulmonary artery) that occurs simultaneously with the a wave of the pulmonic valve echogram.[31]

Recently, we have evaluated Doppler flow velocity patterns in a group of 10 patients with pulmonary hypertension. All exhibited a rapid initial ejection of blood in early systole (increased average acceleration), a rapid decrease of flow in midsystole, and a secondary, lower flow in late systole—i.e., a "spike and dome" contour.[32] Further studies are necessary to determine whether Doppler flow patterns have prognostic significance in pulmonary hypertension.

Tucker and coworkers[33] have utilized saccharide-encapsulated, pressurized carbon dioxide microbubbles in conjunction with an external ultrasonic transducer to estimate right ventricular pressures in open-chest dogs. This non-Doppler technique involves intravenous injection of 100-μ bubbles and ultrasonic detection of the transient compression oscillations produced when the saccharide is dissolved and the microbubble released during intracardiac flow. The oscillation frequency, known as the bubble ultrasonic ringing pressure (BURP), is proportional to the surrounding pressure. In 12 right ventricular pressure determinations, ultrasonic and catheter pressures correlated well (r = 0.84). This preliminary investigation raises the possibility of estimating pressure in the pulmonary artery noninvasively utilizing Doppler echocardiography. Presumably, the frequency shifts of the ultrasound backscattered from microbubbles released from their capsule in the pulmonary artery should be related to pulmonary artery pressure. Pulmonary pressure could thus theoretically be estimated if the resonant frequency characteristics of the particular size and type of microbubble and the frequency of the emitted ultrasound are known. Encapsulated microbubbles, however, are not generally available at present, even for experimental use.

Multi-Gate Doppler Technique

Investigators at the University of Washington have reported the development of a prototype multi-gate, digital Doppler instrument that permits simultaneous examination of flow signals at up to 120 sites.[34] The system utilizes a single crystal high-frequency transducer that detects echo and Doppler shift signals simultaneously at multiple sites. A time–motion tracing including simultaneous echocardiographic and Doppler information can be recorded on an oscilloscopic screen; the anatomic image is depicted in gray scale, while flow features are superimposed and displayed in color. The initial experience indicates the utility of this approach in detecting different valvular lesions and intracardiac shunts in children. More recently, Bommer and associates[35] have described preliminary work with a prototype instrument capable of producing real-time two-dimensional images along with superimposed color-coded Doppler flow velocity information. With further development, such a multi-gate technique should be capable of providing detailed intracardiac flow information superimposed on real-time two-dimensional images of the heart.

DOPPLER STUDIES IN CARDIAC DISEASE STATES

Dilated (Congestive) Cardiomyopathy

In a group of 12 patients with dilated cardiomyopathy, peak aortic flow velocity reportedly ranged from 35 to 62 cm/second (mean 47 cm/second)—significantly different ($p < 0.001$) from the peak flow velocities (range 72 to 120 cm/second; mean 92 cm/second) reported in 20 normal subjects.[16,22] There was no overlap in data between the two groups. Similarly, aortic flow velocity integral was able to distinguish patients with dilated cardiomyopathy (mean 6.7 cm, range 3.5 to 9.1 cm) from normal subjects (mean 15.7 cm, range 10.7 to 22.5 cm) ($p < 0.001$). Aortic peak flow velocity correlated relatively well ($r = 0.83$) with M-mode echocardiographic measurements of left ventricular percentage fractional shortening. Both measurements appeared to be equally useful in discriminating patients with normal left ventricular function from those with global dysfunction (dilated cardiomyopathy).

Hypertrophic Cardiomyopathy

Doppler echocardiographic studies have been performed in patients with hypertrophic cardiomyopathy with and without left ventricular outflow obstruction.[36–40] We evaluated patients with M-mode echocardiographic evidence of asymmetric septal hypertrophy and marked systolic anterior motion (SAM) of the mitral valve. Utilizing a suprasternal notch transducer for recording ascending aortic flow velocity and a two-dimensional transducer from an apical two-chamber view to record left atrial flow velocity, we found that aortic flow velocity decreased sharply at the onset of mitral valve–septal contact but did not cease entirely. Furthermore, regurgitant flow into the left atrium peaked after mitral valve–septal contact. It appears that the left ventricle continues to shorten after mitral valve–septal contact (SAM) by ejecting blood into the left atrium, in addition to the markedly diminished ejection into the aortic root.[37]

In another study, comparison of Doppler ascending aortic flow velocities in patients with nonobstructive and obstructive hypertrophic cardiomyopathy revealed that the patterns differed in the two groups.[39] The mean ejection time was greater in the obstructive hypertrophic cardiomyopathy patients (348 milliseconds) than in both the nonobstructive hypertrophic cardiomyopathy patients (288 milliseconds, p < 0.05) and 20 normal subjects (294 milliseconds, p < 0.01). Aortic flow velocity showed a rapid decrease in midsystole—i.e., a "spike and plateau" contour—in all obstructive cardiomyopathy patients but in none of the nonobstructive patients or normal subjects. These studies support the concept that left ventricular ejection is impeded in patients with obstructive hypertrophic cardiomyopathy[37] and are in agreement with previous case report observations by Boughner and associates.[40]

Coronary Artery Disease

Some progress has been made in identifying patent aortocoronary bypass vein grafts noninvasively as well as in studying native coronary artery flow directly at the time of coronary artery surgery.[41-45] In addition, Doppler flow studies have been used in evaluating global left ventricular function in patients with apical left ventricular aneurysms.[46]

Gould and associates[41] used a pulsed Doppler technique from the suprasternal and parasternal positions to determine noninvasively the patency of saphenous vein coronary bypass grafts. A visible dot was stored on an oscilloscopic screen at a point corresponding to the location of any flow detected in the anterior mediastinum. A composite picture of a proximal segment of the saphenous vein bypass graft was developed by repeated sampling at various depths. Flow velocity signals from coronary arteries distal to patent saphenous vein grafts were recorded during diastole; these flow signals could therefore be distinguished from other arterial systolic flow signals. In a preliminary evaluation of the technique, distinct arterial flow signals during diastole were recorded from 24, or 59 percent of the 41 grafts proven to be patent by angiography. An additional 10 grafts, or 24 percent, were judged probably patent from audible diastolic arterial flow signals that could not be recorded due to a low signal-to-noise ratio. Although this approach is interesting, it lacks sufficient accuracy for generalized clinical application to the detection of graft patency. Problems with this Doppler technique included the fact that the position of the patient and the orientation of the transducer were critical in locating the grafts, as no images were available.

In another study, Diebold et al[42] evaluated bypass graft patency in 120 consecutive patients at the time of postoperative coronary angiography. Without imaging the grafts, a range-gated pulsed Doppler technique was used to record diastolic flow velocity in the grafts. After the aorta was located by M-mode echocardiography the transducer was moved anteriorly and to the left to locate the right ventricular outflow tract. Identifying graft flow in front, or to the left of, the right ventricular outflow tract was accomplished by moving the Doppler sample volume anteriorly, by changing the sample volume depth, or by tilting the transducer laterally. When both the left anterior descending and circumflex arteries were grafted, the left anterior descending graft was usually anterior and to the right of the circumflex graft. Bypass graft flow to the right coronary artery was recorded to the right of the aorta with the patient lying in the right lateral position (Figure 15-7). In this study 127 patent and 14 occluded grafts were correctly identified when compared with coronary angiog-

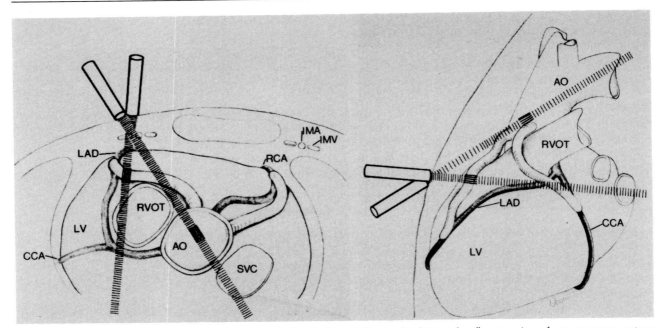

Figure 15-7. One method of recording pulsed Doppler flow tracings from coronary artery bypass grafts described by Diebold and coworkers (see text for details). Ao denotes aorta; CCA, circumflex coronary artery; IMA, internal mammary artery; IMV, internal mammary vein; LAD, left anterior descending coronary artery; RCA, right coronary artery; SVC, superior vena cava. (From Diebold B, Theroux T, Bourassa MG, et al: Noninvasive assessment of aortocoronary bypass graft patency using pulsed-Doppler echocardiography. Am J Cardiol 43:10, 1979. With permission.)

raphy. Eleven patent grafts could not be recorded and 11 occluded grafts were falsely diagnosed as patent. The method had an overall sensitivity of 92 percent but a specificity of only 56 percent. The high sensitivity level could be increased to almost 100 percent by improvement in technical skills. The low specificity level, however, was a persistent problem and emphasized the importance of correctly identifying other sources of diastolic blood flow—i.e., the superior vena cava, internal mammary veins, tricuspid valve, mitral valve, and right ventricle—by careful adjustment of the depth, site, and size of the pulsed Doppler sample volume. In contrast to these findings, Fabian and coworkers[43] found in a comparison of Doppler ultrasound to coronary angiography in a study of aortocoronary bypass grafts that the Doppler technique had greater specificity (90 percent) than sensitivity (77 percent) in detecting graft patency.

The utility of a 20-MHz crystal mounted on a silicone cup has been examined in recording Doppler flow in the native coronary arteries at the time of surgery. Coronary reactive hyperemia measured after periods of occlusion was found to be helpful in assessing the physiologic significance of coronary obstruction. Measurements of reactive hyperemia significantly altered the operative plan for coronary bypass surgery in approximately 20 percent of patients studied.[45]

To date, it has not been possible to reliably record flow in the coronary arteries in the clinical laboratory using the Doppler technique. Two problems that remain to be solved before this Doppler application becomes a reality are the need for improving two-dimensional imaging of coronary arteries so that greater lengths can be imaged with better resolution and the need for developing a tracking device that will permit the Doppler sample volume to remain within the moving coronary artery once it is properly positioned.

Doppler aortic flow velocity measurements can be used to estimate stroke volume as well as other parameters of left ventricular systolic function—such as aortic peak flow velocity, flow velocity integral, and ejection time (see preceding discussion). In addition, Doppler aortic flow velocity measurements are useful in detecting depressed global left ventricular function in patients who have apical aneurysms with normal basal left ventricular fractional shortening.[46] The application of Doppler echocardiography to the detection of ventricular septal defects and mitral regurgitation, which may be seen after infarction, is discussed in following sections.

DETECTION AND VALVULAR AND SHUNT LESIONS

A number of investigators have demonstrated that pulsed Doppler echocardiography may be useful in detecting and estimating the severity of valvular stenosis and regurgitation. This technique has also been shown to be of benefit in localizing various shunt lesions and the origin of murmurs.

Valvular Regurgitation

Detection of valvular regurgitation by Doppler echocardiography is based on alterations in flow pattern (turbulent as opposed to laminar flow), timing (systolic versus diastolic), and location and direction of regurgitant flow. Figure 15-8 depicts Doppler flow velocity tracings recorded in patients with aortic regurgitation in the ascending aorta from the suprasternal notch (Figure 15-8A) and in the left ventricular outflow tract from the apical two-chamber approach (Figure 15-8B). Note that in diastole there is spectral broadening of the flow pattern consistent with the presence of turbulent flow. The diastolic flow is also negative when compared to the zero-flow line—i.e., directed away from the aortic root toward the left ventricle. In addition, there is spectral broadening of the systolic pattern consistent with turbulent flow, which may be present even in the absence of aortic stenosis. These characteristics are typical of aortic regurgitation. Figure 15-8A also demonstrates how aliasing can be a problem with the pulsed Doppler technique. Typically in aortic insufficiency, systolic peak flow velocity is high and the range–velocity product is exceeded, resulting in a "fold-over" of the top portion of the spectral pattern. In this figure the fold-over is displayed at the bottom of the velocity scale during systole.

Figure 15-9A is a pulsed Doppler flow recording at the level of the mitral valve in a patient with combined mitral stenosis and regurgitation. The recording was made with the Doppler sample volume just inside the left atrium in the apical four-chamber view. In this case the presence of a stenotic lesion is reflected by a reduced diastolic flow rate across the mitral valve (the equivalent of the reduced E-F slope on the M-mode echocardiogram), as well as diastolic spectral broadening, indicating disturbed diastolic flow. The presence of mitral regurgitation is indicated by systolic flow in a direction opposite to diastolic flow—i.e., from left ventricle to left atrium— and by spectral broadening (Figure 15-9B).

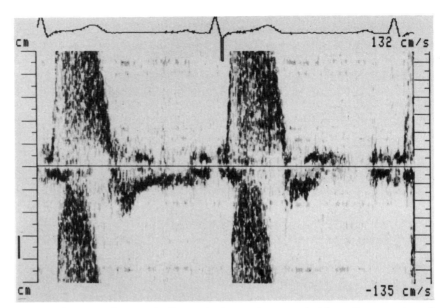

Figure 15-8A. Doppler ascending aortic flow velocity tracing recorded from the suprasternal notch in a patient with aortic insufficiency. Note the relatively high peak flow velocity and turbulent flow above the baseline (toward the transducer) in systole and the turbulent flow away from the transducer during diastole. Note also that there is systolic flow displayed below the baseline at the bottom of the scale which appears as if it has been "decapitated" from the top of the systolic flow curve. This flow pattern results from aliasing, i.e., exceeding the range–velocity product for this pulsed Doppler recording (see text for details).

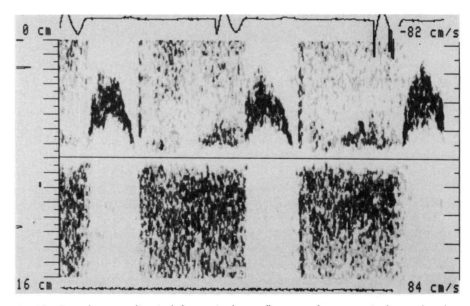

Figure 15-8B. Doppler recording in left ventricular outflow tract from an apical two-chamber view in a patient with aortic insufficiency. Note the marked diastolic turbulent (regurgitant) flow below the baseline—i.e., into the left ventricular outflow tract.

344

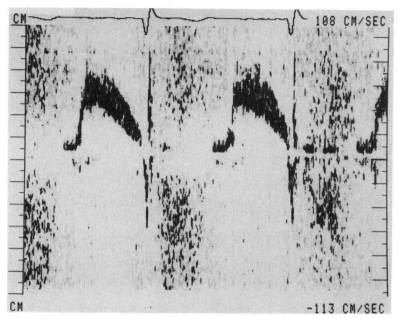

Figure 15-9A. Pulsed Doppler flow velocity recording in the left atrium near the mitral valve level in a patient with combined mitral stenosis and regurgitation. Note the reduced diastolic flow rate and diastolic spectral broadening, as well as turbulent systolic flow in the opposite direction (toward the left atrium).

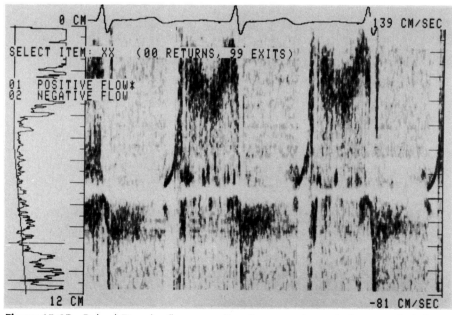

Figure 15-9B. Pulsed Doppler flow recording demonstrating turbulent systolic left atrial flow in a patient with mild mitral regurgitation. Although there is also some turbulence in diastole, there is no reduction in diastolic flow rate or in the a wave as was recorded in the patient in Figure 15-9A.

Aortic Regurgitation

The sensitivity of the Doppler technique in detecting aortic regurgitation, even in the presence of aortic stenosis, has been reported to be in the range of 85 to 96 percent; the specificity has been reported to be in the range of 82 to 90 percent.[47–50] Ciobanu and associates have utilized a parasternal approach to detect the presence of diastolic turbulent flow in the left ventricular outflow tract or apical portions of the left ventricle. They noted that it is sometimes difficult when using this approach to differentiate the presence of aortic insufficiency from mitral stenosis.[49] Other associated lesions, such as mitral regurgitation and aortic stenosis, should not interfere with the detection of aortic insufficiency.[50]

Three basic methods have been proposed to estimate the severity of aortic regurgitation. The first method, proposed by Veyrat and associates, involves recording flow velocity by pulsed Doppler from multiple sample volumes in the ascending, transverse, and descending aorta.[47] The more distal from the aortic valve that turbulent retrograde diastolic flow could be recorded, the more severe the regurgitation. These investigators also noted an early onset of systolic flow in the ascending aorta when the left ventricular end-diastolic and aortic pressures were almost equal.

A second approach, proposed by Ciobanu and associates, utilizes M-mode echocardiography to locate multiple Doppler sample volumes from a region just below the aortic valve leaflets to the apex of the left ventricle. These workers demonstrated a correlation of r = 0.88 between angiographic estimates of severity of aortic regurgitation and the distance below the aortic valve (within the left ventricle) that Doppler diastolic turbulence could be recorded. Utilizing two-dimensional echocardiography, Bommer and associates applied a similar approach to mapping Doppler flow in the left ventricle.[51]

A third approach in estimating the severity of aortic regurgitation has used planimetry of the area under the systolic and diastolic flow tracings recorded from the ascending aorta[47] or proximal descending aorta.[52] The ratio of diastolic flow (regurgitant flow) to systolic flow (forward flow) has shown good correlation with angiographic estimates of severity of regurgitation.

Mitral Regurgitation

In the detection of mitral regurgitation the Doppler technique has shown a specificity in the range of 89 to 96 percent.[47,53–55] As in aortic regurgitation, three approaches have been useful in estimating the severity of mitral regurgitation. Kalmanson, Abassi and associates have utilized methods similar to those they proposed for assessing aortic regurgitation in detecting the distribution of abnormal systolic spectral dispersion (turbulence) within the left atrium (Figure 15-10).[53,55] Minimal mitral regurgitation was diagnosed if abnormal systolic flow was localized immediately posterior to the mitral valve, whereas severe mitral regurgitation was diagnosed when systolic flow was present diffusely within the entire left atrium. Utilizing both M-mode and two-dimensional echocardiography to locate the pulsed Doppler sample volumes, these Doppler studies correlated well with angiographic estimates of the severity of mitral regurgitation.

A second approach to estimating the severity of mitral regurgitation involves analyzing flow velocity obtained from the ascending aorta or aortic arch.[56] Nichol and associates noted that the aortic blood flow velocity recording in normals was parabolic during systole, with about equal areas under the first and second half of the curve. With increasingly severe mitral regurgitation, the systolic curve skewed left-

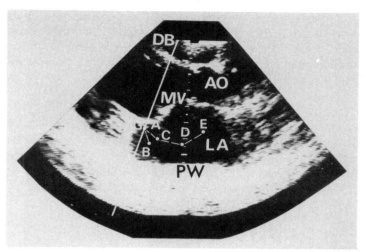

Figure 15-10. Method for "geographic mapping" of Doppler flow in the left atrium to estimate the severity of mitral regurgitation. In general, the more severe the regurgitation, the more widespread the area of turbulent flow. A, B, C, D, and E denote various mapping sites in the left atrium. (From Kalmanson D, Veyrat C, Abitbol G, et al: Doppler echocardiography in valvular regurgitation, with special emphasis on mitral insufficiency: Advantages of two-dimensional echocardiography with spectral analysis, in Rijsterborgh H (ed): Echocardiology. The Hague, Martinus Nijhoff, 1981, pp 279–290. With permission.)

ward so that the percentage of the area in the first half of the curve ranged from 53 to 79 percent.

In a third approach investigators utilized continuous wave Doppler (pulsed Doppler could also be used) to record the ascending aortic flow velocity curve from which cardiac output (forward flow) was estimated. Doppler-estimated forward flow was subtracted from total cardiac output, which was estimated from M-mode echoocardiography. This difference estimated mitral regurgitant flow well in comparison to angiography.[57]

Tricuspid and Pulmonic Regurgitation

When compared with angiography, Doppler recordings in the right atrium have been found to be 83 to 94 percent sensitive and 86 percent specific in detecting tricuspid regurgitation.[55,58,59] The Doppler technique was also found to be very sensitive in the detection of pulmonic valve regurgitation.[55,58] However, the absence of diagnostic physical findings in many of the patients with tricuspid or pulmonic valvular regurgitation detected by Doppler indicates that the hemodynamic severity of the Doppler-detected regurgitation in these patients was probably insignificant. One interesting approach for semi-quantitating the degree of tricuspid insufficiency employs continuous wave Doppler estimates of the maximum velocity in the regurgitant jet to measure the right ventricular–right atrial pressure difference during systole.[60] This technique is based on the same principle used to estimate transvalvular gradients in stenotic lesions (see following discussion). Another interesting method for semi-quantitation of tricuspid regurgitation employs two-dimensional echocardiography from a subcostal approach to position a pulsed Doppler sample volume in a hepatic vein. Degree of tricuspid regurgitation was estimated by dividing the area under the systolic regurgitant (backwash) flow by the area representing net forward flow.[60a] This technique has some theoretical advantage over recording Doppler flow in the inferior vena cava since it is easier to position a sample volume parallel to flow in a hepatic vein. At least one group has suggested that recording tricuspid or pulmonic regurgitation by the Doppler method is superior to M-mode echocardiography in detecting pulmonary hypertension.[58]

Limitations

Estimation of the severity of valvular regurgitation by geographic mapping of Doppler turbulence has a number of limitations. First, the regurgitant jet may be small or eccentric and not detected by the flow sampling method. Second, a reduced flow rate, as in congestive heart failure, may result in an erroneous underestimation of the severity of valvular insufficiency. Finally, in mitral regurgitation, marked left atrial enlargement may lead to underestimation of the severity of the condition.[50,55]

Valvular Stenosis

The appearance of flow velocity patterns in the presence of valvular stenosis is dependent upon a number of factors, which include (1) the angle of incidence of the ultrasound beam relative to the angle of blood flow in the stenotic jet and surrounding turbulent areas; (2) the area in which flow velocity is recorded—i.e., within the stenotic jet, distal to the jet, or around the jet[47,61–65]; and (3) the presence of a "watershed" effect resulting in different flow velocity patterns recorded distal to the stenotic lesion.[64]

Pulsed Doppler

Criteria described for estimating the severity of mitral stenosis by the pulsed Doppler technique have included an indentation of the diastolic flow curve, a decreased rate of rise of diastolic flow velocity, and a large "a" (atrial) wave.[65] Other investigators have noted a loss of the a wave in the mitral diastolic flow pattern in severe stenosis.[66] In aortic stenosis increased severity has been associated with delay in systolic wave appearance in the arch of the aorta, spectral broadening, and early indentations on the ascending limb of the analog flow velocity curve. In addition, severe prolongation of the ejection time has been noted in some cases.[46] Utilizing the pulsed Doppler technique to estimate the severity of aortic stenosis, Young and associates[63] recorded flow velocity in the ascending aorta from either the left sternal border, the cardiac apex, or the suprasternal notch. They analyzed the amplitude and duration of turbulence on the time interval histogram with a grading score based on five parameters. This score yielded an excellent separation ($p < 0.001$) of patients with aortic valve areas greater and less than 1.0 cm^2.

Continuous Wave Doppler

An even more promising quantitative approach to evaluating the degree of valvular stenosis involves continuous wave Doppler recording of the maximum flow velocity in the stenotic jet.[61,62] With the Bernoulli equation as a theoretical basis, the pressure gradient in mm Hg across the stenotic valve in aortic and mitral stenosis can be determined from the following formula:

$$P_1 - P_2 = 4 \times V_2^2$$

where V_2 equals maximal velocity measured in the stenotic jet (m/second). Since

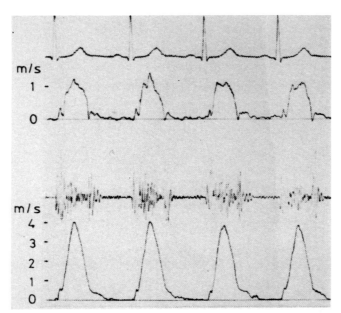

Figure 15-11A. Continuous wave Doppler recordings from the ascending aorta in a patient with aortic stenosis. Note the significant difference between the peak or jet flow velocity (bottom panel) and the mean flow velocity (top panel), this difference being a reflection of the greater-than-normal spectral dispersion. The patient had a peak aortic pressure gradient of 69 mm Hg calculated by the Doppler technique and of 68 mm Hg found at catheterization.

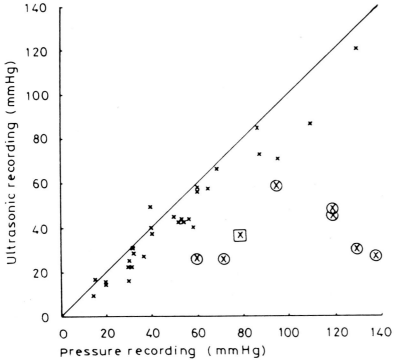

Figure 15-11B. Data comparing aortic valve gradient calculated by the continuous wave Doppler (vertical axis) and invasive pressure measurement techniques (horizontal axis). A circled x represents those cases in which auditory signals from the aorta were inadequate. The x in a square represents a patient in whom the aortic jet signal was easily recorded; nonetheless, significant underestimation of the pressure drop occurred in this patient. (From Hatle L, Angelsen BA, Tromsdal A: Noninvasive assessment of aortic stenosis by Doppler ultrasound. Br Heart J 43:284, 1980. With permission.)

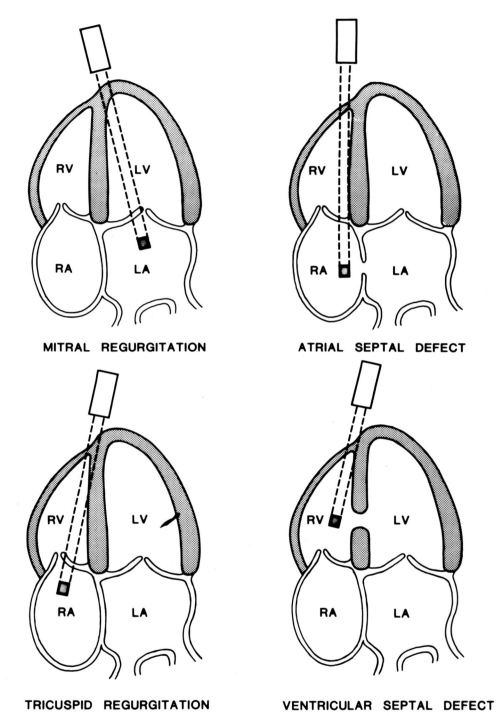

MITRAL REGURGITATION

ATRIAL SEPTAL DEFECT

TRICUSPID REGURGITATION

VENTRICULAR SEPTAL DEFECT

Figure 15-12. Diagrammatic representation of proper placement of pulsed Doppler sample volumes in the apical four-chamber view to detect mitral regurgitation, tricuspid regurgitation, atrial septal defect, and ventricular septal defect. This simplified diagram does not depict the geographic mapping that should be performed in each cardiac chamber and great vessel.

the continuous wave Doppler technique as described does not use imaging to aid in placing the sample volume, locating the maximum flow velocity within the stenotic jet requires experience. Hatle and associates[61] reported excellent sensitivity and specificity in 55 patients with mitral stenosis. They also reported a good correlation between transvalvular gradients estimated from Doppler and those found at cardiac catheterization. In aortic stenosis patients less than 50 years old, the aortic jet flow velocity could be recorded reproducibly (Figure 15-11). Although Doppler underestimated the aortic valve gradient calculated at cardiac catheterization, it was within 25 percent in 17 of 18 patients. In patients over age 50, however, there was considerably more difficulty in recording Doppler signals from the stenotic jet; the pressure gradient across the valve was significantly underestimated by the Doppler technique in one-third of patients.[62]

Shunt Lesions

The Doppler technique has been shown to be useful in differentiating ventricular septal defect from other lesions, such as mitral regurgitation[67,68] (Figure 15-12). "Mapping" the flow velocity along the right side of the interventricular septum may record turbulent systolic flow at, and somewhat distal to, the level of the ventricular septal defect. A pulsed Doppler sample volume in the right ventricle can generally differentiate the turbulent flow of ventricular septal defect from the turbulent systolic flow of mitral regurgitation recorded in the left atrium (Figure 15-13).

A number of Doppler techniques have been described for estimating the severity of the shunt in patients with an atrial septal defect. One method involves analyzing Doppler recordings of jugular flow velocity curves.[69] Another pulsed Doppler ap-

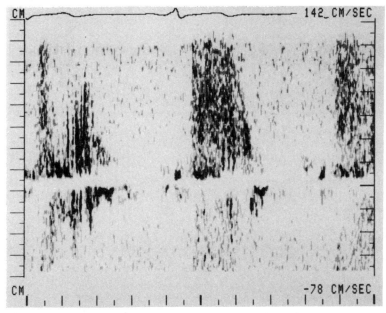

Figure 15-13A. Pulsed Doppler flow recording from the right ventricle demonstrating turbulent systolic flow near the area of a ventricular septal defect.

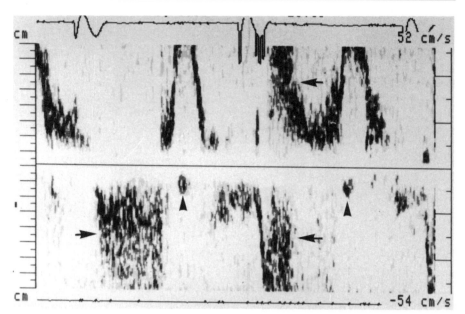

Figure 15-13B. Pulsed Doppler flow recording from the right atrium demonstrating turbulent systolic retrograde flow (arrows) in a patient with tricuspid regurgitation. In diastole there is mild aliasing, with the "decapitated" portion of the top of the flow curve being displayed just beneath the zero-flow line (arrowheads).

proach to detect left-to-right interatrial shunts involves recording diastolic dispersion in the right atrial outflow tract.[70] Quantitation of left-to-right shunts by comparing the areas under the flow velocity curves (flow velocity integrals) in the pulmonary artery[71–75] and the aorta appears to be feasible. The ratio of the pulmonary to aortic flow velocity should give an estimate of the ratio of pulmonary to aortic volume flow and, hence, of the degree of left-to-right shunt. Alternatively, a multi-gate flow profiling technique should one day be capable of providing quantitative information relative to intracardiac shunts.

REFERENCES

1. Baker DW, Daigle RE: Non-invasive ultrasonic flowmetry, in Hwang NHC, Normann NA (eds): Cardiovascular Flow Dynamics and Measurements. Baltimore, University Park Press, 1977, pp 151–190

2. Wells PNT: Ultrasonic Doppler equipment, in Fullerton GD, Zagzebski JA (eds): Medical Physics of CT and Ultrasound: Tissue Imaging and Characterization. New York, American Institute of Physics, 1980, pp 343–366.

3. Atkinson P: A fundamental interpretation of ultrasonic velocimeters. Ultrasound Med Biol 2:107–111, 1976

4. Light H, Cross G: Cardiovascular data by transcutaneous aorto velography, in Roberts C (ed): Blood Flow Measurement. London, Sector, 1972, pp 60–63

5. Light LH: Initial evaluation of transcutaneous aortovelography—A new non-invasive technique for haemodynamic measurements in the major thoracic vessels, in Reneman RS (ed): Cardiovascular Application of Ultrasound. Amsterdam and London, North Holland, 1974, pp 325–360

6. Angelsen BAJ, Brubakk AO: Transcutaneous measurement of blood flow velocity in the human aorta. Cardiovasc Res 10:368–379, 1976

7. Holen J, Aaslid R, Landmark K, et al: Determination of pressure gradient in mitral stenosis with a non-invasive ultrasound Doppler technique. Acta Med Scand 199:455–460, 1976

8. Wells PNT: A range-gated ultrasonic Doppler system. Med Biol Eng 7:641–652, 1969

9. Baker DW: Pulsed ultrasonic Doppler blood-flow sensing. IEEE Trans Sonics Ultrasonics SU-17(3):170–185, 1970

10. Baker DW, Rubenstein SA, Lorch GS: Pulsed Doppler echocardiography: Principles and applications. Am J Med 63:69–80, 1977

11. Baker DW: The present role of Doppler techniques in cardiac diagnosis. Prog Cardiovasc Dis 21(2):79–91, 1978

12. Johnson SL, Baker DW, Lute RA, et al: Doppler echocardiography: The localization of cardiac murmurs. Circulation 48:810–822, 1973

13. Reneman RS, Hoeks A, Ruissen C, et al: Pulsed Doppler systems in cardiovascular diseases, in Rijstersborgh H (ed): Echocardiology. The Hague, Martinus Nijhoff, 1981, pp 269–278

14. Griffith JM, Henry WL: An ultrasound system for combined cardiac imaging and Doppler blood flow measurement in man. Circulation 57:925–930, 1978

15. Pearlman AS, Stevenson G, Baker DW: Doppler echocardiography: Applications, limitations and future directions. Am J Cardiol 46:1256–1262, 1980

15a. Hatle L, Angelsen B: Doppler Ultrasound in Cardiology. Physical Principles and Clinical Applications. Philadelphia, Lea & Febiger, 1982, pp 211–223

16. Gardin JM, Burn C, Childs WJ, et al: Evaluation of blood flow velocity in the ascending aorta and main pulmonary artery of normal subjects by Doppler echocardiography. Am Heart J (in press)

17. Chetwa P: Blood flow measurement using ultrasonic pulsed random signal Doppler system. IEEE Trans Sonics Ultrasonics SU-22(1):1–11, 1975

18. Ling SC, Atabek HB, Fry DL, et al: Application of heated-film velocity and shear probes to haemodynamic studies. Circ Res 23:789–801, 1968

19. Rockwell RL, Anliker HB, Elsner J: Model studies of the pressure and flow pulses in a viscoelastic arterial conduit. J Franklin Inst 297(5):405–427, 1974

20. Parker KH: Instability of arterial blood flow, in Hwang NCH, Normann NA (eds): Cardiovascular Flow Dynamics and Measurements. Baltimore, University Park Press, 1977, pp 633–663.

21. Buchtal A, Hanson GC, Peisach AP: Transcutaneous aortovelography: Potentially useful technique in management of critically ill patients. Br Heart J 38:451–456, 1976

22. Gardin JM, Iseri LT, Elkayam U, et al: Evaluation of dilated cardiomyopathy by pulsed Doppler echocardiography. Am Heart J (in press)

22a. Gardin JM. Dabestani A, Matin K, et al: Are Doppler aortic blood flow velocity measurements reproducible? Studies on day-to-day and inter-observer variability in normal subjects (Abstract). J Am Coll Cardiol 1:657, 1983

23. Elkayam U, Gardin J, Berkley R, et al: Doppler flow velocity measurements in the assessment of hemodynamic response to vasodilators in patients with heart failure. Circulation 67:377–382, 1982

24. Steingart RM, Miller J, Barovick J, et al: Pulsed-Doppler echocardiographic measurement of beat-to-beat changes in stroke volume in dogs. Circulation 62:542–548, 1980

25. Darsee JR, Mikolich JR, Walter PF, et al: Transcutaneous Doppler method of measuring cardiac output. I. Comparison of transcutaneous and juxta-aortic Doppler velocity signals with catheter and cuff electromagnetic flowmeter measurements in closed and open chest dogs. Am J Cardiol 46:607–612, 1980

26. Darsee JR, Walter PF, Nutter DO: Transcutaneous Doppler method of measuring cardiac output. II. Noninvasive measurements by transcutaneous Doppler aortic flow velocity integration and M-mode echocardiography. Am J Cardiol 46:613–618, 1980

26a. Chandraratna PAN, Nanna M, McKay C: Determination of cardiac output by transcutaneous continuous wave ultrasonic Doppler computer (Abstract). Circulation 66(Suppl II):II-21, 1982

26b. Huntsman LL, Stewart DK, Barnes SR, et al: Noninvasive Doppler determination of cardiac output in man. Clinical validation. Circulation 67:593–601, 1983

27. Magnin PA, Stewart JA, Myers S, et al: Combined Doppler and phased-array echocardiographic estimation of cardiac output. Circulation 63:388–392, 1981

28. Hoenecke HR, Goldberg SJ, Carnahan Y, et al: Controlled quantitative assessment of pulmonary and aortic flow by range gated pulsed-Doppler in children with cardiac disease (Abstract). Circulation 64(Suppl IV):IV-167, 1981

28a. Waters J, Kwan OL, Kerns G, et al: Limitations of Doppler echocardiography in the calculation of cardiac output (Abstract). Circulation 66(Suppl II):II-122, 1982

29. Fisher DC, Sahn DJ, Larson D, et al: The mitral valve orifice method for noninvasive determination of cardiac output by two-dimensional echo/Doppler: Validation and initial clinical trials (Abstract). Am J Cardiol 49:932, 1982

29a. Fisher DC, Sahn DJ, Friedman MJ, et al: The effect of variations on pulsed Doppler sampling site on calculation of cardiac output: An experimental study in open-chest dogs. Circulation 67:370–376, 1983

29b. Gardin JM. Tobis JM, Dabestani A, et al: Superiority of two-dimensional measurement of aortic vessel diameter in Doppler echocardiographic estimates of left ventricular stroke volume (Abstract). Clin Res 31:8A, 1983

30. Kusnick CA, Gardin JM, Johnston WD, et al: Doppler aortic blood flow velocity assessment of the hemodynamic response to supine bicycle exercise in normal subjects (Abstract). Clin Res 30:14A, 1982

30a. Kawanishi D, McKay C, Chandraratna PAN, et al: Circulatory response to excersise in patients with chronic arotic regurgitation: A decrease in aortic regurgitation (Abstract). Clin Res 31:11A, 1983

31. Gardin JM, Childs WJ, Burn CS, et al: Evaluation of pulmonic valve "a" wave by Doppler pulmonary artery blood flow (Abstract). Circulation 62(Suppl III):III-32, 1980

32. Dabestani A, Gardin JM, Burn C, et al: Relationship of pulmonic valve motion and pulmonary artery blood flow in pulmonary hypertension (Abstract). Circulation 66(Suppl II):II-161, 1982

33. Tucker C, Sahines T, Rasor J, et al: Noninvasive right ventricular pressure measurement by micro-bubble oscillation (Abstract). Circulation 64(Suppl IV):IV-65, 1981

34. Stevenson B, Brandestini M, Weiler T, et al: Digital multigate Doppler with color echo and Doppler display-diagnosis of atrial and ventricular septal defects (Abstract). Circulation 60(Suppl II):II-205, 1979

35. Bommer W, Miller L: Real-time two-dimensional color-flow Doppler: Enhanced Doppler flow imaging in the diagnosis of cardiovascular disease (Abstract). Am J Cardiol 49:944, 1982

36. Joyner CR, Harrison FS, Gruber JW: Diagnosis of hypertrophic subaortic stenosis with a Doppler velocity flow detector. Ann Int Med 74:692–696, 1971

37. Glasgow GA, Gardin JM, Burn CS, et al: Echocardiographic and Doppler flow observations in idiopathic hypertrophic subaortic stenosis (IHSS) (Abstract). Circulation 62(Suppl III):III-99, 1980

38. Chandraratna PAN, Aronow WS, Murdock K, et al: Systolic murmur of idiopathic hypertrophic subaortic stenosis: Phonocardiographic, echocardiographic, continuous Doppler and pulsed Doppler ultrasound correlations (Abstract). Clin Res 28:3A, 1980

39. Gardin JM, Dabestani A, Glasgow GA, et al: Doppler aortic blood flow studies in obstructive and non-obstructive hypertrophic cardiomyopathy (Abstract). Circulation 66(Suppl II):II-267, 1982

40. Boughner DR, Schultz R, Persaud JA: Hypertrophic obstructive cardiomyopathy. Assessment by echocardiographic and Doppler ultrasound techniques. Br Heart J 37:917–923, 1975

41. Gould KL, Mozersky DJ, Hokanson DE, et al: A noninvasive technique for determining patency of saphenous vein coronary bypass grafts. Circulation 46:595–600, 1972

42. Diebold B, Theroux T, Bourassa MG, et al: Noninvasive assessment of aortocoronary bypass graft patency using pulsed-Doppler echocardiography. Am J Cardiol 43:10–16, 1979

43. Fabian J, Vojacek J, Grospic A, et al: Noninvasive Doppler ultrasound evaluation of aortocoronary bypass. Jpn Heart J 20:823–830, 1979

44. Fitzgerald DE, Fortescue-Webb CM, Eckestrom S, et al: Monitoring coronary artery flow by Doppler shift ultrasound. Scand J Thorac Cardiovasc Surg 11:119–123, 1977

45. Marcus M, Wright C, Doty D, et al: Measurements of coronary velocity and reactive hyperemia in the coronary circulation of humans. Circ Res 49:877–891, 1981

46. Gardin JM, Childs WJ, Burns CS, et al: Combined Doppler and M-mode echocardiography: A new approach to the noninvasive detection of left ventricular apical aneurysms (Abstract). Clin Res 29:194A, 1981

47. Veyrat C, Cholof N, Abitbol G, et al: Non-invasive diagnosis of aortic valve disease and evaluation of aortic prosthesis function using echo pulsed-Doppler velocimetry. Br Heart J 43:393–413, 1980

48. Ward JM, Baker DW, Rubenstein SA, et al: Detection of aortic insufficiency by pulsed Doppler echocardiography. JCU 5:5–10, 1977

49. Ciobanu M, Abassi AS, Allen M, et al: Pulsed-Doppler echocardiography in the diagnosis and estimation of severity of aortic insufficiency. Am J Cardiol 49:339–343, 1982

50. Quinones MA, Young JB, Waggoner AD, et al: Assessment of pulsed-Doppler echocardiography in detection and quantitation of aortic and mitral regurgitation. Br Heart J 44:612–620, 1980

51. Bommer WJ, Mapes R, Miller L, et al: Quantitation of aortic regurgitation with two-dimensional Doppler echocardiography (Abstract). Am J Cardiol 47:412, 1981

52. Boughner DR: Assessment of aortic insufficiency by transcutaneous Doppler ultrasound. Circulation 52:874–879, 1975

53. Abassi AS, Allen MW, DeCristofaro D, et al: Detection and estimation of the degree of mitral regurgitation by range-gated pulsed-Doppler echocardiography. Circulation 61:143–147, 1980

54. Miyatake K, Kinoshita N, Nagata S, et al: Intracardiac flow pattern in mitral regurgitation studied with combined use of the ultrasonic pulsed-Doppler technique and cross-sectional echocardiography. Am J Cardiol 45:155–162, 1980

55. Kalmanson D, Veyrat C, Abitbol G, et al: Doppler echocardiography in valvular regurgitation, with special emphasis on mitral insufficiency: Advantages of two-dimensional echocardiography with real-time spectral analysis, in Rijsterborgh H (ed): Echocardiology. The Hague, Martinus Nijhoff, 1981, pp 279–290

56. Nichol PM, Boughner DR, Persaud JA: Noninvasive assessment of mitral insufficiency by transcutaneous Doppler ultrasound. Circulation 54:656–661, 1976

57. Darsee JR, Bray DA, Nutter DO: Noninvasive quantification of mitral regurgitation by echo and Doppler stroke volume measurement (Abstract). Circulation 58(Suppl II):II-42, 1978

58. Waggoner AD, Quinones MA, Young JB, et al: Pulsed-Doppler echocardiographic detection of right-sided valve regurgitation. Experimental results and clinical significance. Am J Cardiol 47:279–286, 1981

59. Stevenson G, Kawabori I, Guntheroth W: Validation of Doppler diagnosis of tricuspid regurgitation (Abstract). Circulation 64(Suppl IV):IV-255, 1981

60. Skjaerpe T, Hatle L: Diagnosis and assessment of tricuspid regurgitation with Doppler ultrasound, in Rijsterborgh H (ed): Echocardiology. The Hague, Martinus Nijhoff, 1981, pp 299–304

60a. Dabestani A, French J, Gardin JM, et al: Doppler hepatic vein blood flow in patients with tricuspid regurgitation (Abstract). J Am Coll Cardiol 1:658, 1983

61. Hatle L, Brubakk A, Tromsdal A, et al: Noninvasive assessment of pressure drop in mitral stenosis by Doppler ultrasound. Br Heart J 40:131–140, 1978

62. Hatle L, Angelsen BA, Tromsdal A: Noninvasive assessment of aortic stenosis by Doppler ultrasound. Br Heart J 43:284–292, 1980

63. Young JB, Quinones MA, Waggoner AD, et al: Diagnosis and quantification of aortic stenosis with pulsed Doppler echocardiography. Am J Cardiol 45:987–994, 1980

64. Goldberg SJ, Draelow ZK, Sahn DJ, et al: Echo Doppler (ED) characterization of flow beyond a stenotic aortic valve (Abstract). Circulation 62(Suppl III):III-252, 1980

65. Kalmanson D, Veyrat C, Bouchareine F, et al: Noninvasive recording of mitral valve flow velocity patterns using pulsed Doppler echocardiography: Application to diagnosis and evaluation of mitral valve disease. Br Heart J 39:517–528, 1977

66. Diebold B, Theroux P, Bourassa MG, et al: Noninvasive pulsed-Doppler study of mitral stenosis and mitral regurgitation: Preliminary study. Br Heart J 42:168–175, 1979

67. Stevenson JG, Kawabori I, Dooley T, et al: Diagnosis of ventricular septal defect by pulsed Doppler echocardiography. Sensitivity, specificity and limitations. Circulation 58:322–326, 1978

68. Stevenson JG, Kawabori I, Guntheroth WG: Differentiation of ventricular septal defects from mitral regurgitation by pulsed Doppler echocardiography. Circulation 56:14–18, 1977

69. Kalmanson D, Veyrat C, Derai C, et al: Noninvasive technique for diagnosing atrial septal defect and assessing shunt volume using directional Doppler ultrasound. Correlations with phasic flow velocity patterns of the shunt. Br Heart J 34:981–991, 1972

70. Goldberg SJ, Areias JC, Spitaels SE, et al: Use of time interval histographic output from echo-Doppler to detect left-to-right atrial shunts. Circulation 58:147–152, 1978

71. Goldberg SJ, Sahn DJ, Allen HD, et al: Evaluation of pulmonary and systemic blood flow by two-dimensional echo Doppler using fast Fourier transform spectral analysis. Am J Cardiol (in press)

72. Sahn DJ, Valdes-Cruz LM, Canale JM, et al: Two-dimensional echo/Doppler determination of pulmonary and systemic blood flows and flow ratios in animal models with atrial and ventricular septal defects (Abstract). Proceedings of the Third Congress of the World Federation for Ultrasound in Medicine and Biology, Brighton, England, 1982

73. Sanders SP, Yeager S, Williams RG: Measurement of systemic and pulmonary blood flow and Qp/Qs ratio using echocardiography and Doppler velocimetry (Abstract). Circulation 66(Suppl II):II-231, 1982

74. Meyer RA, Kalavathy A, Korfhagen JC, et al: Comparison of left to right shunt ratios determined by pulsed Doppler/2D-echo (Dop/2D) and Fick method (Abstract). Circulation 66(Suppl II):II-232, 1982

75. Stevenson JG, Kawarobi I: Noninvasive determination of pulmonic to systemic flow ratio by pulsed Doppler echo (Abstract). Circulation 66(Suppl II):II-232, 1982

CHAPTER 16

Three-Dimensional Echocardiography: A Geometric Reconstruction

David J. Skorton and Edward A. Geiser

The ability to describe changes in the size and shape of the heart as it moves through its cycle is exceedingly important in examining experimental and clinical cardiovascular function. As a case in point, left ventricular global and regional myocardial function are currently major variables used to determine prognosis in cardiac disease,[1] suitability of patients for medical and surgical therapy,[2] and the efficacy of these therapies. The shape of the left ventricle is complex and does not precisely fit any idealized geometric model.[3,4] In order to depict this complex shape, several approaches have been used to derive a three-dimensional model of the left ventricle. Perhaps the most widely used clinical and experimental technique is that of single plane or biplane contrast angiography.[5,6] Although supplying clinically useful information on global and regional left ventricular function, there are several drawbacks in using angiography to describe left ventricular shape. Most important among these limitations are the need to presume an ideal geometric shape for volume calculations and inadequate information regarding ventricular wall thickness in all regions throughout the cardiac cycle.[7] Radionuclide angiography has become a widely used technique for the study of left ventricular function in recent years, and it is a technique that does not require any geometric assumptions to calculate global ventricular function.[8,9] However, its relatively poor spatial resolution,[10] coupled with insufficient information on wall thickness, limit its usefulness in quantitative ventricular shape analysis.

Echocardiography gives accurate, high-resolution, real-time images of left ventricular geometry. The extremely high sampling rate of M-mode echocardiography (1000 per second) has made it a benchmark for the study of rapid motion of cardiac walls and valvular structures.[11] The volume of tissue sampled is small, however, and the spatial orientation of the M-mode beam is uncertain. Two-dimensional echocardiography has been successfully used in the clinical and experimental study of left ventricular function, with the advantage of improved spatial orientation.[12] Another advantage of two-dimensional echocardiography is its ability to define regional wall thickening at the rate of 30 frames per second. Finally, the technique is noninvasive and carries no known biologic risk.

Dr. Skorton is a recipient of a Veterans Administration Research Associate Career Development Award. Dr. Geiser is a recipient of a Young Investigator Research Grant from the National Heart, Lung, and Blood Institute.

Despite these inherent advantages of two-dimensional echocardiography in the study of left ventricular size and shape, assessment of performance of the left ventricle is only semi-quantitative at this time. Several independent tomographic cross-sections are obtained using two-dimensional echocardiography. However, the mental "assembly" of these independent sections into a total left ventricular geometric whole must be done without knowing the precise orientation of any particular two-dimensional image with respect to the other images. Volume calculations from two-dimensional echocardiograms have therefore utilized geometric assumptions similar to those used in contrast angiography.[13]

The objective of three-dimensional echocardiographic reconstruction is to spatially relate several two-dimensional images to each other, and to reassemble these sections into a realistic display of left ventricular geometry. In other words, three-dimensional echocardiography consists of the reconstruction of several two-dimensional echocardiographic cross-sections into a three-dimensional display of global and regional left ventricular shape and size. Successful three-dimensional echocardiographic reconstruction would allow improved estimation of left ventricular volume without the necessity of assuming simplified geometric models. It would also allow the study of ventricular volume at the sampling rate of two-dimensional echocardiography, i.e., 30 times each second. From these data, an improved estimation of filling and ejection patterns of the left ventricle, the temporal sequence of regional contraction, and the location and size of wall motion abnormalities could be obtained. In addition, utilizing currently available computer graphics technology, the anatomy of the reconstructed left ventricle (or indeed any cardiac chamber or great vessel) could be viewed from any perspective. Finally, the clinician and physiologist would have the ability to calculate more complex functional indices of left ventricular performance than are currently routinely available, including regional dv/dt and regional myocardial mechanics derived by a noninvasive imaging technique.

Several investigative groups have demonstrated three-dimensional echocardiographic reconstructions using a variety of techniques for acquiring and reassembling the two-dimensional echocardiographic data. In general, all of the methods may be summarized as follows (see Figure 16-1):

• *Data acquisition and spatial registration.* Individual two-dimensional echocardiographic images are obtained in the usual manner, with the addition of one of several devices for spatial registration of the transducer. In this sense, spatial registration refers to recording the position and orientation of the echocardiographic transducer as each two-dimensional image is obtained. This position and orientation information will later be used to reassemble the cross-sections into an overall, three-dimensional model of the left ventricle. Several different approaches have been used to acquire the individual two-dimensional images, some investigators using standard precordial echo views,[14–20] some using apical views,[21,22] and some combining precordial and apical views.[23,24]

• *Digitization of echocardiographic data.* The process of performing a three-dimensional reconstruction from the several two-dimensional images is greatly facilitated by digital computer technology. The two-dimensional echocardiographic data must therefore be converted into numerical form or digitized (analog-to-digital conversion). The process of digitization consists of entering the position of the endocardial and epicardial borders of each individual cross-sectional image into an overall geometric coordinate system. Once these data are entered for each two-dimensional cross-section, they will be combined with the information on transducer position and orientation to reconstruct the three-dimensional geometry.

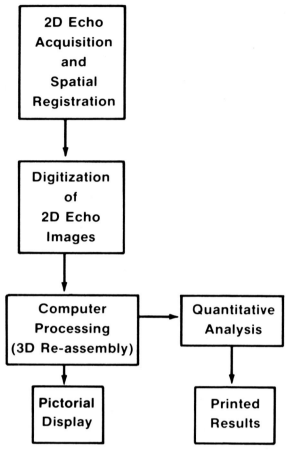

Figure 16-1. An overview of the process of three-dimensional echocardiographic reconstruction. The spatial position of the echocardiographic transducer is recorded while obtaining standard two-dimensional echocardiographic images. The endocardial and epicardial borders in each image are digitized, and the positions of these borders, together with the transducer position and orientation information, are entered into a computer for three-dimensional reassembly. The three-dimensional reconstructions are displayed, and calculated indices concerning cardiac shape and size are printed.

• *Computer processing.* The principles of three-dimensional reconstruction and display by digital computer have been well developed and are commonly used in industrial design and aerospace applications. However, because of the special requirements of three-dimensional echocardiographic reconstruction, adaptations of these methods of reconstruction must be developed expressly for this purpose. Once again, several approaches have been used, and a series of algorithms have been described.

• *Information display.* After reconstruction, the three-dimensional left ventricular model can be displayed using one of several standard computer graphic systems. Visual, qualitative information can then be extracted by the trained observer in much the same way as information is extracted by viewing a left ventricular contrast angiogram.

• *Quantitative analysis.* Since information on chamber size, shape, and wall thickness are contained in the digital computer memory at this point, a variety of calculated indices can be readily derived using this information. For example, volumes may be obtained without the need for geometric assumptions, and sophisticated global and regional left ventricular functional analyses can be accomplished.

What are the computer and display requirements for three-dimensional echocardiography? Although the calculation of complex regional indices of left ventricular performance may require the use of a large, main-frame computer, many of the three-dimensional echocardiographic reconstructions reported so far in the literature have been accomplished using standard minicomputer configurations. For example, the computational capacity used in radionuclide or computed tomography (CT) image processing is adequate to perform basic three-dimensional echocardiographic reconstructions.

In the remainder of this chapter we briefly describe the present status of work in the area of three-dimensional echocardiographic reconstruction. We have tried to supply sufficient technical information to allow those interested in further exploring this exciting area to do so. At the same time we have kept the discussion as relevant to the clinical echocardiographer as possible and related it to other techniques currently available for the description of cardiac size, shape, and function.

SPATIAL REGISTRATION

Spatial registration is the sine qua non of three-dimensional reconstruction. In order to reconstruct the left ventricle from multiple two-dimensional images one must accurately know the orientation of each view with respect to the others. A similar problem exists in an individual two-dimensional echo image, in which each B-mode scan line must be spatially registered with respect to the others in the sector plane. For three-dimensional reconstruction, however, we need to know not only the position of the origin of the sector plane in three-dimensional space but also the orientation of the imaging plane. With this information, the position of any point on any sector plane can be calculated in three dimensions with respect to a fixed external reference point. Several devices for accomplishing this spatial registration have been reported. In general, these fall into the categories of acoustic, mechanical, and laser-based systems.

Acoustic Registration

The sonic devices for spatial registration use the same principle as the sonic digitizing pen. In these devices a spark is produced between two wires close to the tip of the pen. The center frequency of the sound produced by this spark is picked up by microphones. By knowing the time of reception of the sound at each microphone, the position of the origin of the sound can be determined very accurately. In order to calculate both the position and orientation of the transducer for each three-dimensional location, it is necessary to have several sources and several microphones. Usually this is accomplished by using three spark sources attached to the end of the echocardiographic transducer to be received by three microphones.

This type of system very accurately determines the position and orientation of the echo beam in space. It also has the advantage of allowing a great deal of freedom in the use of the transducer, as a fixture to generate the three sparks can be very light. The method has the disadvantage, however, that the microphones are not easily portable and they also present some difficulty in calibrating after movement.

This means that such a system cannot be conveniently moved to the patient's bedside. There may also be some problems with the use of the spark gaps in the presence of oxygen or anesthetic agents. Despite these drawbacks, the accuracy of the system has led to its advocacy and use by several investigators.[23,25,26]

Mechanical Systems

The prototype of the three-dimensional registration arm was first designed by Dekker.[27] This arm had 5 degrees of freedom and allowed movement of a single ultrasound crystal in a random fashion over the precordium to obtain three-dimensional data. More recently, Geiser and coworkers[28] reported the design and use of a mechanical arm with 5 degrees of freedom that allows registration of the origin and orientation of sector planes using a two-dimensional probe. A second-generation design, built by Skorton and coworkers, has 6 degrees of freedom and allows for registration of apical as well as precordial views (Figure 16-2). In the mechanical system the movement through each degree of freedom is monitored by a high-precision potentiometer (which can be cable or gear driven, depending on the design). Each potentiometer is then calibrated so that the change in voltage of the potentiometer is proportional to the angular or linear movement. The position and orientation of the probe can then be calculated using a point on the mounting apparatus of the mechanical arm as the fixed external reference point.

While the accuracy of the calculated spatial position using these mechanical arms does not approach that of the acoustic system, there are other advantages. Once

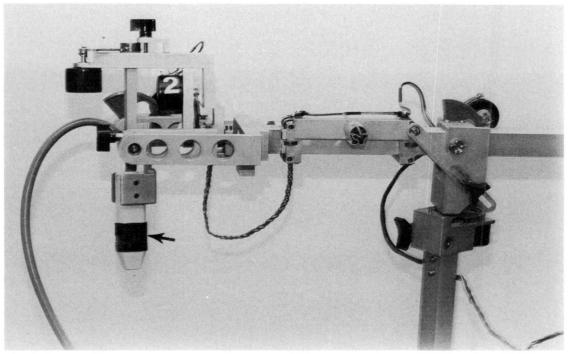

Figure 16-2. A mechanical echocardiographic transducer spatial registration arm with 6 degrees of freedom. The position and orientation of the echocardiographic transducer (arrow) are recorded through the use of six potentiometers and are related to an external reference point.

these arms are calibrated, the whole assembly can be moved quite easily. The arm can be attached to a post on the two-dimensional echo cart and conveniently moved to the patient's bedside. The arm and transducer can then be moved over the patient and the three-dimensional data obtained virtually anywhere in the hospital. Also, because the systems are enclosed, there is virtually no problem in using them in the presence of oxygen or anesthesia.

Laser-Based Registration

This technique of registration has recently been reported by Joskowicz et al.[24] Four small photosensitive elements are mounted on the transducer; its position and orientation are tracked by a laser system. This type of system appears to have excellent accuracy and allow free motion of the transducer for random scanning of the heart.

Relative Accuracy

There is little doubt that the acoustic and laser systems will have greater absolute accuracy than that provided by the mechanical systems of registration. The acoustic system has an accuracy in the range of ±1 mm in repositioning the probe on the chest wall. The accuracy of the mechanical system is likely to be in the range of ±2 mm. Since the cross-plane resolution (thickness of the sector-"slice") of contemporary two-dimensional echo systems is in the range of 2 to 8 mm, it is likely that any of these systems will provide adequate spatial registration. The specific use, cost, and portability will more likely determine which registration system is used than will the absolute accuracy.

Selection of Views

The selection of which views to incorporate into a three-dimensional reconstruction must be based on several considerations, including the complexity of the mathematics necessary for the reconstruction, the type of data one wishes to derive from the reconstruction, and the complexity of the spatial registration system. For the purpose of this discussion, we can examine three different reconstruction frameworks: those based on primarily apical, on precordial, and on randomly obtained two-dimensional echo views.

Apical View Reconstruction

This type of reconstruction has been used extensively by several investigators.[21,22] This framework is attractive because it requires a relatively simple spatial registration device which must only hold the transducer at the apex of the heart and allow it to be rotated incrementally through 180°. Most of these reconstructions use a 30° increment so that in addition to the apical four-chamber view, only five other views are required. These three long-axis views lend themselves very well to a Simpson's rule calculation of ventricular volume.

The difficulties with this system arise because of the position and motion of the apex of the heart relative to the chest wall, and because of the additional problem of visibility of the endocardial surface from the apical views. It is generally accepted that the apical views may produce some shortening of the long axis and that the variability in the long-axis measurement may be in the range of 1 cm.[14,29] To base an entire reconstruction solely on apical views would therefore theoretically maximize this error. Additional work suggests that the endocardium is not routinely visualized on the apical views.[30,31] This would seriously compromise the ability to reconstruct the realistic geometry of the chamber using only apical views. The principal advantage of selecting only apical views to perform the reconstruction is that the entire ventricle is usually seen. When the parasternal long-axis or multiple precordial short-axis views are used, the apex is usually not well visualized.

Precordial View Reconstruction

Multiple precordial views in long- and short-axis have been used by several observers. Matsumoto and coworkers used multiple long-axis views spaced 5 mm apart to reconstruct three-dimensional stereoscopic pictures of the entire heart.[15,16] Geiser and coworkers used five short-axis views realigned on a single parasternal long-axis view to reconstruct the left ventricular chamber and walls (Figure 16-3).[14,17] Similar techniques for reconstruction using cross-sections have also been used by Nixon and Saffer[18] and by Eaton and coworkers.[19] The work of the latter group was performed in beating isolated canine hearts. Initially, short-axis cross-sections were taken every 3 mm in the test tank. Subsequent analysis showed that excellent correlation between calculated and measured volume could be maintained with as few as four or five short-axis sections.[20] The inference from these test tank observations, as well as from those in patients, is that short-axis views appear to be superior to apical views for identification of the endocardium and wall thickening. The greatest difficulty arises when only short-axis views near the base of the heart can be obtained (i.e., no apex-level views) or when it is impossible to identify all of the entire short-axis views adequately. This reconstruction technique is somewhat more difficult than the apical because of the spatial registration device needed. In addition, the calculation of ventricular volume and mass is more difficult because the sections are not parallel and require more complex algorithms, as will be described.

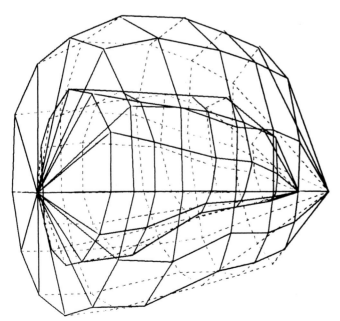

Figure 16-3. A three-dimensional echocardiographic reconstruction of the in vitro left ventricle using short-axis (parasternal equivalent) two-dimensional echocardiographic images, realigned onto a common long-axis.

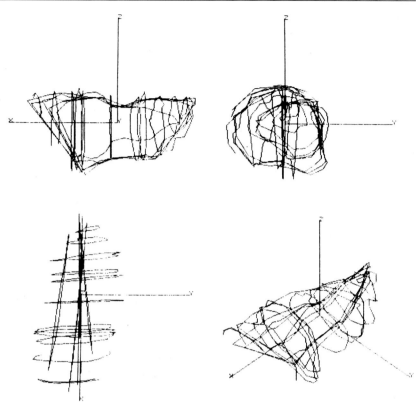

Figure 16-4. Four perspective views of a three-dimensional echocardiographic reconstruction of the in vitro left ventricle using randomly acquired two-dimensional echocardiographic images. (Courtesy of Drs. Alan Pearlman and William Moritz, University of Washington.)

Random View Reconstruction

A three-dimensional reconstruction that incorporates multiple randomly obtained views from the apex and parasternal cross-sectional positions has been described by Moritz and coworkers[23] (Figure 16-4) and by Joskowicz et al.[24] The capability to do these reconstructions is largely due to the freedom of the registration device. The mechanical arm with 6 degrees of freedom (see Figure 16-2) also allows this random type of reconstruction.

QUANTITATIVE ANALYSIS OF THREE-DIMENSIONAL DATA

As noted above, three-dimensional reconstruction can be defined as the calculation of the X, Y, and Z coordinates of any point in a two-dimensional image with respect to a single common reference point. The specific algorithms utilized to accomplish this depend upon the type of registration system used and where the origin of the three-dimensional coordinate system is placed. The mathematical relationships vary in complexity but in general require only calculations in simple spherical or Cartesian space trigonometry.

If the endocardium on a given cross-section were to be considered in three-dimensional space, this endocardium could conceivably consist of an infinite number of points and require an infinite number of calculations for the X, Y, and Z position of each point. Thus, in any practical three-dimensional reconstruction, a certain amount of "down-sampling" (i.e., selection of fewer pertinent points) is necessary. While there is still some question as to how many points are necessary to accurately describe the shape of the endocardium in any given view, recent evidence reported by Ariet and coworkers[32] suggests that the area of a single two-dimensional echo image calculated from 48 points is very close to that calculated from continuous tracing of even complex borders. It thus appears that a three-dimensional surface such as that of the left ventricular endocardium could be adequately represented by selecting approximately 48 equally spaced points on the endocardium from each of the two-dimensional views obtained.

Calculation of the volume enclosed by this described surface can be performed by several means. Moritz and coworkers[23] have calculated the volume by using a polar integration between the adjacent views. This type of approach can be used even though several of the two-dimensional views may cut across each other (see Figure 16-4). If multiple cross-sections are used which are not necessarily parallel but do not intercept each other, then the space between adjacent views can be divided into multiple pyramids, the individual volume of each of these pyramids calculated, and the subsequent total volume calculated by summing all of the pyramids in the slice. This approach was designed by Ariet and is used in the reconstruction of Geiser and coworkers[14] (see Figure 16-3). If the reconstruction is formed by multiple apical views, the long-axis length of each of these views is assumed to be equal and the long axis can be divided into numerous equal segments. In this way a Simpson's rule approximation of the volume can be applied.

Another computational approach that may prove useful in the analysis of three-dimensional reconstruction data is finite element analysis. Finite element technique is an approximate numerical method used to solve problems involving complex geometry in engineering mechanics[33] by dividing a complex structure into many "building blocks" of simple geometric shape. Three-dimensional finite element analysis has been applied to the evaluation of left ventricular geometry and muscle properties using angiographic[34,35] computed tomographic,[36] and echocardiographic[37,38] imaging (Figure 16-5).

Automation

It is noted at the beginning of this chapter that among the objectives of three-dimensional reconstruction is the evaluation of the sequences of regional left ventricular contraction. A rapid sampling rate is therefore necessary, and we would like to perform a three-dimensional reconstruction with each new video frame, or 30 times per second. If only five two-dimensional echocardiographic short-axis sections are used to perform each reconstruction, and if one wishes to study both endocardial motion and wall thickening, then the endocardium and epicardium must be manually identified (traced) on 150 separate video frames—an extremely time-consuming process. More disturbing, however, is the interobserver variability in defining these borders.[39,40] One of the major difficulties in the quantitative analysis of standard two-dimensional echocardiograms is the delineation of endocardial and epicardial borders.[30,40] The accurate definition of these borders is an important prerequisite for three-dimensional reconstructions. Therefore, with all methods of three-dimensional echocardiographic reconstruction,[14] border definition or edge detection is an important source of error at present and thus an important area for future research.

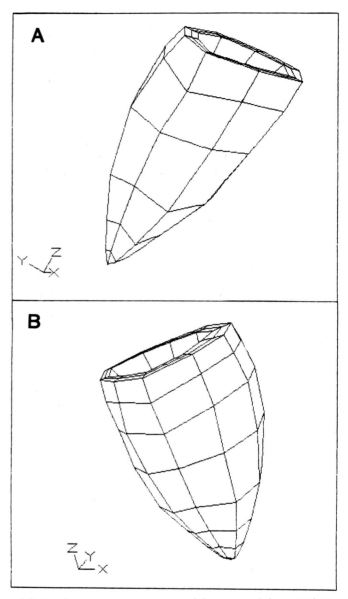

Figure 16-5. Three-dimensional finite element reconstructions of the in vivo left ventricle in early (A) and late (B) diastole. (From Skorton DJ, Chandran KB, Nikravesh PE, et al: Three-dimensional finite element reconstructions from two-dimensional echocardiograms for estimation of myocardial elastic properties, in 1981 Computers in Cardiology. New York, IEEE Computer Society, 1981, pp 383–386. © 1981 IEEE With permission.)

Even if endocardial and epicardial border definition were relatively easily accomplished, the large volume of border tracing necessary to perform three-dimensional echo reconstructions makes a computerized, automated method of border definition extremely important. Preliminary methods for computerized border detection in two-dimensional echocardiography have recently appeared.[41,42,43] One method defines borders by computer in individual echocardiographic frames based on analyzing changes in gray level or image brightness near a border or edge.[41] Left ventricular minor axis and ventricular septal measurements made from the defined endocardial borders using this approach were found to be more accurate than those made from unprocessed echocardiographic stop-frames. Another approach in single frame edge detection utilizes the computer hardware from radioisotope analysis.[42] Another investigative group utilizes cardiac wall motion, which gives important information unavailable in stop-frame analysis to identify and locate cardiac borders.[43] It is our feeling that in the future some combination of the techniques utilizing stop-frame and motion information will optimize automatic border definition.

How close are these automatic techniques to achieving clinically useful computerized border detection in echocardiograms? Most of the work to date has consisted of the definition of the endocardium. Although advances have been made in endocardial definition, this work must still be considered experimental. Unfortunately, epicardial definition has been considerably more difficult, and as yet no reliable methods have been reported. Therefore, automatic edge detection must be considered at present an investigative technique. Computerized border definition will, however, be most important in the future quantitative analysis of two-dimensional echocardiography as well as in clinical three-dimensional echocardiographic reconstruction.

COMPARISON OF OTHER TECHNIQUES OF THREE-DIMENSIONAL CARDIAC RECONSTRUCTION

Several methods in addition to echocardiography are available to describe cardiac shape and size throughout the heart cycle. Chief among these are contrast angiography, radionuclide angiography, and computed tomography (CT). What are the relative advantages and disadvantages of these techniques in the acquisition of three-dimensional cardiac structural information?

As discussed earlier, contrast angiography requires the assumption of an idealized geometric model of left ventricular shape, is invasive, and requires use of a contrast medium and ionizing radiation. Furthermore, adequate information on regional wall thickness throughout the cardiac cycle is not routinely obtained.[7] On the other hand, this is a widely used technique that does supply important information on global and regional left ventricular function. Angiography is the cornerstone of current left ventricular global and regional function analysis, but it is not an ideal method of three-dimensional analysis.

Radionuclide techniques offer the possibility of global and regional left ventricular functional analysis without geometric assumptions. The inherent spatial resolution of radionuclide techniques, however, is relatively poor. In addition, information on regional wall thickness and thickening are not routinely obtained with currently available radionuclide methods.

Computed tomographic scanning has revolutionized the evaluation of the size and shape of stationary organs and has recently been applied to the study of the heart.[44–49] Accurate evaluation of rapid cardiac motion requires gating or referencing of the CT scan to a portion of the cardiac cycle. This rapid motion of the heart, coupled with the relatively long scanning period of most commercial scanners (approximately 2 seconds), makes evaluation of cardiac function by ungated CT scans difficult. However, information on wall thickness and volumes,[45] the patency of saphenous vein bypass grafts,[46] and the presence of myocardial infarction[47,48,49] have all been obtained by investigators using gated or ungated CT scans.[44] Three-dimensional reconstructions of the heart using gated CT should provide extremely accurate shape description, as the cross-sections to be reassembled are all parallel (individual tomographic "slices" are obtained by moving the patient through the CT gantry). However, CT scanning does involve radiation exposure, and furthermore, at present, rapid scanning or gated devices that permit the evaluation of rapid cardiac motion are not widely available. A prototype rapid cardiac CT scanner described by workers at the Mayo Clinic may herald future developments in cardiac CT scanning.[50] The final problem with cardiac CT scanning, also present with contrast angiography and to a lesser extent with radionuclide procedures, is the lack of easy portability of the equipment.

Echocardiography has the potential of being an excellent technique for three-dimensional cardiac reconstructions because of its good spatial resolution, high sampling rate, its ability to analyze regional wall thickness, and the portability of the equipment. The examination is also painless and nonionizing.

CONCLUSION

We have briefly described the current status of three-dimensional echocardiographic reconstruction. Not only can chamber volumes and global left ventricular functional indices be derived by this technique, but three-dimensional echocardiography also improves evaluation of regional wall motion and thickening. Improving regional ventricular functional assessment is a direct result of improving description of cardiac shape and size throughout the heart cycle. Although other methods are available to the clinician and scientist, several inherent characteristics of three-dimensional echocardiographic reconstructions point to a possible increasing role for this technique in the future. The potential accuracy, safety, portability, and cost of such a system may compare favorably to those of other contemporary methods of evaluating ventricular function using radionuclide, CT scanning, or angiographic techniques. It is hoped that such three-dimensional echocardiographic reconstructions will provide a new, sophisticated, and accurate means of noninvasively evaluating cardiac performance.

REFERENCES

1. Nelson GR, Cohn PF, Gorlin R: Prognosis in medically treated coronary artery disease. The value of the ejection fraction compared with other measurements. Circulation 52:408–413, 1975
2. Oldham HN Jr, Kong Y, Bartel AG, et al: Risk factors in coronary artery bypass surgery. Arch Surg 105:918–925, 1972
3. Sandler H, Alderman E: Determination of left ventricular size and shape. Circ Res 34:1–8, 1974
4. Weber KT, Hawthorne EW: Descriptors and determinants of cardiac shape: an overview. Fed Proc 40:2005–2010, 1981
5. Dodge HT, Sandler H, Ballew DW, et al: The use of biplane angiography for measurement of left ventricular volume in man. Am Heart J 60:762–776, 1960
6. Raphael MJ, Allwork SP: Angiographic anatomy of the left ventricle. Clin Radiol 25:95–105, 1974
7. Eber LM, Greenberg HM, Cooke JM, et al: Dynamic changes in left ventricular free wall thickness in the human heart. Circulation 39:455–464, 1969
8. Secker-Walker RH, Resnick L, Kunz H, et al: Measurement of left ventricular ejection fraction. J Nucl Med 14:798, 1973

9. Maddox DE, Holman BL, Wynne J, et al: The ejection fraction image: A noninvasive index of regional left ventricular wall motion. Am J Cardiol 41:1230–1238, 1978

10. Budinger TF, Rollo FD: Physics and instrumentation. Proc Cardiovasc Dis 20:19–53, 1977

11. Feigenbaum H: Echocardiography (ed 3). Philadelphia, Lea & Febiger, 1981, pp 10–21

12. Tajik AJ, Seward JB, Hagler DJ, et al: Two-dimensional real-time ultrasonic imaging of the heart and great vessels: Technique, image orientation, structure identification, and validation. Mayo Clin Proc 53:271–303, 1978

13. Rogers EW, Feigenbaum H, Weyman AE: Echocardiography for quantitation of cardiac chambers, in Yu PN, Goodwin JL (eds): Progress in Cardiology, vol 8. Philadelphia, Lea & Febiger, 1979

14. Geiser EA, Lupkiewicz SM, Christie LG, et al: A framework for three-dimensional time-varying reconstruction of the human left ventricle: Sources of error and estimation of their magnitude. Comput Biomed Res 13:225–241, 1980

15. Matsumoto M, Matsuo H, Kitabatake A, et al: Three-dimensional echocardiograms and two-dimensional echocardiographic images at desired planes by a computerized system. Ultrasound Med Biol 3:163–178, 1977

16. Matsumoto M, Inoue M, Tamura S, et al: Three-dimensional echocardiography for spatial visualization and volume calculation of cardiac structures. JCU 9:156–165, 1981

17. Geiser EA, Ariet M, Conetta DA, et al: Dynamic three-dimensional reconstruction of the human left ventricle *in vivo:* technique and initial observation in patients. Am Heart J 103:1056–1065, 1982

18. Nixon JV and Saffer SI: Three-dimensional echocardiography (Abstract). Circulation 57,58:II-157, 1978

19. Eaton LW, Maughan WL, Shoukas AA, et al: Accurate volume determination in the isolated ejecting canine left ventricle by two-dimensional echocardiography. Circulation 60:320–326, 1979

20. Eaton LW, Maughan WL, Weiss JL: Accurate volume determination in the isolated ejecting canine heart from a limited number of two-dimensional echocardiographic cross-sections (Abstract). Am J Cardiol 45:470, 1980

21. Ueda K, Kuwaki K, Inone K: Three-dimensional display and volume determination of the left ventricle by two-dimensional echocardiography (Abstract). Am J Cardiol 45:471, 1980

22. Maurer G, Ghosh A, Nanda NC: Volume determination and three-dimensional reconstruction of echocardiographic images using rotation method (Abstract). Circulation 64:IV-206, 1981

23. Moritz WE, Medema DK, Ainsworth M, et al: Three-dimensional reconstruction and volume calculation from a series of nonparallel, real time ultrasonic images (Abstract). Circulation 62:III-143, 1980

24. Joskowicz G, Klicpera M, Pachinger O, et al: Computer supported measurements of 2-D echocardiographic images, in 1981 Computers in Cardiology, IEEE Computer Society No. 81CH1750-9, 1982, pp 13–17

25. King DL, Al-Banna S, Larach D: A new three-dimensional random scanner for ultrasonic/computer graphic imaging of the heart, in White D, Barnes R (eds): Ultrasound in Medicine, vol 2, New York, Plenum Press, 1975, pp 363–372

26. Garrison JB, Weiss JL, Maughan WL, et al: Quantifying regional wall motion and thickening in two-dimensional echocardiography with a computer-aided contouring system, in IEEE Computer Society: Proceedings of Computers in Cardiology. Long Beach, Calif, 1977, pp 25–35

27. Dekker DL, Piziali R, Dong E: A system for ultrasonically imaging the human heart in three dimensions. Comput Biomed Res 7:544–553, 1974

28. Geiser EA, Christie LG, Conetta DA, et al: A mechanical arm for spatial registration of two-dimensional echocardiographic sections. Cathet Cardiovasc Diag 8:89–101, 1982

29. Parisi AF, Moynihan PF, Feldman CL, et al: Approaches to determination of left ventricle volume and ejection fraction by real time two-dimensional echocardiography. Clin Cardiol 2:257–263, 1979

30. Meister SG, Casey PR, Jacobs L, et al: 2-D echo definition of endocardium (Abstract). Circulation 62:III-132, 1980

31. Schnittger I, Fitzgerald PJ, Daughters GT, et al: Accurate assessment of left ventricular volumes by two-dimensional echocardiography (Abstract). Circulation 64:IV-129, 1981

32. Ariet M, Geiser EA, Lupkiewicz SM, et al: Evaluation of a three-dimensional reconstruction to compute LV volume and mass (Abstract). Am J Cardiol 49:896, 1982

33. Belytschko T, Osias JR, Marcal PV (eds): Finite Element Analysis of Transient Nonlinear Structural Behavior. American Society of Mechanical Engineers, New York, 1975

34. Vinson CA, Gibson DG, Yettram AL: Analysis of left ventricular behavior in diastole by means of finite element method. Br Heart J 41:60–67, 1979

35. Ray G, Chandran KB, Nikravesh PE, et al: Estimation of the local elastic modulus of the normal and infarcted left ventricle from angiographic data. Proceedings of the Fourth New England Bioengineering Conference, 1976, pp 173–176

36. Heethar RM, Pao YC, Ritman EL: Computer aspects of three-dimensional finite element analysis of stresses and strains in the intact heart. Comput Biomed Res 10:271–285, 1977

37. Nikravesh PE, Chandran KB, Skorton DJ, et al: 3-D finite element reconstruction of left ventricular geometry from cross-sectional echocardiographic recordings, in Van Buskirk WC (ed): Proceedings of 1981 Biomechanics Symposium, New York, American Society of Mechanical Engineers. AMD 43:15–18, 1981

38. Skorton DJ, Chandran KB, Nikravesh PE, et al: Three-dimensional finite element reconstructions from two-dimensional echocardiograms for estimation of myocardial elastic properties, in 1981 Computers in Cardiology. New York, IEEE Computer Society, 1981, pp 383–386

39. DeMaria AN, Kwan OL, Bommer W, et al: Accuracy of echocardiographic measurements of the left ventricle: comparison of reproducibility of two-dimensional and M-mode techniques (Abstract). Circulation 59,60(Suppl II):II-203, 1979

40. Meltzer RS, Bastiaans OL, McGhie J, et al: Normal values and interobserver variability for two-dimensional echocardiographic measurements of the left ventricle (Abstract). Clin Res 28:616A, 1980

41. Skorton DJ, McNary CA, Child JS, et al: Digital image processing of two dimensional echocardiograms: identification of the endocardium. Am J Cardiol 48:479–486, 1981

42. Garcia E, Gueret P, Bennet M, et al: Real time computerization of two-dimensional echocardiography. Am Heart J 101:783–792, 1981

43. Geiser EA, Tou JT, Nawaz A, et al: 2-D echo border extraction by analysis of pixel motion in sequential video fields (Abstract). Circulation 62(Suppl III):III-131, 1980

44. Lackner K, Thurn P: Computed tomography of the heart: ECG-gated and continuous scans. Radiology 140:413–420, 1981

45. Mavroudis C, Skioldebrand C, Lipton M, et al: Myocardial computed tomography can determine left ventricular mass and differentiate left ventricular hypertrophy. Curr Surg 38:216–219, 1981

46. Brundage BH, Lipton MJ, Herfkens RJ, et al: Detection of patent coronary bypass grafts by computed tomography. Circulation 61:826–831, 1980

47. Scanlan JG, Gustafson DE, Chevalier PA, et al: Evaluation of ischemic heart disease with a prototype volume imaging computed tomographic (CT) scanner: Preliminary experiments. Am J Cardiol 46:1263–1268, 1980

48. Doherty PW, Lipton MJ, Berninger WH, et al: Detection and quantitation of myocardial infarction in vivo using transmission computed tomography. Circulation 63:597–606, 1981

49. Higgins CB, Siemers PT, Schmidt W, et al: Evaluation of myocardial ischemic damage of various ages by computerized transmission tomography: Time dependent effect of contrast material. Circulation 60:284–291, 1979

50. Ritman EL, Harris LD, Kinsey JH, et al: Computed tomographic imaging of the heart: The dynamic spatial reconstructor. Radiol Clin North Am 18:547–556, 1980

CHAPTER 17

Ultrasound Tissue Characterization of Myocardium

David J. Skorton, Natesa G. Pandian, and Richard E. Kerber

Standard clinical echocardiography consists of imaging the bright, smooth (specular) reflectors of the heart, such as the endocardium and epicardium. By studying the position and motion of these structures throughout the cardiac cycle, alterations in global and regional cardiac function, such as those due to myocardial ischemia, can be detected. In addition to indirectly identifying ischemic myocardium by displaying abnormalities in regional left ventricular contraction, ultrasound is able to identify directly abnormal tissue regions on the basis of altered acoustic properties. Specifically, ultrasound has been shown to interact differently with ischemic or infarcted muscle than with normal myocardium. This altered ultrasound–tissue interaction, if routinely detectable, would be a powerful technique for direct identification of regional cardiac ischemia. The past 10 years have seen a growing interest in the study of altered acoustic properties of abnormal tissue, and this area of study has been referred to as "ultrasound tissue characterization."[1] In this chapter we will direct our attention chiefly to studies of ultrasound tissue characterization in ischemic or infarcted myocardium.

DEFINITIONS

Ultrasound tissue characterization may be defined as the evaluation of the physical characteristics of a volume of tissue based upon its acoustic properties. The acoustic properties of interest might include the velocity, attenuation,[2-4] and backscatter[5,6] of ultrasound. Although incompletely defined, the physical characteristics responsible for alterations in these acoustic properties may include tissue architecture, elasticity, and relative content of collagen and water.[2,5]

APPROACHES

Three basic approaches have been used in ultrasound tissue characterization studies. Each has inherent advantages and drawbacks, and investigation into each is being actively pursued at the present time.

Supported in part by National Heart, Lung, Blood Institute Grant 14388, American Heart Association—Iowa Affiliate Grant 80-G-36, and by the Veterans Administration.
Dr. Skorton is a recipient of a Veterans Administration Research Associate Career Development Award.

• Direct visualization of regions with abnormal acoustic properties is a qualitative approach to tissue characterization. This approach is based on the display of regional abnormalities in myocardial acoustic properties, as well as on the observer's pattern recognition abilities. In order to display acoustically abnormal regions, the ultrasound imaging system must be capable of accurately transforming a variable of interest (e.g., backscatter) into an image display parameter (e.g., gray level). Current research utilizing this approach is directed at hardware or signal processing developments aimed at accurately displaying acoustic variables of interest in a real-time fashion.

• Alterations in certain displayed features or patterns in a two-dimensional ultrasound study may be more easily appreciated after digital image processing and analysis, using pattern recognition or other, statistical approaches. For example, the texture apparent in most B-mode scans of soft tissue regions (in part, an interference pattern sometimes referred to as "speckle") may be difficult to describe or categorize visually. Several investigative groups have attempted to apply texture analysis and statistical techniques to this problem, with encouraging results.[7,8] This approach to ultrasound tissue characterization depends upon high-resolution analog-to-digital conversion of the ultrasound data and subsequent digital computer analysis.

• The most rigorous approach to ultrasound tissue characterization is the direct measurement of the acoustic parameters of interest. This approach is most easily performed in vitro or in organs that may be studied using transmission techniques (e.g., breast). Several problems unique to echocardiography have limited the application of measurement approaches to myocardial characterization. Chief among these are the complex translational and rotational movements of the heart during the cardiac cycle and the presence of chest wall tissue between the transducer and the area of interest. Despite these difficulties, significant strides have been made toward the goal of regional quantitation of acoustic parameters of myocardium.[2–6]

Having briefly reviewed these three basic approaches to ultrasound tissue characterization, we now review examples of work done using each method and attempt to indicate the probable direction of future research.

DIRECT VISUALIZATION OF INFARCTED MYOCARDIUM

Areas of myocardial infarction may occasionally be visualized directly in echocardiograms performed with currently available ultrasound systems. Rasmussen and coworkers have noted brighter echoes returning from areas of chronic myocardial infarction seen on M-mode echocardiograms[9] (Figure 17-1). This appreciation of myocardial infarction by direct visualization is not, however, predictable. The many signal processing manipulations performed during routine ultrasound studies (e.g., changing gain, reject, or time–gain compensation settings) could probably mask or mimic regional abnormalities of tissue acoustic properties.[10] However, as in other conditions (such as amyloid heart disease[11] and hypertrophic cardiomyopathy[12]), the occasional appreciation of unusual tissue texture on two-dimensional echocardiograms may be clinically useful. That these changes may be seen early in the course of infarction is suggested by demonstrations presented by vonRamm and Smith[13] in 5-day-old infarctions in dogs (Figure 17-2). Hardware developments now being pursued may in the future allow routine direct visualization of regional differences in backscatter in real time.[14]

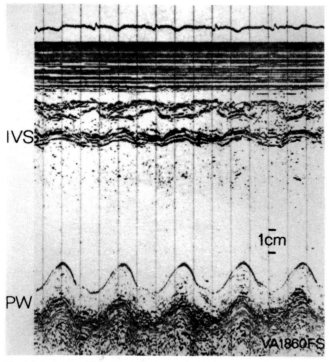

Figure 17-1. M-mode echocardiogram from a patient with ventricular septal scar. Echoes from the interventricular septum (IVS) appear brighter than those from the posterior wall (PW). (From Rasmussen S, Corya BC, Feigenbaum H, et al: Detection of myocardial scar tissue by M-mode echocardiography. Circulation 57:230–237, 1978. By permission of the American Heart Association, Inc.)

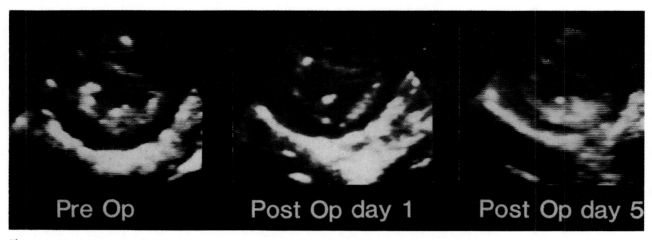

Figure 17-2. Direct visualization of myocardial infarction by two-dimensional echocardiography. An area of increased echo intensity is seen in the posterior wall on the short-axis echocardiogram at far right, recorded 5 days after experimental myocardial infarction. (From vonRamm OT, Smith SW: Prospects and limitations of diagnostic ultrasound. Proc SPIE 206:6–18, 1979. With permission.)

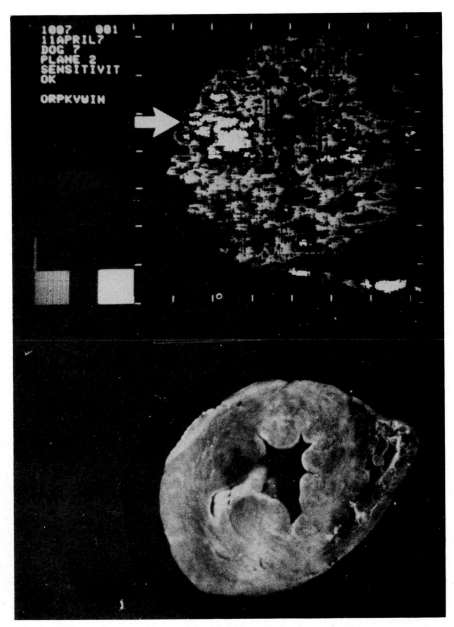

Figure 17-3. Display of region of 30-minute-old myocardial infarct after image processing. The upper panel shows a processed image, with the arrow indicating an area of increased echo amplitude. The lower panel is a thioflavin S fluorescence image with the corresponding perfusion deficit in black. (From Gramiak R, Waag RC, Schenk EA, et al: Ultrasonic detection of myocardial infarction by amplitude analysis. Radiology 130:713–720, 1979. With permission.)

IMAGE AND SIGNAL PROCESSING

The science of image processing (or picture processing) consists of the systematic manipulation and analysis of pictorial data in order to (1) render features of interest more apparent (enhancement), (2) allow recognition of prominent patterns in the picture, and (3) extract statistical or other numerical information. Sophisticated image processing techniques have been used extensively in the fields of satellite photography and remote sensing,[15] terrain mapping,[16] and nuclear medicine,[17] and in various ultrasonic applications.[18] Efforts to utilize these approaches to analyze echocardiographic data have centered on enhanced edge definition,[19–21] improved apparent resolution,[22] and tissue characterization.[23,24] All of these approaches required conversion of the pictorial data to digital form to allow computer processing. As an example, Gramiak and coworkers have used an image processing technique to accentuate the appearance of increased local echo amplitudes from infarcted regions of hearts studied in vitro.[23] This technique rendered the increased amplitude visible as a region of brighter gray levels (Figure 17-3). Another somewhat similar approach has consisted of studying regional gray level distributions in two-dimensional echocardiograms of closed-chest dogs subjected to acute coronary occlusion.[24] Regions of acute infarction exhibited altered gray level distributions compared to those of normal regions.

A different set of approaches involves processing and analyzing the electronic signals from which pictorial data are generated, before the two-dimensional image is produced. That is, the signal representing ultrasound echoes along a single, specific line of sight is analyzed. This signal, usually in the form of a time-varying voltage (which is analogous to echo amplitude) is converted to digital form and processed using a digital computer.

An example of this approach can be found in the studies of Franklin and coworkers.[25] These investigators subjected A-mode ultrasound signals from myocardium to rigorous statistical analysis. They found that the statistical characteristics of the A-mode echoes of infarcted myocardium differed significantly from those of normal tissue. No specific acoustic parameters (e.g., attenuation or backscatter) were measured—the overall characteristics of the signal "shapes" differentiated normal from infarcted myocardium.

Another unique approach that also utilized statistical analysis was that of Joynt and coworkers.[26] From real-time two-dimensional echocardiographic studies, radiofrequency (similar to A-mode) signals from individual ultrasound lines of sight were digitized, stored, and analyzed. A stochastic analytic approach was undertaken, which characterized the distribution of echo amplitudes from specific regions of interest. The amplitude data from infarcted and normal myocardium were characterized by different probability density functions. This approach has also been found effective in the differentiation of mural thrombus from artifact.[27]

MEASUREMENT OF ACOUSTIC PARAMETERS

A conceptually different approach to tissue characterization is to attempt direct measurements of acoustic variables in local regions of interest. This method has the advantage of yielding information on the basic mechanisms of the abnormal image characteristics noted in the methods just discussed. Major difficulties in cardiac tissue characterization (motion, intervening chest wall tissue) have made this a

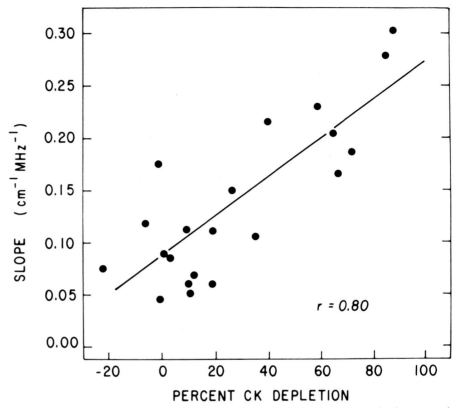

Figure 17-4. Relationship between an ultrasonic index of attenuation, labeled "slope," and the percentage of depletion of creatine kinase (CK), an enzymatic estimator of myocardial necrosis. This linear correlation was found in excised samples of dog myocardium 4–6 weeks after myocardial infarction. (From Mimbs JW, Yuhas DE, Miller JG, et al: Detection of myocardial infarction in vitro based on altered attenuation of ultrasound. Circ Res 41:192–198, 1977. By permission of the American Heart Association, Inc.)

challenging approach, but a number of extremely important observations have already been made in this fashion.

One of the early reports employing measurement of acoustic parameters was that of Namery and Lele,[28] who noted a difference between the acoustic impedance of normal and infarcted samples of myocardium studied in vitro. Miller and coworkers[2–4] studied the frequency dependence of attenuation in myocardium by examining excised samples of tissue in vitro in transmission mode (i.e., using separate transmitting and receiving crystals positioned on opposite sides of the tissue specimen). Differences between the attenuation (versus frequency) slope of normal and ischemic myocardium were detectable as soon as 15 minutes after coronary occlusion and were also present several weeks later.[3,4] The attenuation slope correlated linearly with the percentage of creatine kinase depletion 4–6 weeks after infarction (Figure 17-4). This group later studied experimental infarction using reflected ultrasound and calculated an index of integrated backscatter[5,6] based in part on a method suggested earlier by Sigelmann and Reid.[29] Infarcted tissue was found to exhibit increased levels of backscatter compared to normal myocardium. In attempting to study the physical or biochemical basis of these findings, a series of studies was done to examine the dependence of attenuation and backscatter on tissue collagen

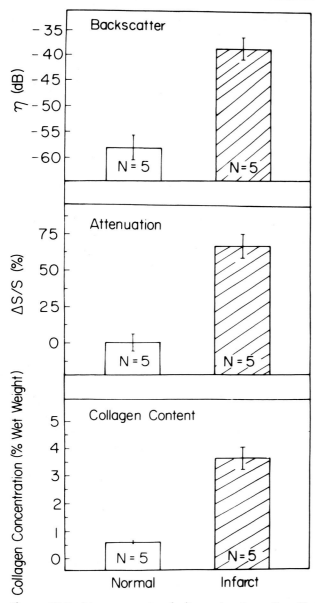

Figure 17-5. Measurements of ultrasonic attenuation (Δs/s), backscatter (η), and collagen concentration are shown for normal and infarcted samples of rabbit heart. The collagen concentration and the acoustic properties were significantly different in the infarcted samples compared to normal. (From Mimbs JW, O'Donnell M, Bauwens D, et al: The dependence of ultrasonic attenuation and backscatter on collagen content in dog and rabbit hearts. Circ Res 47:49–58, 1980. By permission of the American Heart Association, Inc.)

content.[5] Both attenuation and backscatter were found to be related to hydroxyproline concentrations (Figure 17-5). Of interest was the observation that, after perfusion of the tissue with collagenase solution, the backscatter level fell, but attenuation and hydroxyproline concentration were unchanged.[5] This suggested the dependence of backscatter on intact collagen.

This initial series of observations were made in vitro, or in open-chest animals, thereby avoiding interference by tissue intervening between the transducer and the region of interest. This intervening tissue attenuates the ultrasound beam, changes the frequency spectrum, and therefore must be taken into account in order to utilize these measurement techniques in intact subjects. Preliminary investigations into the acoustic properties of chest wall tissue have been performed and are an important step toward clinical applications of measurement techniques.[30]

CLINICAL IMPLICATIONS

Ultrasound myocardial tissue characterization must at this time be considered an investigational technique. However, the interest in this area and the important preliminary contributions noted suggest future progress toward the goal of evaluation of myocardial viability and structure using acoustic analysis. This would obviously be of immense value both to the clinician caring for patients with ischemic heart disease and to the investigator studying cardiac pathophysiology.

REFERENCES

1. Linzer M (ed): Ultrasonic Tissue Characterization II. National Bureau of Standards spec publ 525. US Government Printing Office, 1979
2. Miller JG, Yuhas DE, Mimbs JW, et al: Ultrasonic tissue characterization: Correlation between biochemical and ultrasonic indices of myocardial injury. IEEE Ultrasonics Symposium, Washington, DC, 1976, 76 CH 1120–5SU:33–37
3. Mimbs JW, Yuhas DE, Miller JG, et al: Detection of myocardial infarction in vitro based on altered attenuation of ultrasound. Circ Res 41:192–198, 1977
4. O'Donnell M, Mimbs JW, Sobel BE, et al: Ultrasonic attenuation in normal and ischemic myocardium, in Linzer M (ed): Ultrasonic Tissue Characterization II, National Bureau of Standards spec publ 525. US Government Printing Office, 1979, pp 63–71
5. Mimbs JW, O'Donnell M, Bauwens D, et al: The dependence of ultrasonic attenuation and backscatter on collagen content in dog and rabbit hearts. Circ Res 47:49–58, 1980
6. Mimbs JW, Bauwens D, Cohen RD, et al: Effects of myocardial ischemia on quantitative ultrasonic backscatter and identification of responsible determinants. Circ Res 49:89–96, 1981
7. Lerski RA, Barnett E, Morley P, et al: Computer analysis of ultrasonic signals in diffuse liver disease. Ultrasound Med Biol 5:341, 1979
8. Skorton DJ, Collins SM, Nichols J, et al: Quantitative texture analysis in two-dimensional echocardiography: Application to the diagnosis of experimental myocardial contusion. Circulation (in press)
9. Rasmussen S, Corya BC, Feigenbaum H, et al: Detection of myocardial scar tissue by M-mode echocardiography. Circulation 57:230–237, 1978
10. Jaffe CC, Harris DJ: Physical factors influencing numerical echo-amplitude data extracted from B-scan ultrasound images. JCU 8:327, 1980
11. Siqueira-Filho AG, Cunha CLP, Tajik AJ, et al: M-mode and two-dimensional echocardiographic features in cardiac amyloidosis. Circulation 63:188, 1981
12. Martin RP, Rakowski H, French J, et al: Idiopathic hypertrophic subaortic stenosis viewed by wide-angle, phased-array echocardiography. Circulation 59:1206, 1979
13. vonRamm OT, Smith SW: Prospects and limitations of diagnostic ultrasound. Proc Photo-optic Instrument Eng (SPIE) 206:6–18, 1979
14. Melton HE Jr, Skorton DJ: Rational gain compensation for attenuation in ultrasonic cardiac imaging. IEEE Ultrasonics Symposium, Denver, 1981:81CH 1689–9:607–611
15. Castleman KR: Digital Image Processing. Englewood Cliffs, Prentice-Hall, 1979, p 384
16. McNary CA, Conti DK, Eckhardt WO: Segmentation-based boundary modeling for natural terrain scenes. Proceedings SPIE 23rd International Symposium and Industrial Display, San Diego, 1979.
17. Douglas MA, Ostrow HG, Green MV: A computer processing system for ECG-gated radioisotope angiography of the human heart. Comput Biomed Res 9:133, 1976

18. Keating PN, Sawatari T, Zilinskas G: Signal processing in acoustic imaging. Proc IEEE 67:496, 1979
19. Skorton DJ, McNary CA, Child JS, et al: Digital image processing of two-dimensional echocardiograms: Identification of the endocardium. Am J Cardiol 48:479–486, 1981
20. Garcia E, Gueret P, Bennet M, et al: Real time computerization of two-dimensional echocardiography. Am Heart J 101:783, 1981
21. Geiser EA, Tou JT, Nawaz A, et al: 2-D echo border extraction by analysis of pixel motion in sequential video fields. Circulation 62:III-493, 1980
22. Nathan R: High resolution echocardiography. National Aeronautics and Space Administration tech brief 4(1), item 68, 1979
23. Gramiak R, Waag RC, Schenk EA, et al: Ultrasonic detection of myocardial infarction by amplitude analysis. Radiology 130:713–720, 1979
24. Skorton DJ, Melton HE Jr, Pandian NG, et al: Detection of acute myocardial infarction in closed-chest dogs by analysis of regional two-dimensional echocardiographic gray-level distributions. Circ Res 52:36–44, 1983
25. Franklin TD Jr, Cuddeback JK, Sanghyi NT, et al: Differentiation of A-mode ultrasound signals from normal and ischemic myocardium by multivariate discriminant analysis of waveform parameters. Am J Cardiol 45:403, 1980
26. Joynt LF: A stochastic approach to ultrasonic tissue characterization. Stanford Electronics Laboratories tech report No. G557–4, Stanford University, 1979.
27. Joynt LF, Green SE, Fitzgerald PJ, et al: In vivo ultrasound characterization of mural thrombi using amplitude distribution analysis. Ultrasonic Imaging 3:191, 1981
28. Namery J, Lele PP: Ultrasonic detection of myocardial infarction in dogs. IEEE Ultrasonics Symposium, 1972, 72 CHO 708–8SU:491–494
29. Sigelmann RS, Reid JM: Analysis of measurement of ultrasound backscattering from an ensemble of scatterers excited by sinewave bursts. J Acoust Soc Am 53:1351, 1973
30. Cohen RD, Mottley JG, Miller JG, et al: Successful quantification of myocardial acoustic properties through the chest wall. Circulation 64:IV-204, 1981

Comparison of Two-Dimensional Echocardiography with Cardiac Nuclear and Other Imaging Techniques

Joel Morganroth and Gerald Pohost

Noninvasive cardiac imaging can provide considerable information about cardiac structure and function, some of which is not available by any other means. While cardiac catheterization is the diagnostic standard that has been used to define cardiac pathophysiologic processes, in recent years its limitations have rendered it a less dominant role. These limitations include added expense and the risk of morbidity and mortality inherent in this invasive technique. Several technical problems inherent in cardiac angiography are rotation and structural distortion due to magnification with an imprecise reference system, cardiac motion, and superimposition of underlying structures containing radiopaque contrast medium. Physiologic and pathophysiologic function can also be disturbed by induced arrhythmias and the hemodynamic effects of contrast medium. Furthermore, angiographic studies of the coronary artery provide structural information that cannot be directly related to functional consequences.

The introduction of echocardiographic and nuclear cardiologic imaging techniques in the 1970s and the subsequent advances in their sophistication and diagnostic capability have led to a change in diagnostic practices in the 1980s. In certain cases the clinician can considerably reduce some of the diagnostic uncertainties of the conventional clinical evaluation (i.e., the history, physical examination, resting/exercise ECG, and chest x-ray) in patients with suspected heart disease. Now, at relatively low cost and without risk, echocardiography provides high-resolution information. For example, cardiac valvular structure and motion, ventricular wall thickness and motion during the cardiac cycle, and cardiac chamber size can be evaluated echocardiographically. Occult disease can be identified with this technique before symptoms develop, and cardiac conditions once thought rare have become more commonly appreciated, e.g., mitral valve prolapse and hypertrophic cardiomyopathy.

Radionuclide imaging of the heart has permitted clinical evaluation of myocardial perfusion and integrity, infarct size, and global ventricular function without the geometric assumptions inherent in the angiocardiographic approach.

Dr. Pohost is an established investigator of the American Heart Association.

The purpose of this chapter is to compare the technical advantages and limitations inherent in echocardiography and radionuclide cardiac imaging. These techniques, though noninvasive, can be costly; therefore, care must be exercised in selecting the proper technique for the particular clinical question being asked. Before comparing echocardiography to cardiac nuclear imaging with respect to the major cardiac diagnostic categories, a general discussion of their relative merits and limitations is warranted.[1]

ADVANTAGES AND LIMITATIONS OF ECHOCARDIOGRAPHY

Echocardiography provides a relatively inexpensive noninvasive means of obtaining excellent axial and lateral resolution of cardiac structures and of evaluating cardiac function. We believe that, in light of their complementary roles, both M-mode and two-dimensional echocardiography should be obtained in each patient under study. Echocardiography depicts valve motion in "real time" and provides a means for quantitation of ventricular wall thickness and motion characteristics with the highest resolution available of any present imaging method. It is without known biologic hazard and can be repeated for serial determinations even in the most critically ill patient.

Echocardiography suffers from the limitations noted in Table 18-1. The most important limitation of echocardiography is the inability to obtain a technically adequate study in certain patient groups, e.g., elderly subjects or patients with severe pulmonary disease, since bone and lung provide structural barriers to ultrasound transmission. Technical limitations also exist in the ideal identification of endocardial echoes and tomographic planes. Furthermore, artifacts may occur because of inappropriately high gain settings. Accordingly, when interpreting an ultrasound study, technical issues must be constantly considered.

Nuclear cardiology provides diagnostic data at a moderately higher cost but also involves little risk to the patient. The bone and lung barriers for ultrasound do not substantially affect radionuclide gamma photon trasmission, although substantial breast tissue might lead occasionally to attenuation of the low energy photons of thallium 201. Furthermore, while echocardiography can evaluate regional ventricular wall motion or proximal coronary artery anatomy, nuclear cardiology offers the advantage of allowing evaluation of regional myocardial perfusion. Cardiac nuclear imaging techniques also have limitations; these are listed in Table 18-2.

In addition to being more costly and associated with a potential biologic hazard, cardiac nuclear imaging also has a considerably lower spatial and time resolution of cardiac structures compared to ultrasound. A first-pass function study using technetium 99m requires three cardiac cycles for accurate determination of ejection

Table 18-1
Limitations of Echocardiography

Technically inadequate data in certain patient groups

Distortions due to off-axis plane orientation of cardiac rotational motion

"Dropout" of echoes, resulting in poor endocardial definition in some patients

Artifact production and gain sensitivities with information loss in video format displayed in stop motion

Table 18-2
Limitations of Nuclear Cardiology Imaging Techniques (Gamma Methods)

Intrinsic low resolution

Nontomographic, with inherent difficulties in distinguishing underlying cardiac structures

Inability to obtain data representing one cardiac cycle

Ionizing radiation exposure

Moderate cost

fractions, whereas the gated blood pool scan requires at least 2 minutes of cardiac cycles. The presence of atrial fibrillation, ventricular tachycardia, or frequent premature beats are additional technical limitations of radionuclide angiography.

While limitations exist, both noninvasive approaches have great technical utility. Table 18-3 compares the specific advantages and disadvantages of echocardiographic and radionuclide imaging techniques. The indications for the use of these tests must be understood before appropriate application can provide the most cost-effective approach. Accordingly, the indications for each of these two techniques in various cardiac disease states are considered in Table 18-4 and in the following paragraphs.

COMPARISONS AND CONTRASTS

Global and Regional Ventricular Function

When good image quality is obtained, two-dimensional echocardiography coupled with the M-mode technique allows high-resolution assessment of chamber size, wall thickness, and wall motion. However, echocardiographic imaging produces only narrow field tomographic views of the heart; assessment of global function in the face of abnormalities of regional function is more difficult.[2,3] First-pass and equilibrium-gated radionuclide studies provide an accurate but low-resolution quantitative analysis of global left and right ventricular function without the geometric assumptions required for the ultrasonic determination.[4,5] Radionuclide methods have also permitted ready evaluation of ventricular function during exercise, whereas ultrasound methods are more difficult to perform routinely during exercise. Either ultrasonic or radionuclide techniques are useful to detect left ventricular aneurysm formation. The ultrasound method allows high-resolution evaluation of both wall excursion and wall thinning, while radionuclide methods allow for a more global view but with lower resolution and evaluation of wall excursion but not thinning (see Figure 18-1). In summary, gated or first-pass radionuclide techniques appear to be the best approach at this time for quantitative analysis of global ventricular function. Echocardiography, on the other hand, provides a finely resolved assessment of regional wall motion and thickening.

Valvular Heart Disease

Echocardiography provides the most precise technique for the clinical evaluation of valve motion characteristics. Criteria for valve stenosis and regurgitation are specific and indications for surgical intervention are emerging based on two-dimensional and Doppler echocardiographic findings.[6] Direct detection and quantitation of stenotic lesions of cardiac valves are virtually limited to the echocardiographic approach.

Table 18-3
Technical Comparisons Between Echocardiography and Cardiac Nuclear Imaging

Method	Real-Time Data	Resolution (mm)	Valves	RWM*	Wall Thickness	Usefulness in Depicting: Global VF†	Chamber Size	Blood Flow	Tissue Integrity	Technical Interference	Biologic Hazard
Echocardiography											
M-mode	+	2	Excellent	Excellent‡	Excellent	Poor	Good	None	Fair	Bone, lung	None
Two-dimensional	+	3	Excellent	Excellent	Good	Good	Good	None	Fair	Bone, lung	None
Radionuclide imaging											
Cineangiography§	+	10	None	Good	Poor	Excellent	Fair	None	None	Arrhythmias	Ionizing radiation
Myocardial perfusion	+	12	None	None	Poor	None	Poor	Excellent	Excellent	Breast tissue	Ionizing radiation
Infarct avid	+	10	None	None	None	None	None	Excellent	Excellent	Bone	Ionizing radiation

*Regional wall motion.
†Ventricular function.
‡For areas seen.
§Gated-equilibrium or first-pass studies.

Table 18-4

Comparative Clinical Usefulness of Echocardiography and Radionuclide Imaging

Detection and Evaluation of Patients with:	Echocardiography		Radionuclide Imaging		
	M-Mode	2D	Cineangiography*	Myocardial "Perfusion"	Infarct Avid
Ventricular dysfunction	2	1	1	2	NR
Ventricular aneurysm	2	1	1	2	NR
Valve disease	1	1	2	NR	NR
Stable coronary artery disease	2	2	2(1)	1(2)	NR
Acute myocardial infarction	NR	1	2	2	2
Hypertrophic cardiomyopathy	1	1	2	2	NR
Congenital heart disease	2	1	2(1†)	2	NR
Intracardiac clots or myxoma	1	1	2	NR	NR
Vegetations	1	1	NR	NR	NR

1 = recommended in the initial evaluation; 2 = may be relevant after initial evaluation; NR = not recommended.
*Gated-equilibrium or first-pass techniques.
†Shunt size can be determined by first-pass method.

Cardiac radionuclide techniques can provide indirect information about ventricular function by depicting chamber sizes and response of ventricular function to exercise.[7] Mitral valve prolapse is identified by echocardiographic criteria. Cardiac nuclear imaging has a secondary role in evaluating patients with this disorder in whom concomitant coronary artery disease is suspected.[8] Unfortunately, radionuclide studies demonstrate a high incidence of false positivity for coronary disease in patients with valvular disease.

Coronary Artery Disease

Echocardiographic studies allow direct noninvasive visualization of the proximal coronary arteries in humans and have been used to identify the presence of left main coronary artery disease.[9] Of course, low resolution does not permit radionuclide studies to directly assess coronary artery anatomy, although thallium 201 allows us to evaluate the impact of arterial disease on myocardial perfusion.

M-mode and two-dimensional echocardiograpbic studies can detail regional wall motion abnormalities that often provide evidence of acute or remote myocardial ischemia and/or infarction; however, they cannot easily distinguish between them. Detailed evaluation of the extent and degree of such wall motion abnormalities is possible with echocardiography. An exercise-induced abnormality of regional wall motion detected by two-dimensional echocardiography is highly specific for angiographic coronary artery disease. The sensitivity of this finding is, however, poor. In contrast, exercise radionuclide studies have shown a high degree of accuracy, sensitivity, and specificity in predicting the presence of occult or clinical coronary artery disease. After intensive conventional clinical evaluation, the radionuclide techniques still remain the first approach for answering this clinical question.[10]

In patients with suspected acute myocardial infarction, echocardiography allows evaluation of regional wall motion in selected tomographic planes.[11,12] Radionuclide cineangiography provides similar information with better assessment of global function but with lower resolution of regional wall motion (Figure 18-1). In addition,

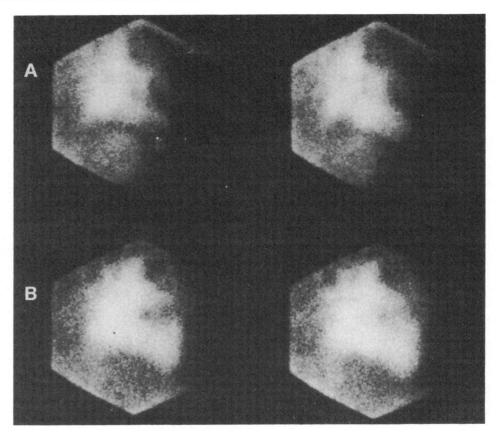

Figure 18-1. A: Normal gated radionuclide ventricular cineangiogram in 30° right anterior oblique projection demonstrating normal systolic (left panel) and diastolic (right panel) frames. B: Gated radionuclide ventriculogram in 30° right anterior oblique projection in a patient with an extensive previous antero-apical infarction. Note the apical aneurysm (dyskinetic region) in the systolic frame (left panel). (Courtesy of Dr. Stewart Spies.)

thallium 201 studies allow immediate assessment of regional myocardial perfusion; and delayed thallium images allow assessment of myocardial viability (Figure 18-2). Technetium 99m pyrophosphate allows specific detection of myocardial infarction by the appearance of a "hot spot" at least 24 hours after the event [13] (Figure 18-3). This study can be helpful in diagnosing myocardial infarction when other clinical parameters are ambiguous.

Prognostication after myocardial infarction can be aided by both echocardiographic and radionuclide studies. In the acute syndromes of coronary artery disease, radionuclide studies have been more widely applied and provide a larger spectrum of clinically relevant information. They remain the first approach when available. Echocardiography, however, remains the procedure of choice for the detection of complications of acute infarction, such as the existence of mural thrombus, rupture of the interventricular septum or papillary muscle, and the detection of left ventricular aneurysm or pseudoaneurysm. Radionuclide techniques provide only secondary evidence of these complications, such as the appearance of a left-to-right shunt or enlargement of the left atrium. Right ventricular infarction is probably detected with equal certainty using either technique.

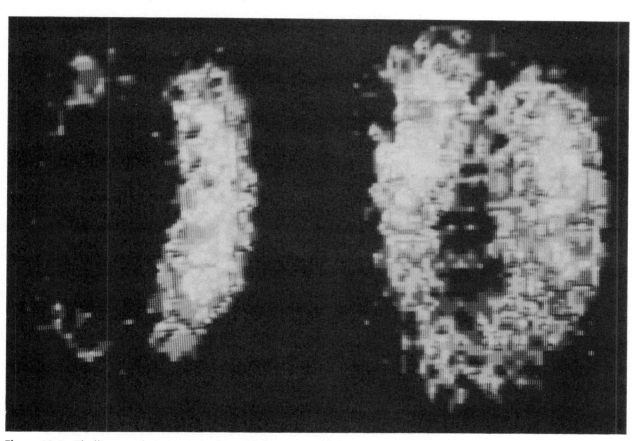

Figure 18-2. Thallium perfusion scan in the 45° left anterior oblique projection demonstrating a large reversible perfusion defect in the anteroseptal region immediately postexercise (left panel). Four hours after exercise (right panel), blood flow is restored to the ischemic portion of the septum. (Courtesy of Dr. James V. Talano.)

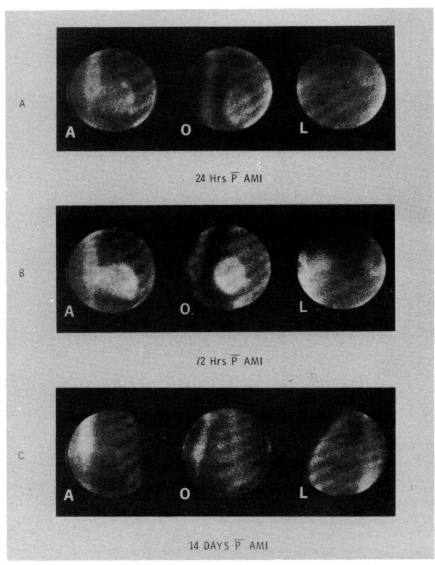

24 Hrs P̄ AMI

72 Hrs P̄ AMI

14 DAYS P̄ AMI

Figure 18-3. Serial technetium 99m pyrophosphate myocardial scintigrams in a patient with an acute anterior wall myocardial infarction. A: A diffusely positive scintigram at 24 hours after the onset of infarction. B: A high-grade localized abnormality at 72 hours after infarction. C: A negative scintigram at follow-up 14 days after infarction. (From Lyons KP, Olson HG: Nuclear cardiology, in Baum S, Vincent NR, Lyons KP, et al (eds): Atlas of Nuclear Medicine Imaging. East Norwalk, Conn, Appleton-Century-Crofts, 1981, pp 339–384. With permission.)

388

Cardiomyopathy

The pathophysiologic principles in congestive, hypertrophic, and restrictive cardiomyopathies have been delineated in recent years with the aid of echocardiography. In fact, echocardiography has replaced cardiac catheterization as the standard of diagnosis for these conditions, not only in terms of safety and cost but also in its ability to provide high-resolution details of valvular myocardial structure and function.[14,15] Serial evaluation performed without risk has provided a greater understanding of the natural history and role of therapy in these conditions. Cardiac nuclear imaging techniques are useful in the differential diagnosis of the cardiomyopathies whenever echocardiography is unavailable, technically inadequate, or equivocal.[16,17] Furthermore, thallium 201 may be helpful in the differential diagnosis of ischemic from idiopathic congestive cardiomyopathy by demonstrating localized perfusion defects in the former.[17]

Congenital Heart Disease

The excellent ability to image the cardiac structural relationships and the lack of reliance on ionizing radiation have made echocardiography the first approach in evaluating patients (especially children) with congenital heart disease. Complex congenital heart disease can be detailed noninvasively using deductive two-dimensional echocardiography in which accurate depiction of the spatial relationships of the great arteries, atrioventricular and semilunar valves, interatrial and interventricular septa, and situs of the ventricles lead to a specific diagnosis.[18,19] Congenital valvular disease can be readily diagnosed and septal defects can be appreciated directly or with the additional use of contrast and Doppler echocardiography (see Chapters 14 and 15). Aortic coarctation and other great vessel abnormalities can also be identified.

Cardiac nuclear imaging provides useful additional information by depicting myocardial perfusion and the size and configuration of the cardiac chambers. Perhaps most importantly, first-pass radionuclide studies allow for intracardiac shunt detection and quantitation.[20]

Other Conditions

Echocardiography has proven to be extremely valuable in identifying and recognizing conditions that previously were only indirectly or uncommonly noted by other techniques. The recognition of vegetations in infective endocarditis has provided the clinician with a means in many cases to diagnose this condition rapidly and to provide useful predictors of prognosis[21] (see Chapter 12).

The identification of cardiac tumors, especially the atrial myxoma, by echocardiography has eliminated the need for catheterization in recognizing this condition and has provided a diagnostic tool to eliminate incorrect or delayed diagnosis.[22]

The delineation of the presence, size, and location of intracardiac thrombus by two-dimensional echocardiography has provided in recent years a newer understanding of this important problem and allows now for careful studies of natural history and response to therapy[23] (see Chapter 12).

Radionuclide imaging has not proven clinically useful in the detection of cardiac vegetations but can be used as an alternative to echocardiography in the detection of intracardiac masses whenever echocardiography is unavailable or equivocal.[24]

—————————————————————————————————— **FUTURE DIRECTIONS**

Echocardiography

New and better echocardiographic equipment will undoubtedly lead to improved image quality, resolution, and penetration. Reconstructed three-dimensional echocardiography may provide an enhanced appreciation of spatially oriented data (see Chapter 16). The combination of Doppler techniques with two-dimensional echocardiographic systems allows quantitation of blood flow and localization of abnormal flow states (see Chapter 15). Tissue identification and characterization by assessing ultrasound reflections should allow differentiation between normal, ischemic, and infarcted myocardium (see Chapter 17). Computer developments will allow rapid quantitation of ultrasound data and will help standardize analysis. Future advances using contrast echocardiographic techniques could allow for analysis of hemodynamics, including possibly the estimation of intracardiac pressures using precision microbubbles (see Chapter 14).

Radionuclide Imaging

Advances in computer and gamma camera technology might allow more rapid acquisition of data with better quantitation for improved evaluation of regional wall motion. New radiopharmaceuticals will be developed to improve evaluation of myocardial metabolism and viability. An example of one future radiopharmaceutical direction is the use of labeled antibody to cardiac myosin to detect regions of acutely infarcted tissue.

Other Techniques

Several other techniques will continue to be developed and provide additional means for cardiac imaging. Positron emission tomography using on-site cyclotron-generated radiotracers will allow for evaluation of cardiac metabolic function. However, the expense and space needs militate against positron imaging becoming a widely employed clinical approach. New and faster computerized x-ray tomographic techniques are becoming available to define cardiac structures using only a peripheral venous injection of radiopaque contrast medium. The computer tomographic method may provide an exciting approach in evaluating ventricular function. In the meantime, the technique is being applied clinically in some centers to evaluate coronary artery bypass graft patency[25-28] using a rapid repetitive scanning sequence after the injection of contrast medium into a peripheral vein. Although the sensitivity and specificity of the method has been reported to exceed 90 percent[25] contrast-enhanced computerized tomography has the limitations of not being able to evaluate the patency of multiple distal anastomoses or detect the presence of stenotic or patent grafts. Other current applications for computed tomographic scanning include the evaluation of aortic dissection,[29] the detection and delineation of intracardiac clots[30-32] and neoplasams,[33] and the demonstration of pericardial effusion and cysts.[34] An additional potentially exciting application of contrast-enhanced computed tomography would be in the imaging of acute myocardial infarction. Preliminary studies have demonstrated that infarcts are imaged as areas of reduced density, presumably related to decreased coronary perfusion.[35]

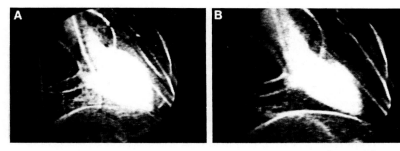

Figure 18-4. End-diastolic (A) and end-systolic (B) images obtained by injecting 10 ml of contrast material over 2 seconds into the left ventricle. The video signals are processed in real time by the method of mask mode subtraction. Images are recorded on videotape and displayed in real time on a television monitor. (From Tobis JM, Nalcioglu O, Johnston WD, et al: Digital angiography in assessment of ventricular function and wall motion during pacing in patients with coronary artery disease. Am J Cardiol 51:668–675, 1983. With permission.)

More likely than widespread application of computed x-ray tomography in cardiac evaluation will be the use of digital angiography, which uses venous injections of low concentration of contrast medium to visualize vessels (Figure 18-4). Fluoroscopic x-ray exposure levels are utilized with significantly less radiation exposure received during cineangiography.[36] This approach applies computer technology to angiography, producing images of high contrast by background subtraction. With this technique, low concentrations of contrast medium can be visualized; the cardiac chambers, great vessels, and, perhaps in the future, the coronary arteries can be imaged after intravenous administration of radiopaque contrast medium.[36,37] Good quality pulmonary angiograms can now be obtained after intravenous injection of contrast material, thus avoiding the necessity of right heart catheterization.[37] In addition, digital intravenous cineangiograms of the left ventricle can be performed with significantly less ventricular irritability than possible with standard cineangiograms.[37]

Instead of the 40 to 50 cc of contrast material utilized in standard ventriculography, multiple intraventricular injections of 5 to 10 cc of contrast material can be performed to obtain left ventriculograms in multiple views. The ability to perform multiple ventriculograms allows better assessment of ventricular function at rest or after interventions such as bicycle exercise or atrial pacing.[38] Aortic root digital angiography appears to be a promising technique to determine the patency of aortic bypass grafts. Perhaps with further developments in computer and electronic technology, the resolution capabilities of digital angiography will improve sufficiently to allow adequate imaging of the native coronary vessels.

Finally, nuclear magnetic resonance imaging uses combined magnetic and radio frequency fields to provide high-resolution structural and metabolic information without the need for tracer injection. This technique is currently being developed at a number of centers and will undoubtedly have greater impact on the field of diagnostic imaging.[39,40]

Noninvasive cardiac imaging will no doubt change during the next decade. One can safely predict that noninvasive or minimally invasive imaging approaches will have an even more important role in diagnosis and management of cardiac disease in the future.

REFERENCES

1. Morganroth J, Pohost GM: Noninvasive approaches to cardiac imaging: Comparisons and contrasts. Am J Cardiol 46:1093–1096, 1980
2. Stack R, Kisslo J: Evaluation of left ventricle with two-dimensional echocardiography. Am J Cardiol 46:1117–1123, 1980
3. Barret MJ, Charuzi Y, Corday E: Ventricular aneurysm: Cross-sectional echocardiographic approach. Am J Cardiol 46:1133–1137, 1980
4. Leitl GP, Buchanan JW, Wagner HN Jr: Monitoring cardiac function with nuclear techniques. Am J Cardiol 46:1125–1132, 1980
5. Winzelberg GG, Strauss HW, Bingham JB, et al: Scintigraphic evaluation of left ventricular aneurysm. Am J Cardiol 46:1138–1143, 1980
6. Kotler MN, Mintz GS, Parry WR, et al: M-mode and two-dimensional echocardiography in mitral and aortic regurgitation: Pre-and postoperative evaluation of volume overload of the left ventricle. Am J Cardiol 46:1144–1152, 1980
7. Boucher CA, Okada RD, Pohost GM: Current status of radionuclide imaging in valvular heart disease. Am J Cardiol 46:1153–1163, 1980
8. Morganroth J, Jones RH, Chen CC, et al: Two dimensional echocardiography in mitral, aortic and tricuspid valve prolapse. The clinical problem, cardiac nuclear imaging considerations and a proposed standard for diagnosis. Am J Cardiol 46:1164–1177, 1980
9. Morganroth J, Chen CC, David D, et al: Echocardiographic detection of coronary artery disease. Detection of effects of ischemia on regional myocardial wall motion and visualization of left main coronary artery disease. Am J Cardiol 46:1178–1187, 1980
10. Okada RD, Boucher CA, Strauss HW, et al: Exercise radionuclide imaging approaches to coronary artery disease. Am J Cardiol 46:1188–1204, 1980
11. Parisi AF, Moynihan PF, Folland ED, et al: Echocardiography in acute and remote myocardial infarction. Am J Cardiol 46:1205–1214, 1980
12. Horowitz RS, Morganroth J, Parrotto C, et al: Immediate diagnosis of acute myocardial infarction by two-dimensional echocardiography. Circulation 65:323–329, 1982
13. Pitt B, Thrall JH: Thallium-201 versus technetium-99m pyrophosphate myocardial imaging in detection and evaluation of patients with acute myocardial infarction. Am J Cardiol 46:1215–1223, 1980
14. DeMaria AN, Bommer W, Lee G, et al: Value and limitations of two dimensional echocardiography in assessment of cardiomyopathy. Am J Cardiol 46:1224–1231, 1980
15. Morganroth J, Chen CC: Noninvasive diagnosis of cardiomyopathies. Med Clin North Am 64:1,33–60, 1980
16. Goldman MR, Boucher CA: Value of radionuclide imaging techniques in assessing cardiomyopathy. Am J Cardiol 46:1232, 1980
17. Bulkley BH, Hutchins GM, Bailey I, et al: Thallium 201 imaging and gated cardiac blood pool scans in patients with ischemic and idiopathic congestive cardiomyopathy: A clinical and pathologic study. Circulation 55:753–760, 1977
18. Kotler MN, Mintz GS, Parry WR, et al: Two dimensional echocardiography in congenital heart disease. Am J Cardiol 46:1237–1246, 1980
19. Henry WL, Maron BJ, Griffith JM: Cross-sectional echocardiography in the diagnosis of congenital heart disease: Identification of the relation of the ventricles and great arteries. Circulation 56:267–273, 1977
20. Treves S, Fogle R, Lang P: Radionuclide angiography in congenital heart disease. Am J Cardiol 46:1247–1255, 1980
21. Mintz GS, Kotler MN, Segal BL, et al: Comparison of two-dimensional and M-mode echocardiography in the evaluation of patients with infective endocarditis. Am J Cardiol 43:738–744, 1979
22. Feigenbaum H: Echocardiography (ed 3). Philadelphia, Lea & Febiger, 1981, p 505
23. De Maria AN, Bommer W, Neuman A, et al: Left ventricular thrombi identified by cross-sectional echocardiography. Ann Intern Med 90:14, 1979
24. Pohost GM, Pastore JO, McKusick KA, et al: Detection of left atrial myxoma by gated radionuclide cardiac imaging. Circulation 55:88–92, 1977
25. Brundage B, Lipton M, Herfkens R, et al: Detection of patent coronary bypass grafts by computed tomography: A preliminary report. Circulation 61:827–831, 1980
26. Moncada R, Salinas M, Churchill R, et al: Patency of saphenous aortocoronary bypass grafts demonstrated by computed tomography. N Engl J Med 303:503–505, 1980

27. Guthaner D, Brody W, Ricci M, et al: The use of computed tomography in the diagnosis of coronary artery bypass graft patency. Cardiovasc Intervent Radiol 3:3–8, 1980
28. Daniel W, Dohring W, Lichtler P, et al: Non-invasive assessment of aortocoronary bypass graft patency by computed tomography. Lancet 1:1024–1032, 1980
29. Godwin J, Herfkens R, Skioldebrand C, et al: Evaluation of dissections and aneurysms of the thoracic aorta by conventional and dynamic CT scanning. Radiology 136:125–133, 1980
30. Godwin J, Herfkens R, Skioldebrand C, et al: Detection of intraventricular thrombi by computer tomography. Radiology 138:717–721, 1981
31. Tomoda H, Mitsumoto H, Furuya H, et al: Evaluation of left ventricular thrombus with computed tomography. Am J Cardiol 48:573–577, 1981
32. Goldstein JA, Lipton MJ, Schiller NB, et al: Evaluation of intracardiac thrombi with contrast enhanced computed tomography and echocardiography (Abstract). Am J Cardiol 49:972, 1982
33. Godwin J, Axel L, Adams J, Computed tomography: a new method for diagnosing tumor of the heart. Circulation 63:448–451, 1981
34. Moncada R, Baker M, Salinas M, et al: Diagnostic role of computed tomography in pericardial heart disease: Congenital defects, thickening, neoplasms, and effusions. Am Heart J 103:263–282, 1982
35. Goldstein JA, Lipton MJ, Kramer PH, et al: Evaluation of acute myocardial infarction by contrast-enhanced computed tomography (Abstract). Clin Res 30(1):10, 1982
36. Kruger RA, Mistretta CA, Houk TL, et al: Computerized fluoroscopy in real time for noninvasive visualization of the cardiovascular system. Radiology 130:49–57, 1979
37. Tobis JM, Nalcioglu O, Johnston WD, et al: Left ventricular imaging with digital angiography using intravenous injection and fluroscopic exposure levels. Am Heart J 104:20–27, 1982
38. Tobis JM, Nalcioglu O, Johnston WD, et al: Digital angiography in assessment of ventricular function and wall motion during pacing in patients with coronary artery disease. Am J Cardiol 51:668–675, 1983
39. Brady TJ, Goldman MR, Pykett IL: Proton nuclear resonance imaging of regionally ischemic canine hearts: Effect of paramagnetic proton signal enhancement. Radiology 144:343–347, 1982
40. Partain CL, Price RR, Rollow FD, et al: Nuclear Magnetic Resonance Imaging. Philadelphia, W.B. Saunders, 1982

Equations

LEFT VENTRICULAR VOLUME

End-systolic volume depends on both the end-diastolic volume and myocardial contractility. Thus it is often ambiguous as an isolated measurement. When both end-diastolic and end-systolic volumes (EDV and ESV) are measured, however, total left ventricular stroke volume (SV) can be estimated:

$$SV_{(cc)} = EDV_{(cc)} - ESV_{(cc)} \tag{1}$$

In the absence of valvular regurgitation, effective cardiac output (CO) can be estimated from stroke volume and heart rate (HR):

$$CO_{cc/min} = HR_{beats/min} \times SV \tag{2}$$

The ejection fraction (EF) can then be calculated as the ratio of stroke volume to end-diastolic volume:

$$EF\% = \frac{SV}{EDV} \times 100\% \tag{3}$$

Models for Volume Determination

Angiographic estimates of left ventricular volume are usually based on the assumption that the left ventricle approximates the geometry of an ellipsoid. The volume of such a figure can be calculated if the lengths of its three hemiaxes, a, b, and c, are known (*ellipsoid method*):

$$Volume = \frac{4}{3} \pi \, a \times b \times c \tag{4}$$

The area of an ellipse is the product of π and its two hemiaxes. Thus if c is the major hemiaxis, a the minor hemiaxis in the anteroposterior plane, b the minor hemiaxis in the lateral plane, and A_{AP} and A_{lat} the respective measured angiographic areas, the minor hemiaxes can be expressed as follows:

$$a = \frac{A_{AP}}{\pi c} \tag{5}$$

$$b = \frac{A_{lat}}{\pi c} \tag{6}$$

Then, by substitution in equation (4), volume can be calculated as follows:

$$\text{Volume} = \frac{4}{3}\pi \times \frac{A_{AP}}{\pi c} \times \frac{A_{lat}}{\pi c} \times c \qquad (7)$$

which can be simplified to *(biplane area–length method)*:

$$\text{Volume} = \frac{4\, A_{AP}\, A_{lat}}{3\pi c} \qquad (8)$$

In applications where angiography is performed in only a single plane, the above formula can be simplified by assuming that both minor hemiaxes (a and b) are equal. Thus volume can be derived from the length and area of the single ventricular silhouette *(single plane area–length method)*:

$$\text{Volume} = \frac{4A^2}{3\pi c} \qquad (9)$$

If D represents the minor axis dimension (at end-diastole or end-systole), the volume can be estimated as follows:

$$\text{Volume} = \frac{4}{3}\pi \times \frac{D}{2} \times \frac{D}{2} \times D \qquad (10)$$

which simplifies to *(cube method)*:

$$\text{Volume} = D^3 \qquad (11)$$

DOPPLER APPLICATION

The Doppler equation relates the flow velocity (V), in cm/second of red blood cells, in the direction parallel to the long axis of blood flow directly to the Doppler frequency shift (Δf) in hertz and inversely to the fundamental frequency of the emitted ultrasound (f_o) in hertz (Hz).

$$V = \frac{\Delta f c}{2\, f_o \cos\theta}$$

where c equals the velocity of sound in tissue (1540 m/second); and θ is the angle between the emitted ultrasound and the long axis of blood flow.

The range–velocity product is derived from the Nyquist equation (sampling rate theorem), which states that the pulse repetition frequency (PRF) of the emitted ultrasound must be at least twice the maximum frequency shift (Δf_{max}) to be sampled:

$$\Delta f_{max} = \frac{PRF}{2}$$

The maximum range (R_{max} in cm) that can be sampled according to the sampling rate theorem is defined by the following equation:

$$R_{max} = \frac{1}{(1.3 \times 10^{-5}) \times PRF}$$

Therefore, the maximum range at which the pulsed Doppler system can function is inversely proportional to the magnitude of the pulse repetition frequency. The maximum Doppler frequency shift (Δf_{max}) that can be detected is related to the maximum depth or range (R_{max}) at which the system can function by the following equation:

$$\Delta f_{max} = \frac{1}{(2.6 \times 10^{-5}) \times R_{max}}$$

The maximum flow velocity that can be detected for a given range (depth), fundamental emitted frequency (f_o), and angle (θ) between the ultrasound beam and the flow velocity vector is computed from the equation:

$$V_{max} = \frac{c}{(5.2 \times 10^{-5}) \times R_{max} \times f_o \times \cos \theta}$$

where V_{max} is the maximum detectable velocity at R_{max}.

BEAM STEERING

The equation for the off-axis angle θ is:

$$\sin \theta = \frac{x}{d}$$

where x is the distance each wavelet propagates before the next element fires and d is the interelement distance.

BEAM WIDTH

The length of the near-field is directly related to the square of the radius (r) of the ultrasound crystal and inversely related to its wavelength (λ). The near-field length (l) can be calculated from the equation:

$$l = \frac{r^2}{\lambda}$$

Normal Two-Dimensional Echocardiographic Measurements for Adults

Table B-1
Chamber Dimensions

View	Chamber	Mean ± SD (cm)	Range (cm or cm²)
PLAX	Aortic dimensions (end-diastole)		
	Aortic annulus	2.1 ± 0.3	1.6–2.6
	Sinus of valsalva	2.9 ± 0.4	2.4–3.9
	Sinotubular junction	2.6 ± 0.3	2.1–3.4
	Ascending aorta	2.6 ± 0.3	2.2–3.4
PLAX	Left atrial dimensions (end-systole)		
	Anterior–posterior (largest)	3.1 ± 0.3	2.5–3.8
	Anterior–posterior (mid)	3.0 ± 0.3	2.4–3.8
	Superior–inferior (largest)	4.4 ± 0.8	3.1–5.5
PSAX	Left atrial dimensions (end systole)		
	Anterior–posterior (mid)	3.0 ± 0.5	2.3–3.7
	Medial–lateral (largest)	4.1 ± 0.7	3.1–5.3
	Medial–lateral (mid)	4.1 ± 0.7	3.0–5.3
Ap 4 Chamber	Left atrial dimensions (end-systole)		
	Superior–inferior (largest)	4.3 ± 0.6	3.3–5.2
	Medial–lateral (largest)	3.6 ± 0.4	2.9–4.4
	Medial–lateral (mid)	3.5 ± 0.5	2.5–4.4
	Mitral valve annulus	2.4 ± 0.3	1.9–3.1
Ap 4 Chamber	Right atrial dimensions (end-systole)		
	Superior–inferior (largest)	4.2 ± 0.4	3.4–4.9
	Superior–inferior (mid)	4.1 ± 0.4	3.4–4.9
	Medial–lateral (largest)	3.7 ± 0.4	3.1–4.5
	Medial–lateral (mid)	3.7 ± 0.4	2.9–4.5
	Tricupsid annulus	2.2 ± 0.3	1.7–2.8
PLAX	Left ventricular internal dimensions		
	Minor axis		
	End-diastole (largest)	4.7 ± 0.4	3.7–5.3
	(mid)	4.6 ± 0.4	3.7–5.1
	End-systole (largest)	3.0 ± 1.0	2.3–3.6
	(mid)	3.0 ± 0.4	2.3–3.6
	Mitral annulus (maximal)	2.7 ± 0.4	2.1–3.4
PSAX	Left ventricular area (cm²)		
	Mitral valve level		
	Diastole	22.5 ± 4.3	16.4–32.3
	Systole	10.7 ± 2.3	6.1–16.8
	Fractional area shortening	53.1 ± 6.1	41.3–69.9

View	Chamber	Mean ± SD (cm)	Range (cm or cm²)
PSAX	Left ventricular area(cm²) (continued)		
	Papillary muscle level		
	Diastole	22.2 ± 4.2	16.0–31.2
	Systole	8.5 ± 2.0	5.2–13.4
	Fractional area shortening	62.0 ± 6.7	50.3–75.8
Ap 4 Chamber	Left ventricular internal dimensions		
	Length (apex to mitral valve)		
	Diastole (mid)	7.6 ± 0.4	7.0–8.4
	Systole (mid)	5.6 ± 0.5	4.6–6.4
	Medial–lateral (minor axis)		
	Diastole (mid)	4.3 ± 0.6	3.3–5.2
	Systole (mid)	3.1 ± 0.4	2.4–4.2
	Papillary muscle to mitral valve		
	Diastole	3.0 ± 0.4	2.2–3.6
	Systole	2.2 ± 0.3	1.6–2.6
Ap 2 Chamber	Left ventricular internal dimensions		
	Length (apex to mitral valve)		
	Diastole (mid)	8.0 ± 0.8	6.8–9.4
	Systole (mid)	5.6 ± 0.9	4.4–7.1
	Medial–lateral (minor axis)		
	Diastole (mid)	4.6 ± 0.6	3.8–5.7
	Systole (mid)	3.2 ± 0.7	2.1–4.6
PSAX	Right ventricular dimensions		
	Largest septal to free wall dimension		
	at tricuspid valve level		
	Diastole	3.1 ± 0.4	2.5–3.8
	Systole	2.7 ± 0.3	2.1–3.4
Ap 4 Chamber	Right ventricular internal dimensions		
	Length (apex to tricuspid valve)		
	Diastole (mid)	6.6 ± 0.6	5.0–7.8
	Systole (mid)	5.0 ± 0.5	4.3–5.9
	Medial–lateral (minor axis)		
	Diastole (mid)	3.3 ± 0.5	2.5–4.2
	Systole (mid)	2.6 ± 0.3	2.0–3.2
PSAX	Pulmonary artery dimensions (end-diastole)*		
	Right ventricular outflow tract	2.7 ± 0.4	1.9–2.2
	Valvular	1.8 ± 0.2	1.1–2.2
	Supravalvular	1.9 ± 0.3	1.5–2.5
	Right pulmonary artery	1.3 ± 0.3	0.8–1.6
	Left pulmonary artery	1.2 ± 0.8	1.0–1.4
Subcostal	Pulmonary artery dimensions (end-diastole)		
	Right ventricular outflow tract	1.9 ± 0.4	1.4–2.4
	Valvular	1.3 ± 0.1	1.1–1.6
	Supravalvular	1.5 ± 0.3	1.2–2.3
	Right pulmonary artery	1.2 ± 0.2	0.9–1.5
	Left pulmonary artery	0.8 ± 0.1	0.8–0.9

Adapted from Triulzi M, Weyman A: Normal cross-sectional echocardiographic measurements in adults, in Weyman A (ed): Echocardiography. Philadelphia, Lea & Febiger, 1982, pp 497–504. With permission.

Ap 2 Chamber denotes apical two-chamber view; Ap 4 Chamber, apical four-chamber view; PLAX, parasternal long-axis view; PSAX, parasternal short-axis view; SD, standard deviation.

*These values are consistently smaller than those obtained from the parasternal transducer location. This is because the pulmonary artery lies in the far field of the scan plane when viewed from the subcostal window and there is significant point-spreading of targets along the vessel walls due to the poor lateral resolution at this level. Therefore, these measurements are more appropriately made from images recorded from the parasternal location, and the subcostal values are included only as a reference for patients in whom the parasternal window is unavailable.

Table B-2
Chamber Volumes

Investigators	Left Atrium		Right Atrium			Right Ventricle
	Vol (cc) Mean ± SD (Range)	Vol Index (cc/m²) Mean ± SD (Range)	Vol (cc) Mean ± SD (Range)	Vol Index (cc/m²) Mean ± SD (Range)	Area (cm²) Mean ± SD (Range)	Area (cm²) Mean ± SD (Range)
Bommer et al[1]						
Plan (n = 25)					13.9 ± 0.7 (—21)	18 ± 1.2 (—27)
Reeves et al[2]						
Plan (n = 45)					16 ± 3.4 (11.4–24)	
Wang et al[3]						
Ap 4 Chamber AL			39 ± 12 (15–58)	21 ± 6 (8–33)	13 ± 3 (6.7–17.7)	
(n = 48)			27 ± 7 (14–44)	17 ± 4 (8–27)		
Schiller et al[4–6]						
Peak of R Wave						
Ap 4 Chamber AL						
Males (n = 23)	38 ± 10 (24–56)	20 ± 6 (11–31)				
Females (n = 25)	34 ± 12 (15–56)	21 ± 8 (10–36)				
Ap 2 Chamber AL						
Males (n = 23)	46 ± 14 (25–77)	24 ± 8 (12–48)				
Females (n = 25)	36 ± 11 (13–59)	22 ± 7 (8–23)				
Simpson						
Males (n = 23)	38 ± 10 (20–57)	20 ± 6 (10–31)				
Females (n = 25)	32 ± 10 (15–49)	20 ± 8 (10–31)				

Table B-2 (continued)

	Left Ventricle						
Investigators	End-Dias Vol (cc) Mean ± SD (Range)	End-Dias Vol Index (cc/m²) Mean ± SD (Range)	End-Sys Vol (cc) Mean ± SD (Range)	End-Sys Vol Index (cc/m²) Mean ± SD (Range)	Ej Fr Mean (%)	LV Mass Mean (g)	LV Mass Index Mean (g/m²)
Schiller et al[4-7]							
Ap 4 Chamber AL							
Males (n = 29)	112 ± 27 (65–193)	57 ± 13 (37–94)	35 ± 16 (13–86)	19 ± 8 (7–44)	68		
Females (n = 23)	89 ± 20 (59–136)		33 ± 12 (13–54)		63		
Ap 2 Chamber AL							
Males (n = 29)	130 ± 27 (73–201)	63 ± 13 (37–101)	40 ± 14 (17–74)	20 ± 7 (7–36)	69		
Females (n = 23)	92 ± 19 (53–146)		31 ± 11 (11–53)		66		
Simpson							
Males (n = 29)	111 ± 22 (62–170)	55 ± 10 (36–82)	34 ± 12 (14–76)	18 ± 6 (8–38)	69		
Females (n = 23)	80 ± 12 (55–101)		29 ± 10 (13–60)		63		
PSAX, Ap 2 Chamber, Ap 4 Chamber							
Males (n = 29)						135	71
Females (n = 23)						99	62
Folland[8]							
Simpson (n = 10)	51 ± 17 (32–83)		19 ± 5 (13–23)		62		

Ap 2 Chamber denotes apical two-chamber view; Ap 4 Chamber, apical four-chamber view; PSAX, parasternal short-axis view; Plan, planimetry; AL, area–length method; Simpson, modified Simpson's rule; Dias, diastolic; Sys, systolic; Vol, volume; Ej Fr, ejection fraction; LV, left ventricle; SD, standard deviation.

1. Bommer W, Weinert L, Neumann A, et al: Determination of right atrial and right ventricular size by two-dimensional echocardiography. Circulation 60:91, 1979
2. Reeves WC, Hallahan W, Schwiter EJ, et al: Two-dimensional echocardiographic assessment of electrocardiographic criteria for right atrial enlargement. Circulation 64:387, 1981
3. Wang Y, Gutman JM, Heilbron D, et al: Atrial volume in a normal population by two-dimensional echocardiography (Abstract). Am J Cardiol 49:905, 1982
4. Schiller NB, Gutman JM: Quantitative analysis of the adult left heart by two-dimensional echocardiography, in Nasser FN, Giuliani ER (eds): Clinical Two-dimensional Echocardiography. Chicago, YearBook (in press)
5. Wahr DW, Wang YS, Schiller NB: Left ventricular volumes determined by two-dimensional echocardiography in the normal adult population. J Am Coll Cardiol (in press)
6. Gutman J, Wang YS, Wahr D, et al: Normal left atrial function determined by two-dimensional echocardiography. Am J Cardiol 51:336, 1983
7. Schiller NB, Skioldebrand CG, Schiller EJ, et al: Canine left ventricular mass estimation by two-dimensional echocardiography. Circulation (in press)
8. Moynihan P, Parisi AF: Unpublished data, VA Medical Center, West Roxbury, Mass

Nomenclature for Myocardial Wall Segments (American Society of Echocardiography)

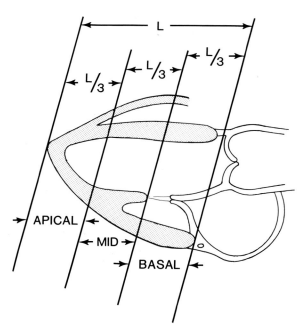

Figure C-1. Parasternal long-axis view demonstrating the method of subdividing the myocardial walls along the long axis (L) into three regions of equal length using the left ventricular papillary muscles as landmarks.

The figures and legends in this appendix are reprinted by permission of the American Society of Echocardiography. The Report of the American Society of Echocardiography Committee on Nomenclature and Standards: Identification of Myocardial Wall Segments, November, 1982.

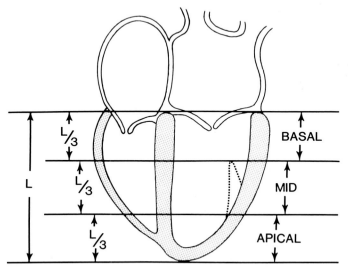

Figure C-2. Apical four-chamber view demonstrating the method of subdividing the myocardial walls into three regions using the left ventricular papillary muscles as landmarks.

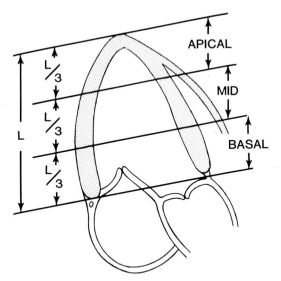

Figure C-3. Apical long-axis view demonstrating the method of subdividing the myocardial walls into three regions of equal length.

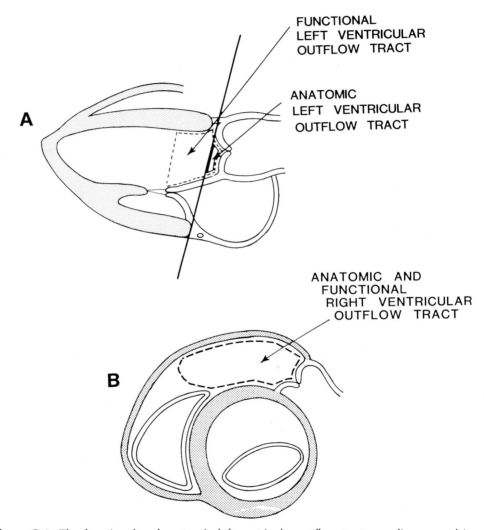

FUNCTIONAL
LEFT VENTRICULAR
OUTFLOW TRACT

ANATOMIC
LEFT VENTRICULAR
OUTFLOW TRACT

A

ANATOMIC AND
FUNCTIONAL
RIGHT VENTRICULAR
OUTFLOW TRACT

B

Figure C-4. The functional and anatomic left ventricular outflow tracts are diagrammed in panel A, and the functional and anatomic right ventricular outflow tract is illustrated in panel B.

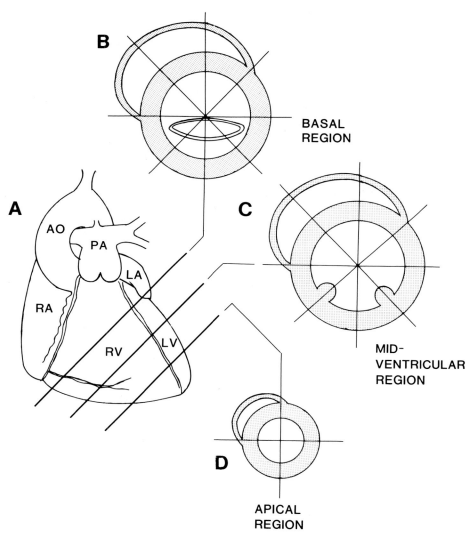

Figure C-5. Diagram of the heart (A) demonstrating where the short-axis views of the basal region (B), midventricular region (C), and apical region (D) are taken.

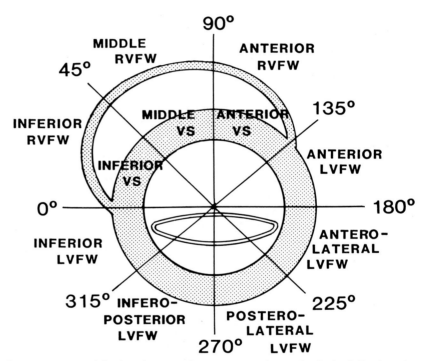

Figure C-6. Short-axis view of the basal region demonstrating the method of subdividing the myocardial walls into segments using a coordinate system consisting of eight lines that are 45° apart. With this system the left ventricular free wall (LVFW) is divided into five segments, whereas the ventricular septum (VS) and right ventricular free walls (RVFW) are subdivided into three segments each.

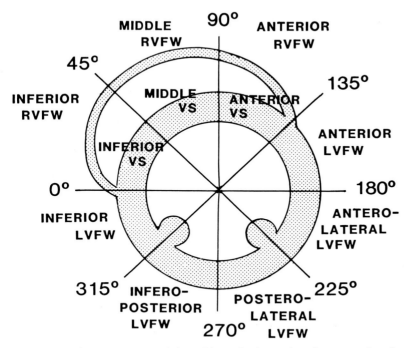

Figure C-7. Short-axis view of the midventricular region demonstrating the method of subdividing the myocardial walls into segments. See Figure C-6 for further details and abbreviations.

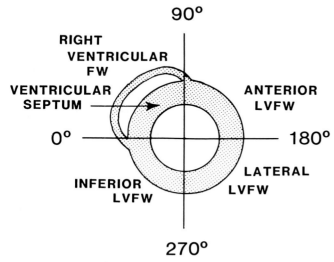

Figure C-8. Short-axis view of the apical region demonstrating the method of subdividing the myocardial walls into segments using a coordinate system consisting of four lines that are 90° apart. With this system the left ventricular free wall (LVFW) is subdivided into three segments, whereas the ventricular septum and right ventricular free wall (FW) are subdivided into one segment each.

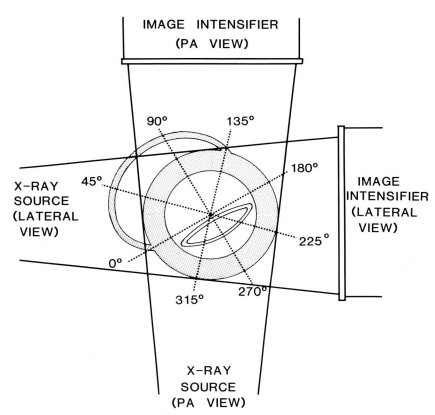

Figure C-9. Short-axis view of the basal region demonstrating the myocardial wall segments that are seen with an x-ray tube and image intensifier in the posterior–anterior (PA) and lateral views. In the PA view, the inferior ventricular septum and anterolateral left ventricular free wall segments are visualized by the x-ray beam. In the lateral view, the anterior ventricular septum and inferoposterior (near the junction of the inferior) left ventricular free wall segments are seen.

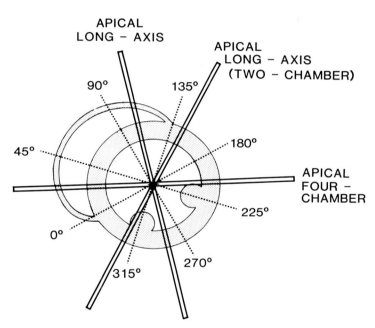

Figure C-10. Short-axis view of the midventricular region demonstrating the myocardial wall segments intersected by the apical long-axis, apical long-axis (two chamber), and the apical four-chamber imaging planes. The exact location of these planes could vary approximately 15° in either direction from the location shown in this diagram.

Index